Intracranial Stereotactic Radiosurgery

Thieme

Intracranial Stereotactic Radiosurgery

L. Dade Lunsford, MD, FACS
Lars Leksell Professor of Neurological Surgery
Distinguished Professor
Director, Center for Image Guided Neurosurgery
University of Pittsburgh
Pittsburgh, Pennsylvania

Jason P. Sheehan, MD, PhD
Assistant Professor
Department of Neurological Surgery and Radiation Oncology
Health Sciences Center
University of Virginia
Charlottesville, Virginia

Thieme
New York • Stuttgart

Thieme Medical Publishers, Inc.
333 Seventh Ave.
New York, NY 10001

Editorial Director: Michael Wachinger
Executive Editor: Kay D. Conerly
Editorial Assistants: Ivy Ip, Lauren Henry
Vice President, Production and Electronic Publishing: Anne T. Vinnicombe
Production Editor: Kenneth L. Chumbley, Publication Services
Vice President, International Marketing and Sales: Cornelia Schulze
Chief Financial Officer: Peter van Woerden
President: Brian D. Scanlan
Compositor: Thomson Digital
Printer: Everbest Printing Company, Ltd.

Library of Congress Cataloging-in-Publication Data

Intracranial stereotactic radiosurgery / [edited by] L. Dade Lunsford, Jason P. Sheehan.
p. ; cm.
Includes bibliographical references.
ISBN 978-1-60406-200-7 (alk. paper)
1. Radiosurgery. I. Lunsford, L. Dade. II. Sheehan, Jason P.
[DNLM: 1. Radiosurgery—methods. 2. Brain Diseases—radiotherapy. 3. Brain Diseases—surgery.
4. Stereotaxic Techniques. WL 368 I6128 2009]
RD594.15.I68 2009
617.4'81059—dc22
2009006986

Printed in China

5 4 3 2 1

ISBN 978-1-60406-200-7

Contents

Foreword

The field of stereotactic radiosurgery continues to expand and mature. Within the space of only a couple of years, I have written both the epilogue for another radiosurgery text[1] and the foreword for this one. Even within this comparatively short interval, an enormous amount of new and updated information has become available.

It has been a pleasure and a privilege to be one of the first to read the manuscripts of all the chapters that are included in *Intracranial Stereotactic Radiosurgery.* The title itself is a reflection of the importance of all the work that, over the past 40 years, has gone into the development of radiosurgery. In the not so distant past, the words *stereotactic radiosurgery* denoted a discipline practiced by a very small number of neurosurgeons who were willing to take some risk with their careers in order to be part of a group of pioneers. More recently, the method has been embraced by radiation oncologists, neuro-otologists, neuro-ophthalmologists, and even spine, chest, and abdominal surgery specialists. Thus, the need to be more specific, by adding *intracranial* to the title of the book, becomes apparent.

In recent years the combined utilization of stereotactic principles, sophisticated and integrated imaging, and advanced treatment planning systems has cross-fertilized both surgical and radiation oncologic thought and practice. The ability to concentrate benefit and reduce risk by focused delivery of cross-fired photons or Bragg peak–delivered protons has revolutionized the concept of treatment using these modalities. There is a progressive blurring between radiation oncologic techniques and surgical principles.

During the first two decades of learning how and when to use radiosurgery, early pioneers were extremely cautious. This philosophy of advancing in small increments was necessary to establish the method, to assess the risks, and to define the long-term benefits. This long period of slow learning laid the foundation for the explosive development that we have witnessed over the last two decades. We have seen one indication after another being added to an ever increasing number of conditions amenable to radiosurgery. We have also seen new technology added to the armamentarium, often seemingly introduced on a fast track, so fast sometimes that one cannot help but wonder if our initial cautiousness was an unnecessary waste of time. Of course, within the four decades of development and application of stereotactic radiosurgery, other fields have come and gone. In contrast, radiosurgery has grown and progressed. The field parallels and incorporates the huge advances that have occurred in imaging, robotics, and minimally invasive surgery, and it has been verified by long-term outcome studies, as well as by risk–benefit analyses.

The reader of this latest addition to the literature on radiosurgery will learn the "tricks of the trade" from some of the field's most experienced practitioners. The chapters on radiobiology and neuropathology of radiosurgery form the basis for all subsequent chapters on the clinical use of radiosurgery for various disease entities. There is a wealth of updated information on the more "established" indications, such as benign tumors, arteriovenous malformations, and metastases. Several chapters explore new and exciting territory; glaucoma, macular degeneration, and epilepsy are some examples.

Interestingly, the revival of functional neurosurgery in the late 1980s and early 1990s, both by neuromodulation and by ablation, seems to increasingly spill over to radiosurgery. Clearly, surgical options need to be compared and evaluated. However, when there are fundamental differences between them, such comparisons can be difficult to make. Different surgical techniques, therefore, over time usually carve out a niche for themselves.

Stereotactic radiosurgical experience worldwide includes over 500,000 Gamma Knife procedures, as well as a significant number of linear accelerator or proton-based procedures. Noninvasive brain surgery has matured to the point where increasingly well-informed patients have come to demand that it be considered as a validated option for them.

This volume, elegantly compiled and edited by L. Dade Lunsford and Jason P. Sheehan, will be mandatory reading for new as well as practicing colleagues who wish to evaluate the role and results of stereotactic radiosurgery.

Dan Leksell
Stockholm, Sweden

1. Lunsford LD. Radiosurgery and pathological fundamentals. In: Progress in Neurological Surgery. Vol. 20.

Preface

In 1951, after observing the difficulties with ether anesthesia and open techniques under Olivecrona, Lars Leksell conceived the principles of radiosurgery. Radiosurgery represented a rapid departure from treatment options at that time, and this creative leap speaks to the genius of Leksell. Although the field of radiosurgery grew slowly at the start, the undeniable successes of the technology attracted an increasing group of radiosurgery disciples. The principles applied today remain grounded in Leksell's original tenets.

Stereotactic radiosurgery has resulted in profound paradigm shifts in neurologic surgery and radiation oncology. Particular intracranial pathologies previously treated with microsurgery or fractionated radiation therapy are now treated more judiciously with radiosurgery. Intracranial and, more recently, extracranial indications for radiosurgery continue to expand.

The past decade has seen rapid improvement in radiosurgical outcomes. Technological advances, including improvements in dose delivery, dose selection, and targeting with multimodality high-resolution neuroimaging, have helped advance the field. Also, a better understanding of the radiobiology of radiosurgery has shed further light on the underlying mechanisms by which radiosurgery achieves success and underscores its differences from fractionated radiation therapy. Long-term clinical data have been thoughtfully analyzed and published by many of the book's contributing authors. Radiosurgical advances have been achieved through the participation and dedication of patients, physicians, and medical physicists alike.

Intracranial Stereotactic Radiosurgery aims to provide a comprehensive understanding of modern-day intracranial radiosurgery. The text includes detailed discussions on radiobiology, indications, methods, outcomes, and complications associated with radiosurgery. In general, contributing authors have chosen literary references based on scientific significance, ease of access, and historical interest. It is our sincere hope that this book will appeal to neurologic surgeons, radiation oncologists, and medical physicists throughout all stages of their learning (i.e., residency, fellowship, and attending physicians). Because medical learning is a lifelong process and is frequently derived from experiences shared by colleagues, we welcome your thoughtful comments regarding this book and any relevant experiences you have had with stereotactic radiosurgery.

Acknowledgments

The completion of this book was the direct result of the diligence of many people. Unfortunately, it is not possible to adequately acknowledge all those who have helped. Nevertheless, we wish to call attention to the assistance of several people. First and foremost, we thank the contributing authors for their efforts. The work of Ivy Ip at Thieme Publishers, Inc., and Kenny Chumbley at Publication Services, proved invaluable.

Finally, we are grateful for the patience and unwavering support of our wives, Julie and Diane, and our children.

L. Dade Lunsford, MD, FACS
Pittsburgh, Pennsylvania
Jason P. Sheehan, MD, PhD
Charlottesville, Virginia

Contributors

John R. Adler Jr., MD
Dorothy and TK Chan Professor
Department of Neurosurgery
Stanford University Medical Center
Stanford, California

Tommy Andersson, MD, PhD
Neurosurgeon and Neuroradiologist
Head of Neurointervention
Department of Neurosurgery
Karolinska University Hospital
Stockholm, Sweden

Yasser Arkha, MD
Department of Stereotactic and
Functional Neurosurgery
Timone University Hospital
Marseille, France

Dave S. Atteberry, MD, MSc
Assistant Professor
Department of Neurological Surgery
University of Pittsburgh
Pittsburgh, Pennsylvania

Erik Olof Backlund, MD, PhD
Department of Neurosurgery
University Hospital
Linkoping, Sweden

Nicholas M. Barbaro, MD
Professor
Department of Neurologic Surgery
University of California, San Francisco
San Francisco, California

Gene H. Barnett, MD, FACS
The Rose Ella Burkhardt Chair in Neurosurgical Oncology
Neurological and Cancer Institutes
Professor and Director
Brain Tumor and Neuro-Oncology Center
Department of Neurological Surgery
The Cleveland Clinic
Associate Dean of Faculty Affairs
Cleveland Clinic Lerner College of Medicine
Case Western Reserve University
Cleveland, Ohio

Joel Bauman, MD
Resident
Department of Neurosurgery
University of Pennsylvania
Philadelphia, Pennsylvania

Stéphanie Bolle, MD
Department of Radiation Oncology
Curie Institute
Orsay, France

Steven D. Chang, MD
Robert C. and Jeannette Powell Professor
Department of Neurosurgery
Stanford University Medical Center
Stanford, California

Lawrence S. Chin, MD, FACS
Professor and Chair
Department of Neurosurgery
Boston University School of Medicine
Neurosurgeon-in-Chief
Boston Medical Center
Boston, Massachusetts

Anne Donnet, MD
Department of Neurology
Timone University Hospital
Marseille, France

Régis Ferrand, Eng-MSc
Project Director
Centre de Protonthérapie d'Orsay
Campus de la Faculte des Sciences
Orsay, France

John C. Flickinger, MD, FACR
Professor
Departments of Radiation Oncology and Neurological Surgery
University of Pittsburgh
Pittsburgh, Pennsylvania

Robert L. Foote, MD
Professor
Department of Radiation Oncology
Mayo Clinic College of Medicine
Rochester, Minnesota

William A. Friedman, MD
Professor and Chairman
Department of Neurosurgery
University of Florida
Gainesville, Florida

Jean-Louis Habrand, MD
Professor
Department of Radiation Oncology
University of Paris
Coordinator, Medical Division
Centre de Protonthérapie d'Orsay
Campus Universitaire
Orsay, France

Jeffrey T. Jacob, MD
Resident
Department of Neurologic Surgery
Mayo Clinic
Rochester, Minnesota

Jay Jagannathan, MD
Radiosurgery Fellow
Department of Neurosurgery
Health Sciences Center
University of Virginia
Charlottesville, Virginia

John A. Jane Jr., MD
Assistant Professor
Department of Neurosurgery
Health Sciences Center
University of Virginia
Charlottesville, Virginia

Mayur Jayarao, MD, MSc
Fellow
Department of Neurosurgery
Boston Medical Center
Boston, Massachusetts

Hideyuki Kano, MD, PhD
Research Assistant Professor
Department of Neurological Surgery
University of Pittsburgh
Pittsburgh, Pennsylvania

Bengt Karlsson, MD, PhD
National University Hospital
Singapore

In-Young Kim, MD
Fellow
Department of Neurosurgery
University of Pittsburgh
Pittsburgh, Pennsylvania

Douglas Kondziolka, MD, MSc, FRCSC, FACS
Peter J. Jannetta Professor and Vice Chairman
Department of Neurological Surgery
University of Pittsburgh
Pittsburgh, Pennsylvania

Edward R. Laws, MD, FACS
Director
Pituitary-Neuroendocrine Center
Professor
Department of Neurosurgery
Brigham and Women's Hospital
Harvard University
Boston, Massachusetts

John Y. K. Lee, MD
Assistant Professor
Department of Neurosurgery
University of Pennsylvania
Philadelphia, Pennsylvania

Marc Levivier, MD, PhD
Professor and Chairman
Department of Neurosurgery
CHUV
Lausanne, Switzerland

Michael J. Link, MD
Associate Professor and Consultant
Department of Neurologic Surgery
Mayo Clinic
Rochester, Minnesota

Bodo Lippitz, MD
Consultant and Professor
Department of Neurosurgery
Karolinska University Hospital
Stockholm, Sweden

Roman Liščák, MD, PhD
Associate Professor
Department of Stereotactic and Radiation Neurosurgery
Na Homolce Hospital
Prague, Czech Republic

Simon S. Lo, MD
Associate Professor
Residency Program Director
Department of Radiation Medicine
Arthur G. James Cancer Hospital
Ohio State University Medical Center
Columbus, Ohio

L. Dade Lunsford, MD, FACS
Lars Leksell Professor of Neurological Surgery
Distinguished Professor
Director, Center for Image Guided Neurosurgery
University of Pittsburgh
Pittsburgh, Pennsylvania

Ricky Madhok, MD
Resident
Department of Neurological Surgery
University of Pittsburgh
Pittsburgh, Pennsylvania

Nicolas Massager, MD, PhD
Professor
Deptartment of Neurosurgery and Gamma Knife Center
University Hospital Erasme
Brussels, Belgium

David Mathieu, MD, FRCSC
Assistant Professor
Division of Neurosurgery/Neuro-oncology
Department of Surgery
Medical Director, Gamma Knife Radiosurgery
University of Sherbrooke and Centre Hospitalier Universitaire de Sherbrooke
Sherbrooke, Quebec, Canada

Gregory J. A. Murad, MD
Assistant Professor
Department of Neurosurgery
University of Florida
Gainesville, Florida

Noriko Murata, MD
Department of Neurosurgery
Timone University Hospital
Marseille, France

Jasvinder Nangiana, BS
Department of Neurosurgery
Stanford University Medical Center
Stanford, California

Ajay Niranjan, MD
Associate Professor
Director of Radiosurgery Research
Department of Neurological Surgery
University of Pittsburgh
Pittsburgh, Pennsylvania

Georges Noel, MD, PhD
Chief
Service de Radiotherapie
Centre Paul Strauss
Strasbourg, France

Rod J. Oskouian Jr., MD
Swedish Neuroscience Institute
Swedish Neuroscience Specialists
Seattle, Washington

Bruce E. Pollock, MD
Professor
Departments of Neurologic Surgery and Radiation Oncology
Mayo Clinic College of Medicine
Rochester, Minnesota

Nader Pouratian, MD, PhD
Chief Resident
Department of Neurosurgery
Health Sciences Center
University of Virginia
Charlottesville, Virginia

Mark Quigg, MD, MSc
Associate Professor
Department of Neurology
Health Sciences Center
University of Virginia
Charlottesville, Virginia

William F. Regine, MD
Isadore and Fannie Schneider Foxman Chair and Professor
Department of Radiation Oncology
University of Maryland
Baltimore, Maryland

Jean Régis, MD
Professor
Department of Stereotactic and Functional Neurosurgery
Timone University Hospital
Marseille, France

Philippe Roussel, MD
Department of Functional Neurosurgery
Timone University Hospital
Marseille, France

David J. Schlesinger, PhD
Assistant Professor
Department of Neurological Surgery
Health Sciences Center
University of Virginia
Charlottesville, Virginia

Jason P. Sheehan, MD, PhD
Assistant Professor
Department of Neurological Surgery and Radiation Oncology
Health Sciences Center
University of Virginia
Charlottesville, Virginia

Gabriela Šimonová, MD, PhD
Department of Stereotactic and Radiation Neurosurgery
Na Homolce Hospital
Prague, Czech Republic

Michael Söderman, MD, PhD
Chief of Neuroangiography and Stereotaxy
Department of Neuroradiology
Karolinska Hospital
Stockholm, Sweden

John H. Suh, MD
Chairman
Department of Radiation Oncology
Cleveland Clinic Foundation
Cleveland, Ohio

György T. Szeifert
National Institute of Neurosurgery
Department of Neurological Surgery
Semmelweis University
Budapest, Hungary

Mary Lee Vance, MD
Professor
Department of Medicine
Health Sciences Center
University of Virginia
Charlottesville, Virginia

Shoji Yomo, MD
Department of Stereotactic and Functional Neurosurgery
Timone University Hospital
Marseille, France

1

Stereotactic Radiosurgery from Notion to Practice

Erik Olof Backlund

A historical account on stereotactic radiosurgery might be given in more than one way. One alternative would be to describe how this new therapeutic conception, arising from and firmly rooted in profound clinical experience, emerged in the minds of the pioneers and, in the same minds, gave rise to seminal driving forces behind technical design processes. Another way of writing radiosurgical history would be just to give a panorama of equipment and machinery, that is, the substantial realization of technical ideas. In this introductory chapter, I will try to use the former of these two narrative approaches.

Radiosurgery as a new therapy was introduced into the clinical setting with the development of the Gamma Knife (GK, Elekta AB, Stockholm, Sweden), invented by professor Lars Leksell in Stockholm, Sweden.[1] In its present design, it is probably still the most sophisticated radiosurgical tool built so far. The launch in 1967 of this first GK prototype represents the "birth" of intracranial radiosurgery, at least in a more limited sense.

◆ The Development of Radiosurgery

Intracranial precision irradiation has been in use since at least the 1940s. Stereotactic, surgical introduction of solid (and liquid) radioactive sources into the pituitary gland and eloquently located brain tumors was more or less routine management at several centers, primarily in Germany and France (for a review, see the reports from a symposium in Paris in 1979).[2] The goal of avoiding these invasive alternatives gave rise to the idea that external cross-firing of intracranial targets, by narrow high-energy ionizing beams, could take the place of these "bloody" techniques, in addition to being completely without surgical risks. Moreover, satisfying—or even better—dose and field parameters would be possible using focused external irradiation.

Beginning in the 1950s, multiportal techniques using protons were explored at several centers (for a thorough review, see Larsson[3]). In Sweden, Lars Leksell and Börje Larsson were conducting such studies using the 185 MeV proton beam at the Gustav Werner Institute in Uppsala. Interestingly, an early key paper from this group[4] became seminal ("a crucial flash of inspiration") in the mind of Allan Cormack when thinking out the computed tomography (CT) technique (for which he later won the Nobel prize together with Godfrey Hounsfield). Thus, the radiosurgical cross-firing concept seems to have fertilized Cormack's thoughts while he was designing the first CT machine.

The Gustav Werner Institute became the cradle of neurosurgical radiosurgery. Irradiation with heavy particles was also practiced by Lawrence's group in Berkeley, California, however, without the use of stereotactic technique in its limited sense. Raymond Kjellberg, a neurosurgeon using the cyclotron at Harvard, started to explore the applicability of the proton beam Bragg peak in pituitary irradiation.

From the standpoint of a practically working neurosurgeon, these early attempts to develop radiosurgery soon necessitated an analysis of possible clinical applications. This gave rise to the formulation of new therapeutic arguments, rationales, and principles, tracks of thought that were less obvious for the great majority of brain surgeons. For example, when it came to advocating radiosurgical treatment of benign intracranial tumors, the new radiosurgical therapeutic principle was not removing but inactivating and possibly obliterating the neoplasm. Such thoughts proved provocative to the devoted supporters of microsurgery as a superior method of management and were even insulting to its great masters.

It is an understatement to claim that the use of high-energy beams, for example, from a synchrocyclotron, in the exclusive clinical setting is a less convenient, if not impossible, technique. Thus, Leksell's idea of a more handy "beam knife" was conceived. In this, a large number (i.e., as many as technically possible) of cobalt 60 radiation sources, distributed in a half-sphere around the patient's head, would safely allow a simultaneous firing of beams from all these sources, collimated as well as possible, and directed to a preselected intracranial target (volume). An absolute prerequisite was that a clinically well-proven stereotactic technique should be employed.

Importantly, Leksell's focus from the very beginning was on the possible destruction (or stimulation) of deeply located tracts and nuclei in the brain, within the functional brain surgery. The development of "psychosurgical procedures without opening the skull" was a first technical goal in his early considerations. Similarly, a "nonbloody" thalamotomy for parkinsonism (or pain) was another beckoning application. Thus, in the first GK, the technical aim was to obtain slit-formed beam apertures, making the composite ionization pattern in the tissue as "cutlike" as possible. Therefore, during the period of the unit's construction, its nickname was "the beam knife."

The Development of Neurosurgical Radiosurgery

There are strong reasons to assume that Leksell, a clinical surgeon himself, made manifest the term *radiosurgery* when inventing the GK. Already in 1951 he had introduced the term.[5] For him, the GK was nothing but "a surgical tool," in many aspects analogous to the cautery loop, the instrument for cutting or digging out tissue, normal or neoplastic, in traditional surgery. This comparison is what he himself often made. Moreover, it fixed his standpoint that radiosurgery should remain surgery, essentially without overlap radiotherapy, except for the fundamental fact that the same physical agent was used, beams of ionizing radiation.

Thus, Leksell maintained that the composition of any operating team responsible for a radiosurgical procedure should be analogous to the group of surgeons performing conventional surgery. This was his absolute conviction. He regretted that, for practical (radiation protection) reasons, he had to give up his aims to have the first GK installed in one of the three operating rooms of the neurosurgical department. According to Leksell, this would be the site for the new machine.

Some uneasiness was raised between the neurosurgical staff at the Karolinska Institute and influential oncologists and radiophysicists. For example, the editor of *Acta Radiologica* refused to accept that the title of one of the first manuscripts from the GK team included the term *radiosurgery.* After tough negotiations between the senior author and the editor, for this particular paper the word combination *radiation surgery* was eventually accepted by both parties (however, under considerable mutual dissatisfaction).[6]

Although the theoretical and practical background—a crossfiring with extremely well-collimated high-energy beams proven as a straightforward and very efficient way to deliver precision radiation therapy (in the central nervous system)—radiosurgery as a clinical discipline was not fully established until the first GK prototype was used in Stockholm in late 1967.[7]

This historical claim is supported by the fact that Leksell and his next coworkers very early and very decisively set the conceptual, and partly provocative, agenda for clinical radiosurgery and formulated the prerequisites for new modes of approaching classical neurosurgical problems. For example, a spin-off from this policy making was that the synchrocyclotron, with its extensive staff of physicists and other laboratory personnel, would never fit into an exclusively clinical setting, as a "surgical tool."

From a conceptual standpoint it became quite clear that basic key words for genuine clinical *radiosurgery* were (1) heavy *single* dose, (2) *small* irradiated volume, (3) *benign* pathology, (4) *functional* surgery, and (5) *stereotactic* technique. Notably, involvement by any oncologist was deemed unnecessary. Corresponding key words for *radiotherapy* were (1) multiple doses/*fractionation*/radiosensitizers, (2) *larger* volumes treated, (3) *malignancies,* and (4) an *oncologist* as principal of the treatment team. With the gradual appearance of more and more sophisticated radiation equipment, however, this orthodoxy over time has partly lost some of its relevance.

But any radiosurgical procedure still has the following traits in common with a common surgical operation: It is limited in time to a few hours and might thus be described in military terms, such as attack, assault, mission, and operation. At the end of the procedure, the commission is performed, the job is done. This should be compared with the long-lasting (weeks) fractionation courses used in radiotherapy. Moreover, as mentioned, the whole surgical procedure is performed by a small, well-defined, tight group of people (typically, the surgeon and assistants), under one team leader with a supreme continuous responsibility for all decisions made during the irradiation procedure. This is in striking contrast to the extended (weeks) course of treatment, not uncommonly including ad hoc decisions, characterizing routine radiotherapy.

The Pilot Cases

The very first case treated with the GK occurred in October 1967.[7] The patient was a young man with a solid craniopharyngioma remaining after previous yttrium 90 installation in a tumor cyst, with rewarding result. The dimensions of the tumor were appropriate for irradiation using a 3×5 mm collimator alternative. A single dose of 20 Gy was given to the center of the tumor.

The second patient had a pituitary tumor, a so-called chromophobe adenoma, recurrent after previous transfrontal surgery. Twenty-eight Gy was given to the center of the sella turcica. The radiation dose level was chosen primarily with regard to the radiation tolerance of the optic apparatus (10 Gy), assumed to be a qualified guess.

It is interesting to follow the team's discussion in connection with the procedure, as noted in the patient's chart. In this, apart from thorough considerations regarding the dose level/distribution in the particular case, the potential risk of postirradiation tumor swelling was discussed. Furthermore, the next possible applications were actualized, thalamotomy for intractable pain and irradiation of hypersecreting pituitary adenomas, respectively.

The pilot cases stimulated the GK team to design protocols for further and systematic studies. For example, over the coming years, Rähn and Thorén presented reports on patients with Cushing disease[8] and vestibular schwannomas,[9] respectively, each in its field seminal for the further progress of a virtually clinical radiosurgery. Ladislau Steiner, together with Leksell, led the most exciting project, the irradiation of intracranial arteriovenous malformations (AVMs). A marvelous disappearance of the AVM could be seen already in the first cases.[10] Leksell himself was strongly involved in the treatment of patients with intractable cancer pain, not least to try to develop perioperative pain tests for assessing the expected radiolesions in the nonspecific pain pathways in the centrum medianum, used as a target area.[11] A project on pinealomas was foreseen and even longed for, as the GK might be optimal to use in a circumscribed and benign pineal neoplasm. Preirradiation stereotactic biopsy would make the case selection safe, thus making obsolete any diagnostic guessing, during this time too commonly practiced in pineal tumors.[6]

The collimator system of the first GK was designed to produce disk-shaped radiolesions. In the first tumor cases, it became obvious that the next edition of GK should be designed for the production of spherical and larger radiation fields, congruent with the most common shape of tumors. The need for cylindrical collimators was obvious, and in 1974 a new machine thus designed was taken into use (the apertures being 4–14 mms wide) (**Fig. 1.1**). Notably, the principle of "clustering" isocenters was introduced already in several of the first patients, the very first one harboring a large pituitary adenoma, irradiated in October 1969, using five isocenters.[12]

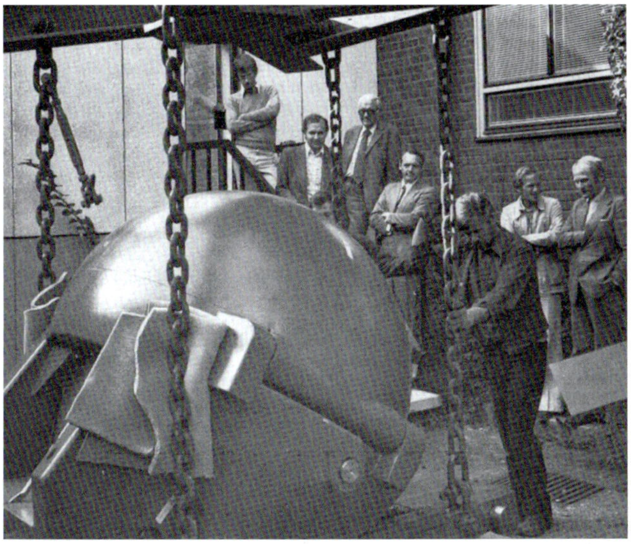

Figure 1.1 The first Gamma Knife for routine use (GK2) under installation at the Karolinska Institute in 1974. Under the supervision of Professor Leksell (in the background), those to be first involved witness the procedure: from left Drs. Norén, Rähn, Melander (oncologist), Backlund, and Sarby (physicist). (Photo Börje Nilsson, courtesy Karolinska Sjukhuset. Used with permission.)

During the first 10 years, 286 patients were treated in Stockholm, with the following diagnoses (in decreasing order of frequency):

1. Pituitary tumor (nonsecreting adenoma, Cushing syndrome, acromegaly)
2. AVM
3. Acoustic neuroma
4. Intractable cancer pain (thalamotomy)
5. Pineal tumor
6. Miscellaneous, including capsulotomy (in obsessive-compulsive disorder) and hypophysectomy (in metastasizing carcinoma)

A comprehensive account of the early work with the first two GKs is given in a recent publication.[12]

The experiences from Stockholm soon fertilized the (already existing) interest among some neurosurgeons worldwide who tried to modify linear particle accelerator (linac) techniques for intracranial stereotactic irradiation. These included Drs. Barcia-Salorio in Valencia, Spain, Betti in Buenos Aires, Argentina, Colombo in Vicenza, Italy, and Sturm in Heidelberg, Germany.

After being used for 5 years, the first GK prototype was donated by the Karolinska Institute to the University of California at Los Angeles, for experimental work under Professor Robert Rand. The first neurosurgeons to use GK outside Sweden were, apart from Rand, Hernan Bunge in Buenos Aires, Argentina (1984), David Forster in Sheffield, United Kingdom (1985), and, after a tedious approval procedure, Dade Lunsford in Pittsburgh, Pennsylvania (1987). It proved to be anything but self-evident to have the GK technique accepted in the United States.[13]

As a new medical technology, stereotactic radiosurgery has undergone an uncomparable development: "Like Pandora's box, the lid on radiosurgery was opened in the 1980s, and an explosion of medical interest spread across the world."[14] Today, this statement by Lunsford even has a vague touch of understatement. Forty years after the introduction of radiosurgery, thousands of patients have profited from the foresight and decisive work of the pioneers in terms of decreased risk taking, increased cure rate, and improved quality of life.

Step-by-step sophistications (of both hard- and software, in the GK as well as in stereotactic irradiation units based on parallel beam/linac concepts), made by various medical-technical companies in the forefront, have over time brought about treatment options that, until just a few decades ago, seemed too marvelous to be anticipated. Surprisingly, it is of utmost interest that in this formidable technical and conceptual progress, a kind of discrete "phenomenological merge" between radiosurgery and radiotherapy may even be perceived.

References

1. Leksell L. Stereotaxis and Radiosurgery: An Operative System. Springfield, IL: Charles C Thomas; 1971
2. Szikla G, ed. Stereotactic Cerebral Irradiation. Amsterdam: Elsevier; 1979
3. Larsson B. The History of Radiosurgery: The Early Years (1950–1970). Vol. 1. Radiosurgery. Basel: Karger; 1996:1–10
4. Larsson B, Leksell L, Rexed P, Sourander P, Mair W, Andersson B. The high-energy proton beam as a neurosurgical tool. Nature 1958;182: 1222–1223
5. Leksell L. The sterotaxic method and radiosurgery of the brain. Acta Chir Scand 1951;102:316–319
6. Backlund EO, Rähn T, Sarby B. Treatment of pinealomas by stereotaxic radiation surgery. Acta Radiol Ther Phys Biol 1974;13:368–376
7. Backlund EO. Stereotaxic treatment of craniopharyngiomas. In: Hamberger CA, Wersäll J, eds. Nobel Symposium 10: Disorders of the Skull Base Region. Stockholm: Almqvist & Wiksell; 1969:237–244
8. Rähn T, Thorén M, Hall K, Backlund EO. Stereotactic radiosurgery in Cushing's syndrome: acute radation effects. Surg Neurol 1980; 14:85–92
9. Norén G, Arndt J, Hindmarsch T. Stereotactic radiosurgery in acoustic neurinoma: further experiences. Neurosurgery 1983;13:12–22
10. Steiner L, Leksell L, Greitz T, Backlund EO. Stereotaxic radiosurgery for cerebral arteriovenous malformations: report of a case. Acta Chir Scand 1972;138:459–464
11. Leksell L. Cerebral radiosurgery, I: Gammathalamotomy in two cases of intractable pain. Acta Chir Scand 1968;134:585–595
12. Backlund EO. Gamma Knife—the early story: memoirs of a privileged man. Progr Neurol Surg 2007;20:21–28
13. Lunsford LD, Flickinger J, Lindner G, Maitz A. Stereotactic radiosurgery of the brain using the first United States 201 cobalt-60 source Gamma Knife. Neurosurgery 1989;24(2):151–159
14. Lunsford LD, Alexander E, Loeffler JS. General introduction: history of radiosurgery. In: Alexander E, Loeffler JS, Lunsford LD, eds. Stereotactic Radiosurgery. New York: McGraw-Hill; 1993:1–4

2

Radiobiology of Stereotactic Radiosurgery

John C. Flickinger

Radiosurgery exploits the ability of small volumes of a normal organ to tolerate much higher radiation doses without injury than large volumes of the same organ. This dose–volume effect for radiation becomes highly pronounced at very small volumes like those treated in radiosurgery. By using stereotactic fixation and localization techniques, radiosurgery allows clinicians to do away with the need to expand radiation treatment volumes by adding margins around well-defined target/tumor volumes to correct for the localization/targeting errors seen with conventional radiotherapy setups. The highly conformal radiation dose distributions delivered through multiple beams using radiosurgery techniques reduce the amount of normal tissue treated to full treatment doses within the intracranial treatment volume and also reduce radiation dose fall-off into surrounding normal tissue outside the target volume. This allows clinicians to change from treating with multiple small dose fractions to total doses that large volumes of surrounding normal tissue can tolerate to treating with high-dose single-fraction radiation doses that markedly smaller, thin rims of normal tissue adjacent to radiosurgical targets can tolerate.

Rationale for Fractionation in Conventional Radiotherapy

Prior to the introduction of radiosurgery, almost all clinical radiation therapy to intracranial targets was fractionated Starting with observation of the reaction of skin that received much higher doses with external beam orthovoltage radiotherapy used before the introduction of megavoltage radiotherapy sources (cobalt 60 and linear particle accelerator [linac]), it became obvious that early and late normal tissue reactions could be limited through fractionation while maintaining high response rates in treating malignant tumors. Radiobiological analysis of a few cell culture lines of fast-growing malignant tumors and analysis of clinical experience of tumor control and complications with some common fast-growing malignant tumors commonly treated with fractionated radiotherapy in the clinic strongly supported this observation. These studies showed that increased fractionation (reducing daily radiation dose fractions to the range of 1.8 to 2.0 Gy per fraction and treating with more fractions to equal or slightly higher total doses) preferentially spared normal tissue from radiation injury without changing tumor control as much. With widespread use of 1.8 to 2.0 Gy fractions, radiation oncologists became most comfortable treating everything that way (both rapidly growing malignant and slow-growing benign tumors), especially because most information about normal tissue tolerance was learned using these fractionation schemes.

Slow-growing benign tumors have been notoriously difficult to study in cell culture or animal models. Their radiobiological responses, particularly how a response changes with different fractionations, are poorly defined. Prior to the advent of radiosurgery, few radiation oncologists had more than limited experience with treating with high doses of single-fraction radiation. Stereotactic radiosurgery provided clinicians the ability to administer high single doses of radiation to intracranial targets with relative safety. Radiosurgery ushered in a new era of understanding of how different approaches to radiation treatment planning and radiobiology may be modified in the clinic to achieve goals previously thought unreachable.

The Mechanics of Tissue Irradiation

When a person undergoes x-ray treatment or cobalt irradiation, the target region is exposed to a high-energy photon beam. That beam interacts with the tissue at the target, producing a cascade of ionizing electrons that in turn cause biochemical damage within the cells exposed to the radiation. Both single- and double-stranded deoxyribonucleic acid (DNA) breaks may occur. Depending on how much biochemical damage occurs and how much of that damage can be repaired by the cell, the consequences lead to necrosis (rapid cell death), apoptosis (slow programmed cell death), or cell survival (with or without survival of abilities such as further mitosis and hormonal secretion). The exact biology of these injury and repair responses is being unraveled to show increasing complexity with potential points of modification.[1–3] Tumor control by radiation treatment comes not only through radiation directly affecting tumor cells, but also through effects on the adventitia, most notably the supporting vasculature.[4] Within the range of doses commonly used for radiosurgery, the dominant mode of cell death in tumors seems to be mediated through radiation effects on endothelial cells in the supporting vasculature.[4] Pathological studies of tumors resected after radiosurgery also indicate that vascular endothelium may be the primary target responding to radiosurgery.[5] This vasculature effect seems to explain why single-fraction radiosurgery provides similarly high tumor rates for very different tumors found to differ widely by being either highly resistant or highly sensitive to radiation either in cell culture models or in clinical experience with conventional fractionated radiotherapy.

Optimizing the outcome of any clinical intervention (radiation, drug therapy, or surgery) usually requires striking a balance between maximizing the desired outcome from the intervention (tumor cure, vascular malformation obliteration, etc.) while minimizing undesired sequelae of the intervention (complications). This balance can be represented in many clinical situations by a pair of dose–response curves representing cure (tumor control or arteriovenous malformation [AVM] obliteration) and complications (radiation injury), as shown in **Fig. 2.1.** The separation between the curves has been referred to as the therapeutic window, and the ratio of cure to complication risk is referred to as the therapeutic ratio. Radiosurgery exploits the radiobiological fact that smaller volumes of normal tissue can withstand much higher doses of radiation than larger volumes of normal tissue. Reducing the volume of tissue irradiated to high doses lessens the complication risk for any dose given to the target, shifting the complication dose–response curve for the treatment to the right, farther away from the complication curve, thereby improving the therapeutic ratio. The effect on both curves must be adequately assessed to evaluate potential radiation dose–response modifications (e.g., altered fractionation, radiation protectors, or radiosensitizing drugs, including some chemotherapy and hypoxic radiation sensitizers) to find if they improve the therapeutic ratio.

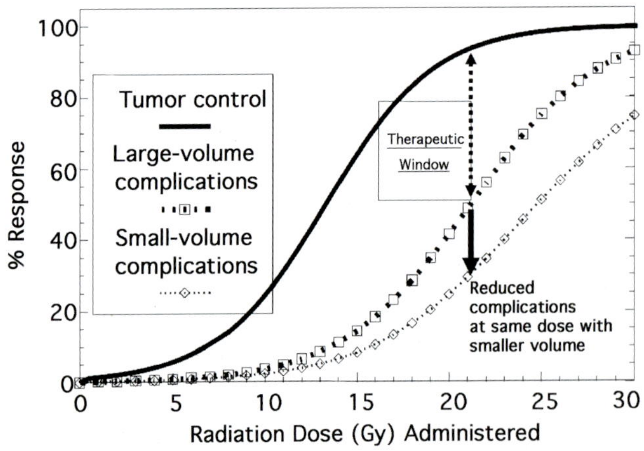

Fig. 2.1 Typical sigmoid dose–response curves for tumor control and complications and the effect of reducing treatment volume on the complication curve.

◆ Estimating the Effects of Fractionating Radiation in Radiosurgery

The linear-quadratic formula is the most widely accepted way to represent fractionation effects in radiotherapy.[6–11] It relates the log of surviving cells after a dose fraction of ionizing radiation as being proportional to a linear function of the dose per fraction (consisting of the dose per fraction multiplied by a coefficient, α) plus a second quadratic function (consisting of the dose per fraction squared multiplied by a second coefficient, β). This formula forms a power series modeling radiation cell killing with a combination of linear, single-hit kinetics (which could mathematically represent double-stranded DNA breaks leading to cell death) and quadratic, double-hit kinetics (which could mathematically represent a critical accumulation of single-stranded DNA breaks leading to cell death). The linear-quadratic formula represents the probability of either tumor cure or normal tissue injury, *P* (cure or complication), from a single fraction of radiation of dose, *d*, by the following probabilistic double-exponential equation:

$$P(\text{cure or complication}) = \exp[-K \times \exp(-\alpha \times d - \beta \times d^2)] \quad (1)$$

where exp represents the number *e* (2.7183, used in natural logarithms) raised exponentially to the power of the terms that follow, *K* represents the number of target clonogens, and α and β are the linear and quadratic coefficients.

This mathematical expression describes sigmoid-shaped dose–response curves with the probability of cure or complications increasing with dose from 0% to a limit of 100% as dose is increased (**Fig. 2.1**). Although used in research, this expression of the linear-quadratic formula is virtually never used in day-to-day clinical radiotherapy practice.

A much more useful calculation in the clinic is the formula to equate the effect of a fractionated course of radiotherapy with one dose per fraction (fr) d_1 and total dose D_1 to a different fractionation scheme with dose per fraction d_2 *and total dose* D_2 according to a given α/β ratio, as follows:

$$\text{Total dose } D_1 \text{ Gy} \times (d_1 \text{ Gy/fr} + a/b) = \text{total dose} - (D_2 \text{ Gy} \times d_2 \text{ Gy/fr} + \alpha/\beta) \quad (2)$$

Another formula useful in the clinic is the expression for NTD_2, the normalized total dose at 2 Gy per fraction,

Table 2.1 Calculation of Radiobiologically Equivalent Dose (Normalized Total Dose) for Fractionated Radiotherapy with 2 Gy Fractions (NTD_2) from Single-Fraction Radiosurgery According to the Linear-Quadratic Equation Using Different Values of α/β (and No Time Correction)

Single-Fraction Dose (Gy)	NTD_2 (α/β = 10) Equivalent Dose (Gy) for Early-Reacting Tissue	NTD_2 (α/β = 2) Equivalent Dose (Gy) for Late-Reacting Tissue	NTD_2 (α/β = 1) Equivalent Dose (Gy) with a Lower Value of α/β = 1	NTD_2 (α/β = 0) Equivalent dose (Gy) for Model with No α Component
4	4.7	6	6.7	8
6	8.0	12	14.0	18
8	12.0	20	24.0	32
10	16.7	30	36.7	50
12	22.0	42	52.0	72
14	28.0	56	70.0	98
16	34.7	72	90.7	128
18	42.0	90	114.0	162
20	50.0	110	140.0	200
22	58.7	132	168.7	242
24	68.0	156	200.0	288

which is the equivalent total dose administered with daily 2 Gy fractions using a given α/β value.[6] NTD_2 for a given α/β ratio can be calculated for a course of radiotherapy given with a dose per fraction of *d* Gy/fr with the following equation:

$$NTD_2 \text{ for } (\alpha/\beta) = \text{total dose at } d \text{ Gy/fr} \times (d \text{ Gy/fr} + \alpha/\beta) / (2 \text{ Gy/fr} + \alpha/\beta) \quad (3)$$

Table 2.1 shows the 2 Gy/fraction equivalent doses predicted for different single-fraction radiosurgery doses with the linear-quadratic formula using different α/β ratios.

Table 2.1, Eq. 2, and Eq. 3 ignore the effect of overall treatment time, which should be negligible for central nervous system tissue and benign tumors in normal circumstances. A time-dependent repopulation term should be added for protracted fractionated treatment of fast-growing malignant tumors. Repopulation of malignant tumors accelerates 2 to 3 weeks after the start of radiotherapy. Because of clinical studies that related poor tumor control from head and neck cancer radiotherapy with increasing overall treatment time, split-course radiotherapy with planned 2-week breaks in the middle to alleviate mucositis are no longer routinely used.

The ratio of the α coefficient divided by the β coefficient (the α/β ratio) provides a useful parameter to quantify fractionation effects in target tissues and tumors. With the α/β ratio for a given organ or tumor, we can estimate the total dose and number of fractions needed to change from treatment with one dose per fraction to another dose per fraction and with the same effect on that tissue or tumor. Because different kinds of tumors, different organs, and even different types of injury reactions in the same organ (e.g., skin redness vs late skin fibrosis) have different α/β ratios, changing to a different fractionation scheme with an equivalent effect calculated for one organ will lead to a different effect on organs or tumors with different α/β ratios. This became apparent when early radiation therapists tried to switch to cheaper and more convenient hypofractionated radiation schemes with larger dose fractions producing similar acute skin reactions and found increased late complications.

Different tissues can be lumped into categories by their α/β ratios as either early-responding tissues (fast growing with injury responses, e.g., mucositis and skin erythema, occurring a relatively short time after radiation) or late-responding tissues (slow-growing tissues that take a longer time after radiation exposure for injury reactions to become apparent). Studies of fractionation effects in radiotherapy clinics and in animal models found the brain and spinal cord to be late-responding tissues, relatively more sensitive to large-dose fractions, with α/β ratios around 2. Faster growing, faster responding tissues such as skin erythema and mucositis reactions have α/β values in the intermediate range of 5 to 8, whereas many fast-growing malignant tumors have α/β values closer to 10.[6] Smaller radiation dose fraction schedules cause proportionally less injury to normal tissues (or a limited number of tumors) with a low α/β ratio (a smaller α or single-hit component to radiation cell-kill kinetics) compared with malignant tumors (or faster responding tissues) with higher α/β ratios.

Because most malignant tumors have a higher α/β ratio than adjacent normal tissue, increasing fractionation for conventional large-field radiotherapy improves the therapeutic window most of the time. This is not the case for all tumors that can be treated by radiation and may not hold for radiosurgery dose distributions. First of all, there is a wide variation of α/β ratios found in malignant tumors. Some malignant tumors, such as melanoma and prostate cancer (or at least some strains of them), have lower α/β ratios than surrounding normal tissues (skin or rectum/bladder), supporting the use of larger dose fractions for treatment.[10] Second, benign tumors should have lower α/β ratios than malignant tumors. Third, and possibly most important for radiosurgery, α/β ratios for the tumor cells themselves do not describe the radiation response of the supporting adventitia such as the endothelial cells within the tumor vasculature, which appear to be responsible for most of the response with high-dose single fractions and appear to have low α/β ratios.[4]

Limitations of the Linear-Quadratic Formula to Estimate Radiation Effects in Radiosurgery

The linear-quadratic formula provides a reasonably good fit to postradiation single-cell culture survival data and is useful in the clinic for limited extrapolations from one course of fractionated radiotherapy to another with different-sized dose fractions, particularly within a dose fraction range of 1 to 8 Gy. Extrapolating from 1.8 to 2.0 Gy fractions used in conventionally fractionated radiotherapy to the high single-fraction doses commonly used in radiosurgery stretches the formula beyond the limits of accuracy.

Table 2.1 takes commonly used single-fraction radiosurgery doses and relates predicted equivalent doses for fractionated radiotherapy with 2 Gy fractions (NTD_2) using α/β values of 10 for early-reacting tissue and 2 for late-reacting tissue (which is the accepted value for brain tissue from large studies of fractionated radiotherapy data). The last column provides dose-equivalent dose calculations using an α/β value of 0 (specifically, $\alpha = 0$), making it a quadratic exponential formula rather than a true linear-quadratic formula. A conservative estimate of the NTD_2 equivalent for brain injury is easily calculated using an α/β value of 0, as it is simply one half the single-fraction dose squared. Using an α/β value of 0 is quite a stretch from the theoretical basis of the formula, which presupposes some contribution with single-hit kinetics (the α component) corresponding to direct double-stranded DNA breakage. From what is known about optic nerve tolerance (discussed in the next section), an α/β ratio somewhere between 0 and 1 seems to fit the data for optic nerve injury risk with radiosurgery doses near 12 Gy.

Optic Nerve Tolerance Doses for Radiosurgery

An early analysis of optic nerve complications in the combined Harvard and University of Pittsburgh experience recommended 8 Gy as a safe dose limit for the optic nerves/chiasm.[12] The lowest optic chiasm dose quoted for radiation-induced optic injury in that study was 9.7 Gy. According to **Table 2.1,** the linear-quadratic formula with values of 0 and 2 for α/β predicts that a 10 Gy single-fraction dose to the optic chiasm should have the equivalent effect of 32 Gy or 50 Gy at 2 Gy per fraction, respectively, for $\alpha/\beta = 0$ or 2. Using an α/β value of 0, the equivalent dose at 2 Gy per fraction for the 9.7 Gy radiosurgery dose that caused optic neuropathy is only 47 Gy. From clinical experience with fractionated radiotherapy of pituitary adenomas and other parasellar tumors, the risk of optic neuropathy for 46 to 48 Gy at 2 Gy per fraction should be ~1/300.[13]

Stafford et al reported a later analysis of the Mayo Clinic experience with four cases of optic neuropathy occurring out of 215 radiosurgery patients receiving a median optic chiasm dose of 10 Gy.[14] One case of optic injury developed after a dose of 12.8 Gy with radiosurgery alone, where the risk seemed to be ~3%. The other cases developed after prior fractionated radiotherapy (7 Gy preceded by 58.8 Gy fractionated, 9 Gy after 45 Gy fractionated, and one case that followed two radiosurgery procedures delivering 9 and later 12 Gy to the optic system after 50.4 Gy of fractionate radiotherapy).

Leber et al from Graz, Austria, analyzed optic neuropathy risks in 50 patients after 24- to 60-month follow-up (median 40 months) following Gamma Knife radiosurgery for benign skull base tumors.[15] They found optic neuropathy risks of 0% with < 10 Gy, 27% with 10 to 15 Gy, and 78% with > 15 Gy. No cavernous sinus nerve injury developed with doses of 5 to 30 Gy. The optic nerve injury risks seen in the Graz and Mayo Clinic series are what would be expected with 2 Gy fraction equivalent values calculated with α/β ratios between 0 and 1 Gy/fraction, rather than the value of 2 Gy/fraction expected from a large body of data for fractionated radiotherapy.[6]

Problems in Assessing Radiobiological Parameters from Radiosurgery Data

Analyzing clinical radiosurgery data from dose–response relationships and defined radiobiological parameters is full of difficulties. Radiosurgery plans typically use inhomogeneous dose distributions, with doses prescribed to 50 to 80% isodose treatment volumes covering anywhere from 90 to 100% of the target volume. Absolute minimum doses within the target volume typically run 5 to 30% lower than the prescription dose, and they are highly dependent on how accurately targets are contoured. Contours of the same tumor/target volume or critical structures can vary slightly from one clinician to another. With the steep dose fall-off at the edge of the tumor contour in most radiosurgery plans, there can be significant variation in absolute minimum dose with subtle differences in tumor contouring, much more than the variation seen for average dose, percent coverage, or other parameters. Early treatment planning programs for the Gamma Knife radiosurgery were not integrated with imaging and tumor-contouring tools. After starting with that approach, many Gamma Knife centers, such as the University of Pittsburgh, did not routinely contour all target volumes until many years later. Single-fraction radiosurgery dose–response data for AVM obliteration and radiation injury to brain parenchyma and cranial nerves can be used to calculate α/β ratios; however, as shown in **Table 2.2,** they yield values of −30 to −60 Gy/fraction rather than 2 to 3 Gy/fraction as would be expected from conventional fractionated radiotherapy data.[6,9,10]

Table 2.2 Calculated α/β Ratios for Different End Points after Radiosurgery at the University of Pittsburgh

Clinical End Point	Number of Subjects	α/β Ratio
Facial weakness	31/218 acoustic schwannomas	−60.8 ± 81.4
Hearing loss	57/138 acoustics with hearing	−39.6 ± 9.2
In-field AVM obliteration	293/355 AVM obliterated	−49.3 ± 5.3
Post-RS imaging changes	87/307 AVMs with changes	−29.7 ± 2.4

Abbreviations: AVM, arteriovenous malformation; RS, radiosurgery.

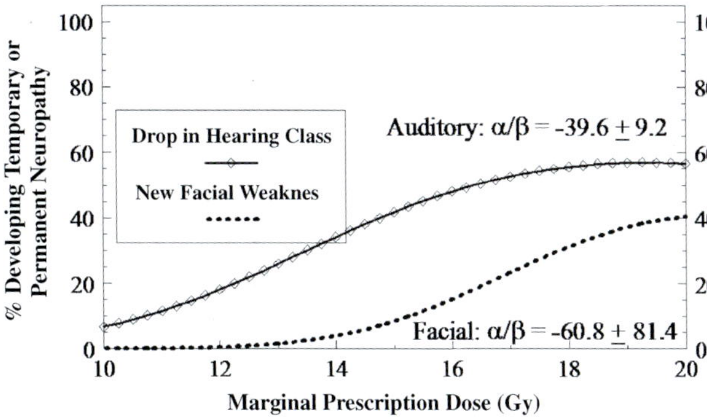

Fig. 2.2 Linear-quadratic (Poisson) dose–response curves for the development of auditory and facial neuropathies according to marginal (minimum tumor) dose. These curves and their corresponding α/β ratio values were obtained from nonlinear regression analysis of 218 acoustic schwannoma patients who underwent radiosurgery at the University of Pittsburgh from 1987 to 1997 with more than 2 years of follow-up.

Attempts to calculate α/β ratios for benign tumor control are further limited by the difficulty defining any clear dose–response using the very small number of failures that occur. The long-term failure rate for vestibular schwannoma radiosurgery is in the range of 1 to 2%. Tumors that have been previously resected have higher marginal failure rates, but there are more difficulties with defining the true target volume because of the difficulty distinguishing gross tumor from postoperative effects and the inability to define microscopic areas of residual tumor that can lead to marginal recurrence. Unresected and unbiopsied meningiomas defined by imaging criteria provide more clearly defined targets for defining a dose–response but without a biopsy, they also have at least a 2% chance of misdiagnosis.[16] After excluding known cases of misdiagnosis in the Pittsburgh unbiopsied meningioma experience, it was not possible to define a significant dose–response by prescription dose. Tumor contours were lacking to test dose–response relationships for absolute minimum dose, and any assessment would be limited by the lack of failures to analyze (because of the 93% tumor control rate). Genetic differences in tumors and/or host adventitia (particularly endothelial cells) can lead to radiobiological heterogeneity that flattens or blurs tumor dose–responses. That could make α/β ratios more difficult or impossible to define from the data, the same way that misdiagnosis could.

Malignant tumors, particularly brain metastases, have higher failure rates that should make dose–responses easier to define. The chief problem with assessing radiobiological parameters from dose–responses for brain metastasis radiosurgery is reliably distinguishing recurrence from radiation injury reactions before patients die from advanced metastatic cancer. Other problems, such as tumor/adventitial heterogeneity and possibly slight variations in tumor definitions, remain.

Neuropathy Models for Acoustic Schwannoma Radiosurgery

The linear-quadratic formula runs into problems in modeling dose–response curves for cranial neuropathies after single-fraction radiosurgery of acoustic schwannomas. We should be able to calculate values of α and β and the α/β ratio from clinical data for the single-fraction dose–response curve. Data for injury to the facial, acoustic, and auditory nerves after acoustic schwannoma radiosurgery should allow calculation of α/β ratios for radiation injury to these nerves. We analyzed 218 acoustic schwannoma patients who underwent radiosurgery at the University of Pittsburgh from 1987 to 1997 with more than 2 years of follow-up.[17] Higher doses used in the early experience in Pittsburgh resulted in higher rates of facial and trigeminal neuropathy and poorer hearing preservation during that time than are seen with marginal doses of 12 to 13 Gy currently in use. This analysis assumed that the dose to the facial and auditory nerves matched the marginal doses prescribed at the time of radiosurgery, as these nerves invariably lie along the capsule of the tumor. This assumption is not as reliable for the trigeminal nerve, so that data will be excluded, although the findings were similar. We found small, negative values for the β coefficients for facial and auditory neuropathy, with best-fitting α/β ratios in the range of −30 to −55 (**Fig. 2.2** and **Table 2.2**). Not only does this clash with the expected value of $\alpha/\beta = 2$ from analysis of conventional fractionated radiotherapy data, but the negative values for β and the α/β ratios that mathematically describe the empirically best-fitting dose–response curves for these data should be disallowed by the theoretical rationale for the linear-quadratic formula.

Radiobiological Analyses of Arteriovenous Malformation Radiosurgery

We found similar problems using the linear-quadratic formula to fit dose–response data for AVM radiosurgery. We analyzed obliteration after Gamma Knife radiosurgery in

351 AVM patients with 3 to 11 years of follow-up imaging after Gamma Knife radiosurgery at Pittsburgh.[18] The median marginal dose range was 12 to 30 Gy (median = 20 Gy) to treatment volumes that varied from 0.26 to 24.00 cc (median = 5.70 cc). We documented obliteration with angiography in 193 of 264 (73%) AVM patients, and with magnetic resonance (MRA) alone in 75 of 87 (86%) AVM patients who refused angiographic follow-up. The overall corrected obliteration rate (assuming 96% accuracy for MR) was 75%.

Because part of the AVM nidus may be unintentionally omitted from the treatment volume due to poor visualization at radiosurgery, it makes more sense to define a radiobiological dose–response analysis for in-field nidus obliteration (whether or not there was obliteration within the treatment volume). The best-fitting values of α/β ratios for in-field obliteration for empirically derived logistic regression models were $\alpha/\beta = -44.4 \pm 12.5$ and $\alpha/\beta = -45.3 \pm 9.8$ for angiographic only and for MR plus angiographic obliteration, respectively. We derived similar values with standard linear-quadratic Poisson models of $\alpha/\beta = -48.1 \pm 5.9$ for angiographic obliteration only and $\alpha/\beta = -49.3 \pm 5.3$ for MRI or angiographic obliteration. **Figure 2.3** shows the dose–response curve for in-field MR or angiographically defined obliteration. The negative α/β ratio was necessary to mathematically describe the plateau in the in-field dose–response curve (at <23 Gy).

We also derived an alternative maximum obliteration rate model for the dose–response of AVM obliteration using data for overall obliteration, rather than in-field obliteration as the end point. This model added an empirically fitted maximum obliteration rate to the dose–response function to account for marginal misses or any unknown factor that could limit the maximum obliteration rate from reaching 100%. Because it required only overall obliteration data, it avoided any potential error in determining whether failures with persistent AVM nidus were inside or outside the original radiosurgery treatment volume. We found a maximum obliteration rate for cases treated without embolization of $87.9 \pm 4.9\%$ ($p < .0001$). The additional failure rate due to embolization (probable increased marginal miss) was $16.4 \pm 7.6\%$ ($p = .03$). This model had less sensitivity to the α/β value, so its value could not be precisely defined aside from seeing a poor fit with any positive values. A negative value for the α/β ratio could not be precisely defined when negative values were allowed. The α/β ratio value converged to 0 when constrained to positive values, but unlike the data for in-field obliteration, an adequate fit was achieved at that value.

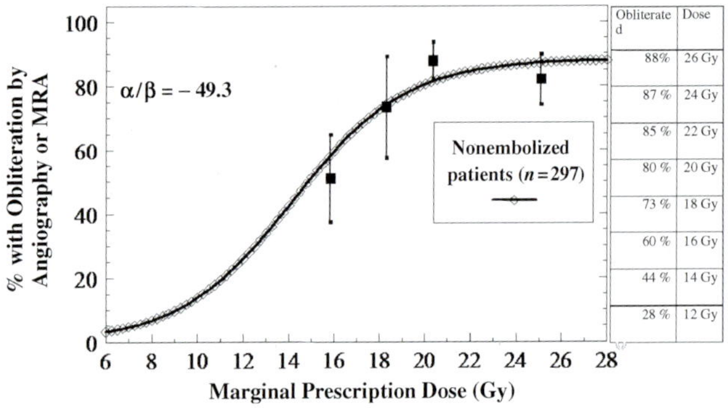

Fig. 2.3 Standard linear-quadratic (Poisson) dose–response curve for postradiosurgery, magnetic resonance, or angiographic arteriovenous malformation obliteration of 297 patients who underwent Gamma Knife radiosurgery at the University of Pittsburgh from 1987 to 1997 without embolization. Each square and associated error bar represent the percent obliteration rate with the respective 95% confidence interval for each marginal dose groups at the mean marginal dose value for each group. MRA, magnetic resonance angiography.

Radiation injury reactions after AVM radiosurgery also provide excellent data to test radiobiological models. New areas of increased signal develop on T2-weighted MRI sequences in brain adjacent to AVM in <30% of patients within 2 years of radiosurgery. These postradiosurgery imaging changes represent a radiation injury reaction involving surrounding brain. These signal changes are symptomatic in one third of patients developing this reaction (10% of all AVM radiosurgery patients). The chance that these changes produce noticeable symptoms varies dramatically with location in the brain. Because modeling the influence of location on symptomatic sequelae is extremely complex,[19] postradiosurgery imaging changes (which do not seem to vary with location) represent a better end point for radiobiological analysis of parenchymal brain injury.

We tested the fit of the linear-quadratic equation with data for postradiosurgery imaging changes in 307 AVM patients with more than 2 years of follow-up after radiosurgery at Pittsburgh. We identified postradiosurgery imaging changes in 87 of 307 (28%) of these patients; 32 (37%) of these 87 were symptomatic. We used marginal dose (minimum AVM nidus dose prescribed) to represent the dose. As shown in **Table 2.2,** the best-fitting α/β value with nonlinear regression analysis using a Poisson model (Eq. 1) was $\alpha/\beta = -29.7 \pm 2.4$. Although marginal dose is a simplified way to represent the inhomogeneous dose distribution to the surrounding normal tissue, we obtained a negative α/β value that was consistent with those for AVM obliteration and facial and auditory neuropathies.

Radiation Injury Reactions Aren't Limited to Surrounding Tissue

Except for functional radiosurgery, where the target is normal tissue, it seems intuitive that radiation injury reactions should depend only on the dose distribution of radiation received by the normal tissue surrounding a radiosurgery target volume, the same tissue that manifests that injury. Normal tissue complication probablity models calculate chances of radiation injury from dose distribution to normal tissue outside the target/tumor. If this is true, then there should be no difference in complications between different targets (AVM and benign or malignant

Table 2.3 Multivariate Logistic Regression Models Comparing Postradiosurgery Imaging Changes (Symptomatic or Asymptomatic Edema) in 307 AVM Patients and 291 Meningioma Patients with 2 or More Years of Follow-Up

Variable	*p* Value	Odds Ratio	95% Confidence Interval
AVM vs meningioma	$<.0001$	7.502	3.43–16.40
Marginal dose*	.0143	2.457 per Gy	1.197–5.043
Marginal dose squared*	.0148	0.9789 per Gy^2	0.9624–0.9958
Volume	$<.0001$	1.142 per mL	1.217–3.431

* Approximate value of $\alpha/\beta = -42.21 \pm 17.22$.
Abbreviation: AVM, arteriovenous malformation.

tumor) after accounting for the effects of dose and volume. To test this, we modeled postradiosurgery imaging changes (symptomatic or asymptomatic edema) that developed in 27 of 307 AVM patients and compared them to those developing in 14 of 291 meningioma patients, all of whom had 2 or more years of follow-up. **Table 2.3** shows the results of the multivariate logistic regression model comparing postradiosurgery imaging sequelae for AVM versus meningioma while controlling for the effects of dose (in a linear-quadratic expression with marginal dose and marginal dose squared) and for treatment volume in the model. The probability of postradiosurgery imaging sequelae was significantly higher ($p < .0001$) for AVM patients by a factor of 7.5 (95% confidence interval: 3.4 – 16.4). The ratio of the regression coefficients for marginal dose and marginal dose squared gave an α/β ratio of -42.2 ± 17.2 for these postradiosurgery imaging changes for the combined dataset.

Reanalyzing these data using symptomatic postradiosurgery injury as the end point gave similar results, despite the fact that location was not incorporated into the analysis to keep it as simple as possible. AVM had a significantly higher ($p = .04$) risk of symptomatic postradiosurgery sequelae by a factor of 2.58 (95% confidence interval: 1.04 – 6.41). The approximate α/β value calculated using symptomatic postradiosurgery sequelae as an end point was -42.0 ± 26.7.

These comparisons of postradiosurgery imaging changes and of symptomatic sequelae in AVM versus meningioma radiosurgery targets demonstrate that the target tissue can have a substantial effect on the chance of developing a radiation injury reaction and should not be ignored in radiobiological models. The higher risk of an injury reaction in treating AVM compared with meningioma suggests that the injury reaction of the target vasculature may affect the surrounding normal tissue and its supporting vasculature and contribute to radiation injury reaction outside the target.

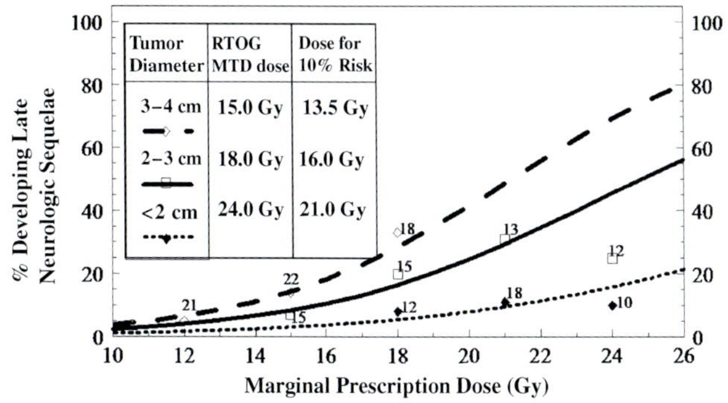

Fig. 2.4 Logistic dose–response curves fit to the late toxicity data reported for the Radiation Therapy Oncology Group (RTOG) Radiosurgery Dose-Escalation Study. The numbers refer to the number of tumors treated at each dose level for each size category (stars < 20 mm, squares 21–30 mm, diamonds 31–40 mm). The doses where 10% late toxicity occurs in the fitted curves are shown next to the legend. MTD, maximum tolerated dose.

Radiation Therapy Oncology Group Radiosurgery Dose-Escalation Study

The Radiation Therapy Oncology Group (RTOG) phase 1 Radiosurgery Dose-Escalation Study (95–05) provided several important findings.[20] In the study, 156 patients who failed prior conventional radiotherapy for either brain metastasis or primary tumors were enrolled and treated according to a dose-escalation protocol stratified by lesion diameter.[16] Brainstem tumors were excluded from the study because of higher risks of symptomatic injury expected that could have confounded the analysis. Starting with marginal doses of 18, 15, and 12 Gy for diameters < 20, 21 to 30, and 31 to 40 mm, respectively, the study escalated doses in 3 Gy intervals in successive patient cohorts until unacceptable toxicity was reached, defined as irreversible RTOG grade 3, 4, or 5 neurologic toxicity within 3 months of radiosurgery in > 30% of patients. The researchers defined maximum tolerated dose (MTD) as the next lowest dose level before reaching unacceptable (> 30%) toxicity. The cohort with tumors ≤ 20 mm never exceeded 30% grade 3 or greater toxicity despite dose escalation to 24 Gy, and investigators balked at escalating to higher doses. **Figure 2.4** shows the reported late neurologic toxicity data at each size category fitted to logistic dose–response curves.

◆ Summary

Radiobiological analysis of clinical data from radiosugery leads to several conclusions:

1. The linear-quadratic equation cannot reliably extrapolate from data for conventional fractionated radiotherapy to estimate equivalent radiation effects for the high-dose (12–25 Gy) single-fraction radiosurgery. We consistently found high negative values for α/β ratios calculated from radiosurgery responses that conflict with values seen with conventional fractionated radiotherapy.
2. Radiation injury models need to take into account contributions from the target or tumor affecting radiation injury reactions in the surrounding normal tissue.
3. Much of the radiation response of a radiosurgical target and surrounding tissue from radiosurgery appears to be mediated through the response of the supporting vasculature.

References

1. Richard DJ, Bolderson E, Cubeddu L, et al. Single-stranded DNA-binding protein hSSB1 is critical for genomic stability. Nature 2008;453(7195): 677–681
2. Ayoub N, Jeyasekharan AD, Bernal JA, Venkitaraman AR. HP1-beta mobilization promotes chromatin changes that initiate the DNA damage response. Nature 2008;453(7195):682–686
3. Greenberger JS, Epperly MW. Antioxidant gene therapeutic approaches to normal tissue radioprotection and tumor radiosensitization in vivo [Review]. 2007;21(2):141–163
4. Garcia-Barros M, Paris F, Cordon-Cardo C, et al. Tumor response to radiotherapy regulated by endothelial cell apoptosis. Science 2003; 300(5622):1155–1159
5. Szeifert GT, Massager N, DeVriendt D, et al. Observations of intracranial neoplasms treated with Gamma Knife radiosurgery. J Neurosurg 2002;97:623–626
6. Barendsen GW. Dose fractionation, dose rate and iso-effect relationships for normal tissue responses. Int J Radiat Oncol Biol Phys 1982; 8(11):1981–1997
7. Dale RG. The application of the linear-quadratic dose-effect equation to fractionated and protracted radiotherapy. Br J Radiol 1985;58(690): 515–528
8. Fowler JF. The linear-quadratic formula and progress in fractionated radiotherapy. Br J Radiol 1989;62(740):679–694
9. Hall EJ, Brenner DJ. The radiobiology of radiosurgery: rationale for different treatment regimes for AVMs and malignancies. Int J Radiat Oncol Biol Phys 1993;25(2):381–385
10. Brenner DJ, Hall EJ. Fractionation and protraction for radiotherapy of prostate cancer. Int J Radiat Oncol Biol Phys 1999;43:1095–1101
11. Flickinger JC, Kalend A. Use of normalized total dose to represent the biological effect of fractionated radiotherapy. Radiother Oncol 1990;17:339–347
12. Tishler RB, Loeffler JS, Lunsford LD, et al. Tolerance of cranial nerves of the cavernous sinus to radiosurgery. Int J Radiat Oncol Biol Phys 1993;27:215–221
13. Flickinger JC, Rush SC. Linear accelerator radiotherapy of pituitary adenomas. In: Landolt AM, Vance ML, Reilly PL, eds. Pituitary Adenomas: Biology, Diagnosis and Treatment. Edinburgh, UK: Churchill Livingstone; 1996:475–483
14. Stafford SL, Pollock BE, Leavitt JA, et al. A study on the radiation tolerance of the optic nerves and chiasm after stereotactic radiosurgery. Int J Radiat Oncol Biol Phys 2003;55(5):1177–1181
15. Leber KA, Berglöff J, Pendl G. Dose–response tolerance of the visual pathways and cranial nerves of the cavernous sinus to stereotactic radiosurgery. J Neurosurg 1998;88(1):43–50
16. Flickinger JC, Kondziolka D, Maitz AH, Lunsford LD. Gamma Knife radiosurgery of imaging-diagnosed intracranial meningioma. Int J Radiat Oncol Biol Phys 2003;56(3):801–806
17. Flickinger JC, Kondziolka D, Lunsford LD. Dose and diameter relationships for facial, trigeminal, and acoustic neuropathies following acoustic neuroma radiosurgery. Radiother Oncol 1996;41(3): 215–219
18. Flickinger JC, Kondziolka D, Maitz AH, Lunsford LD. An analysis of the dose–response for arteriovenous malformation radiosurgery and other factors affecting obliteration. Radiother Oncol 2002;63: 347–354
19. Flickinger JC, Kondziolka D, Lunsford LD, et al. Development of a model to predict permanent symptomatic post-radiosurgery injury for arteriovenous malformation patients. Int J Radiat Oncol Biol Phys 2000;46:1143–1148
20. Shaw E, Scott C, Souhami L, et al. Single dose radiosurgical treatment of recurrent previously irradiated primary brain tumors and brain metastases: final report of RTOG protocol 90–05. Int J Radiat Oncol Biol Phys 2000;47(2):291–298

3

How Brain Tumors Respond to Stereotactic Radiosurgery

György T. Szeifert, Dave S. Atteberry, Douglas Kondziolka, and L. Dade Lunsford

Tumor radiosurgery has become an effective and widely used procedure during the past 4 decades.[1–10] The first Gamma Knife radiosurgery patient had a craniopharyngioma. The radiobiological effect of radiosurgery is not well understood.[11,12] Although more than 200,000 patients with benign or malignant intracranial neoplasms have undergone Gamma Knife radiosurgery worldwide, the histopathologic response leading to tumor control or continued growth has received limited attention.[13–17] The purpose of this study was to define the types of histopathological changes as determined by analysis of tumor specimens from patients who required resection for either tumor progression or delayed intratumoral hemorrhage.

◆ Patients and Methods

From a series of 5,000 brain tumors in the University of Pittsburgh Gamma Knife program, surgical pathology material was reviewed from 19 patients who underwent 24 tumor resections at 2 to 82 months (median 13 months) after radiosurgery. All patients had radiological and clinical progression that warranted removal of the lesion via craniotomy. Tumors included metastases ($n = 15$), anaplastic astrocytoma,[2] atypical meningioma,[2] vestibular schwannoma,[2] and one meningioma, jugular foramen schwannoma, and hemangioblastoma. Radiosurgery was performed using the Gamma Knife (Elekta Instruments AB, Stockholm, Sweden) models U, B, or C. Dose planning was based on magnetic resonance (MR) and computed tomography (CT) imaging. Tumor volumes varied between 0.266 and 25.600 mL (median 4.7 mL). Tumors received 12 to 20 Gy as the margin dose (median 16 Gy) at the 30 to 60% isodose line (median 50%), with a 24 to 40 Gy maximal dose (median 32 Gy).

Histopathological investigations were performed on all available surgical pathology materials. Resected specimens were fixed in 10% neutral buffered formaldehyde and embedded in paraffin. Hematoxylin-eosin, Masson's trichrome, and Luxol-fast blue stains were used. Immunohistochemical reactions included glial fibrillary acidic protein (GFAP), vimentin, S100, neurofilament, synaptophysin, EMA, pankeratin, CK7, CK20, CAM5.2, CD3, CD20, CD31, and CD68 (PGM1) antigens to characterize the reactive cell population around/or infiltrating neoplastic tissues. Ki67 and p53 reactions were used to assess the proliferative activity of tumor cells. Biotin-streptavidin-peroxidase complex methods were performed according to standard protocols on 5 μm paraffin sections.

◆ Results

Acute Changes

Histopathological changes attributable to radiosurgery were observed within the tumor parenchyma, adjacent connective tissue stroma, and vessels (**Table 3.1**).

Table 3.1 Histological Responses after Radiosurgery

Timing of Resection	Histological Response (number of cases)		
	Acute	Subacute	Chronic
0–6 months	3 (B:1; M:2)	3 (B:0; M:3)	0
6–12 months	2 (B:0; M:2)	3 (B:0; M:3)	0
12–24 months	2 (B:1; M:1)	4 (B:0; M:4)	1 (B:1; M:0)
> 24 months	0	2 (B:0; M:2)	4 (B:2; M:2)

Abbreviations: B, benign; M, malignant.

Table 3.2 Histopathological Characteristics of Gamma Radiolesions

Type	Parenchymal Changes	Stromal Alterations	Vasculopathy	Temporal Development
Acute	Sharply demarcated coagulation necrosis	No cellular reaction/or scattered apoptotic cells and polymorphonuclear leukocytes around the necrosis	Dilated small venules; endothelial destruction, undulation of internal elastic membrane, fibrinoid changes in vessels' wall, vacuolar degeneration	Early or delayed
Subacute	Well-circumscribed coagulation necrosis	Macrophage reaction around the necrosis; granulation tissue; mild reactive gliosis	Proliferative vasculopathy with narrowing of the lumen	Early or delayed
Chronic	Replaced by scar tissue	Focal lymphocytic infiltration; hyaline degenerated scar tissue, calcification	Subendothelial cell proliferation; subtotal or complete lumen obliteration; hyaline degeneration in the wall, focal calcification	Delayed

These changes were either degenerative or proliferative. The main histopathological characteristics are summarized in **Table 3.2.** Degenerative alterations occurred mostly in the parenchyma of different tumors, whereas proliferative processes were realized first of all in the connective tissue stroma and vessels of neoplasms. The basic histopathological alteration evoked by the ionizing energy of high-dose radiation was recognized as a well-circumscribed lesion with sharp demarcation toward surrounding tissues according to the steep radiation fall-off (**Fig. 3.1A**). Regarding the histological and cellular composition of these gamma radiolesions, three main types were realized following radiosurgery (**Table 3.2**). In the acute-type reaction, coagulation necrosis constituted the center with a network of acidophilic fibrinoid material and amorphous homogeneous tissue or cellular debris (**Fig. 3.1B**). No cellular reaction or scanty basophilic hyperchromatic apoptotic cells characterized by nuclear fragmentation and pyknosis intermingled with scattered polymorphonuclear leukocytes and some dilated postcapillary venules surrounded this necrotic core (**Fig. 3.1C**). There was no prominent macrophage or lymphocytic infiltration, reactive gliosis, or scar tissue formation. The necrosis in this targeted volume was usually circumscribed, homogeneous, and sharply demarcated from surrounding remaining tumor tissue (**Fig. 3.1A**) as compared with other necrotic tumor areas outside the focused irradiation, which had an irregular multifocal appearance and entrapped tumor islands (**Fig. 3.1D**). A similar histological picture of the acute-type lesion could be observed at either an early or a delayed time interval after radiosurgery. These parenchymal changes were accompanied by alterations of stromal vessels around the necrotic core characterized by endothelial destruction, fibrinoid necrosis, undulation of the internal elastic membrane, and vacuolation and accumulation of eosinophilic material (transudation) in the vessel wall (**Fig. 3.1E,F**).

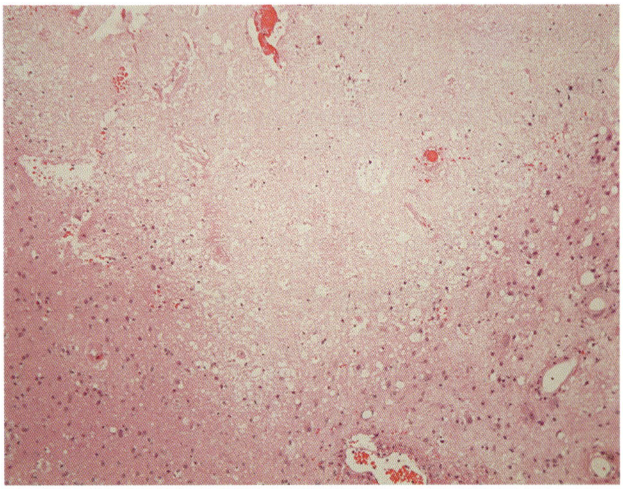
A

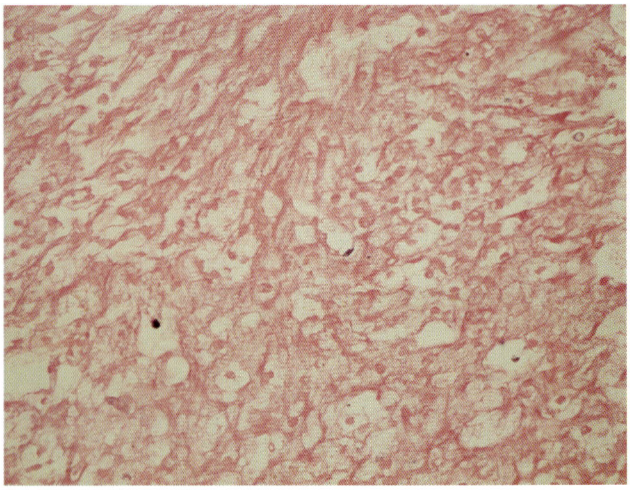
B

Fig. 3.1 (A–D) Histological characteristics of acute-type gamma radiolesions from a metastatic non–small cell carcinoma 4 months after Gamma Knife radiosurgery. **(A)** A sharply demarcated coagulation necrosis in the tumor parenchyma (hematoxylin-eosin [H. & E.], ×100). **(B)** Fibrinoid mesh in the center of the radiolesion (H. & E., ×300).

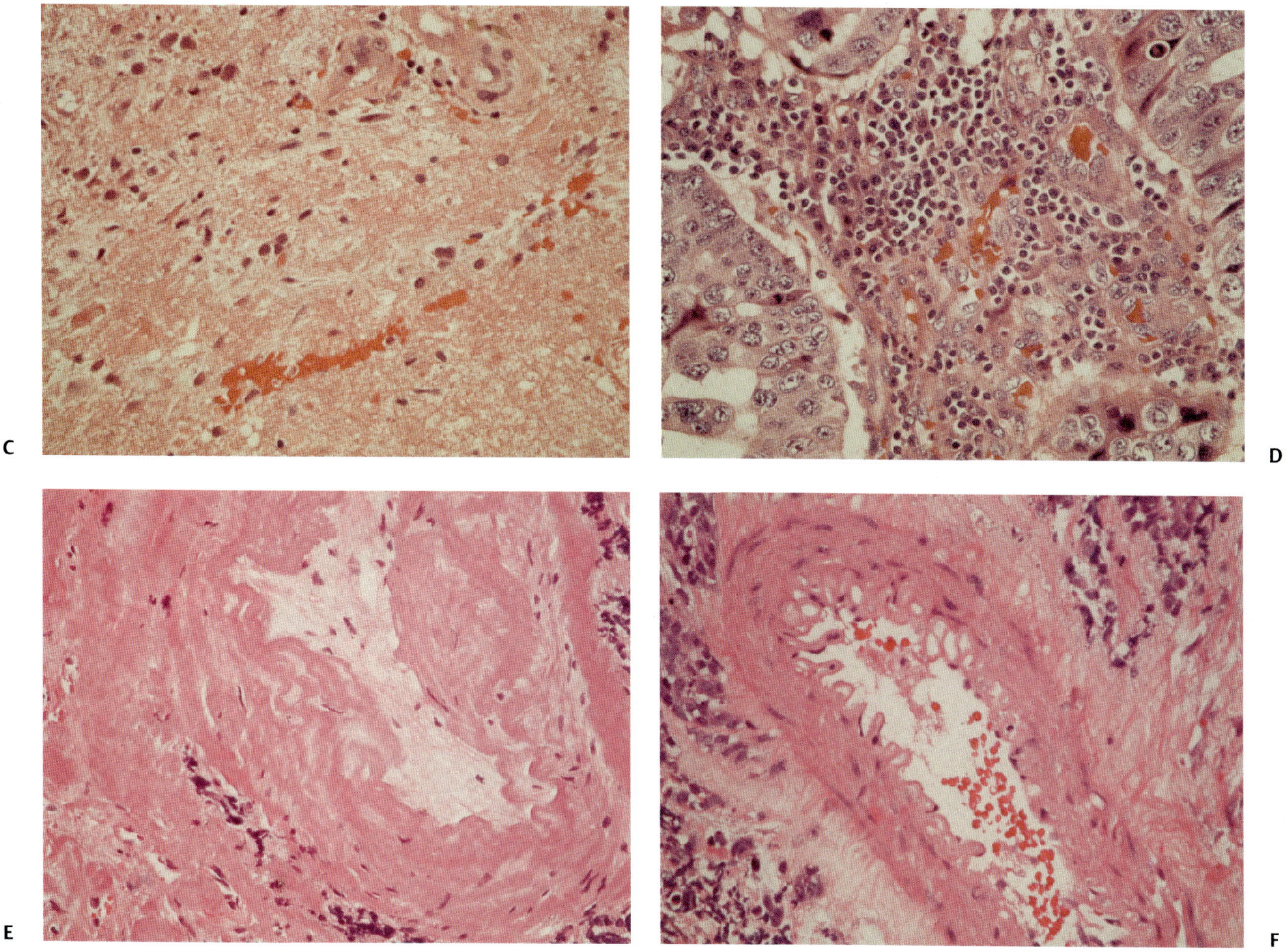

Fig. 3.1 *(Continued)* **(C)** Scattered pyknotic cells at the periphery of the lesion (H. & E., ×300). **(D)** Irregular tumor necrosis outside the irradiated target volume (H. & E., ×300). **(E)** Fibrinoid necrosis in the vessel's wall (H. & E., ×300). **(F)** Endothelial destruction, undulation of internal elastic membrane, and vacuolar degeneration of the vessel's wall (H. & E., ×300). (**E** and **F** are from a metastatic small cell lung carcinoma 3 months following Gamma Knife radiosurgery.)

Subacute Changes

The second group of gamma radiolesions had the characteristics of subacute-type pathological reactions that were observed several months to years after radiosurgery. The main histological feature of these lesions was an inflammatory tissue response. The central coagulation necrotic core was surrounded by a macrophage rim (**Fig. 3.2A**). These macrophages revealed phagocytotic activity and mainly CD68 (PGM1) but sometimes CD31 immunohistochemical reactivity as well (**Fig. 3.2B**). A granulation tissue zone was situated outside the macrophage layer containing abundant small vessels, capillaries, arterioles, and venules accompanied by inflammatory cells, fibrocytes, and fibroblasts expressing vimentin positivity (**Fig. 3.2C,D**). Postirradiation vasculopathy was also observed at the periphery of the central necrotic region (**Fig. 3.2E.F**). A reactive gliotic scar mantle formed by astrocytic elements and abundant glial filaments coated and constituted the outer border of the radiolesion as it was demonstrated by GFAP immune reaction (**Fig. 3.2G,H**).

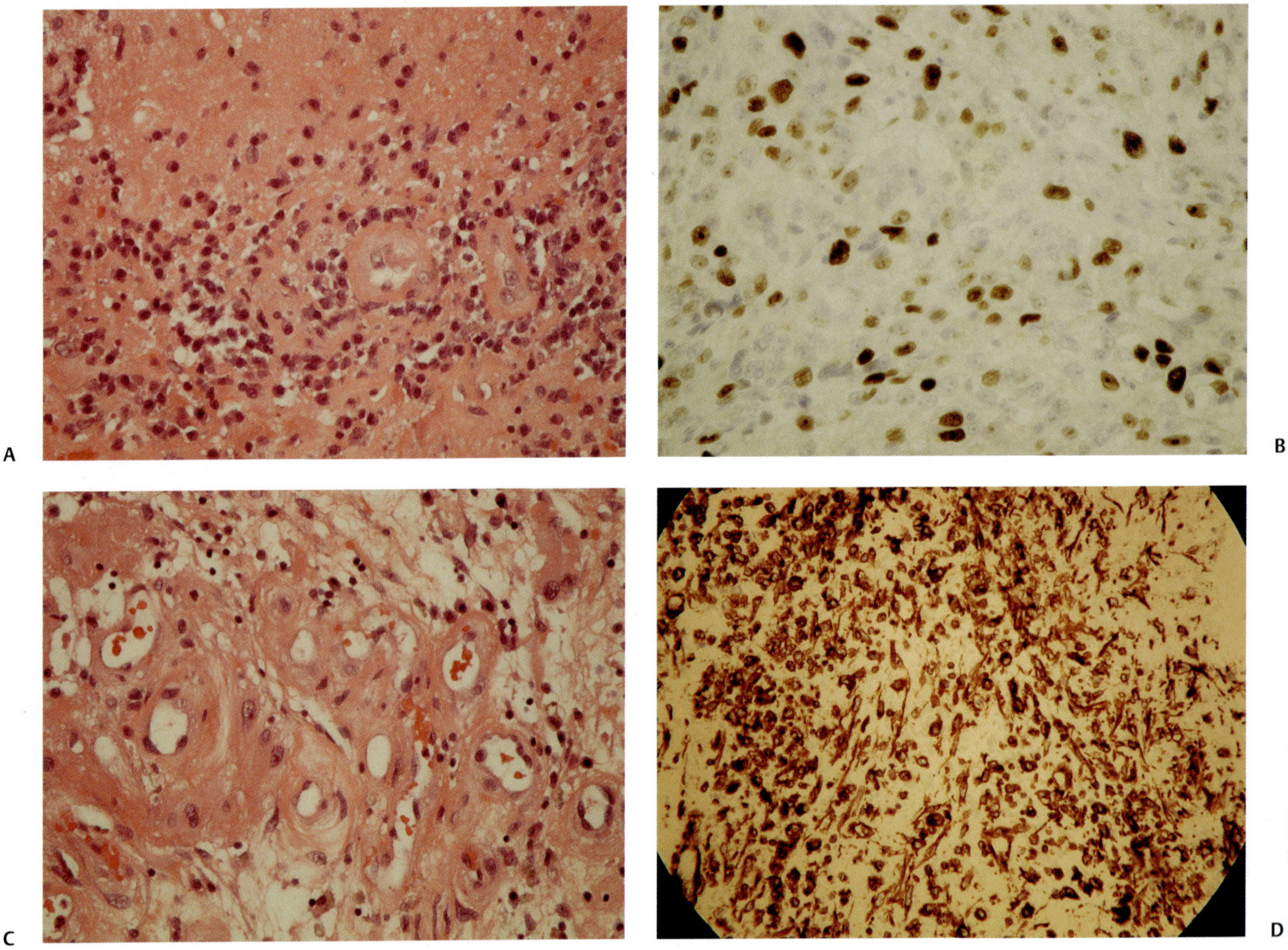

Fig. 3.2 (A–D) Subacute-type histological changes in gamma radiolesions from a metastatic renal cell carcinoma 10 months after Gamma Knife radiosurgery. **(A)** Intense macrophage reaction at the periphery of the necrotic core (hematoxylin-eosin [H. & E.], ×300). **(B)** CD68 (PGM1) immune reactivity demonstrates active macrophages (×300). **(C)** Granulation tissue with inflammatory cells surrounding and organizing the necrosis (H. & E., ×300). **(D)** Vimentin positivity indicates fibroblasts and fibrocytes in granulation tissue (×300).

Chronic Changes

The third, so-called chronic-type or "end-stage" pathological reaction appeared several years after radiosurgery. The central part of the radiolesion was replaced by hypocellular scar tissue with degenerative changes that included hyaline deposition and/or focal calcification that demarcated sharply toward the remaining surrounding tumor tissue (**Fig. 3.3A**). Scattered fibrocytes, fibroblasts, and sporadic focal lymphocytic infiltration were disclosed around dense collagen bundles (**Fig. 3.3B**). Immunohistochemical markers for tumor antigens like S100 or neurofilament reactions demonstrated considerable decrease in these areas (**Fig. 3.3C,D**). Advanced postirradiation vasculopathy with subendothelial spindle-shaped cell proliferation and hyaline degeneration resulted in subtotal or even complete luminal obliteration (**Fig. 3.3E,F**).

Acute-type histological changes were found in eight tumors (two anaplastic astrocytomas, one non–small cell lung metastasis, one small cell lung metastasis, one breast carcinoma metastasis, one meningioma, one atypical meningioma, and one hemangioblastoma) at 2 to 17 months (median 11 months) following radiosurgery. The subacute-type histological reaction developed in 12 tumors (8 non–small cell metastases, 2 renal cell metastases, 1 metastatic breast carcinoma, and 1 metastatic melanoma). These alterations were observed at 4 to 59 months (median 16 months) after radiosurgery. The chronic-type tissue response occurred in five neoplasms (one sporadic vestibular schwannoma, one neurofibromatosis 2 (NF2) vestibular schwannoma, one jugular foramen schwannoma, one atypical meningioma, and one metastatic breast carcinoma). These were noted 18 to 82 months (median 32 months) following radiosurgery.

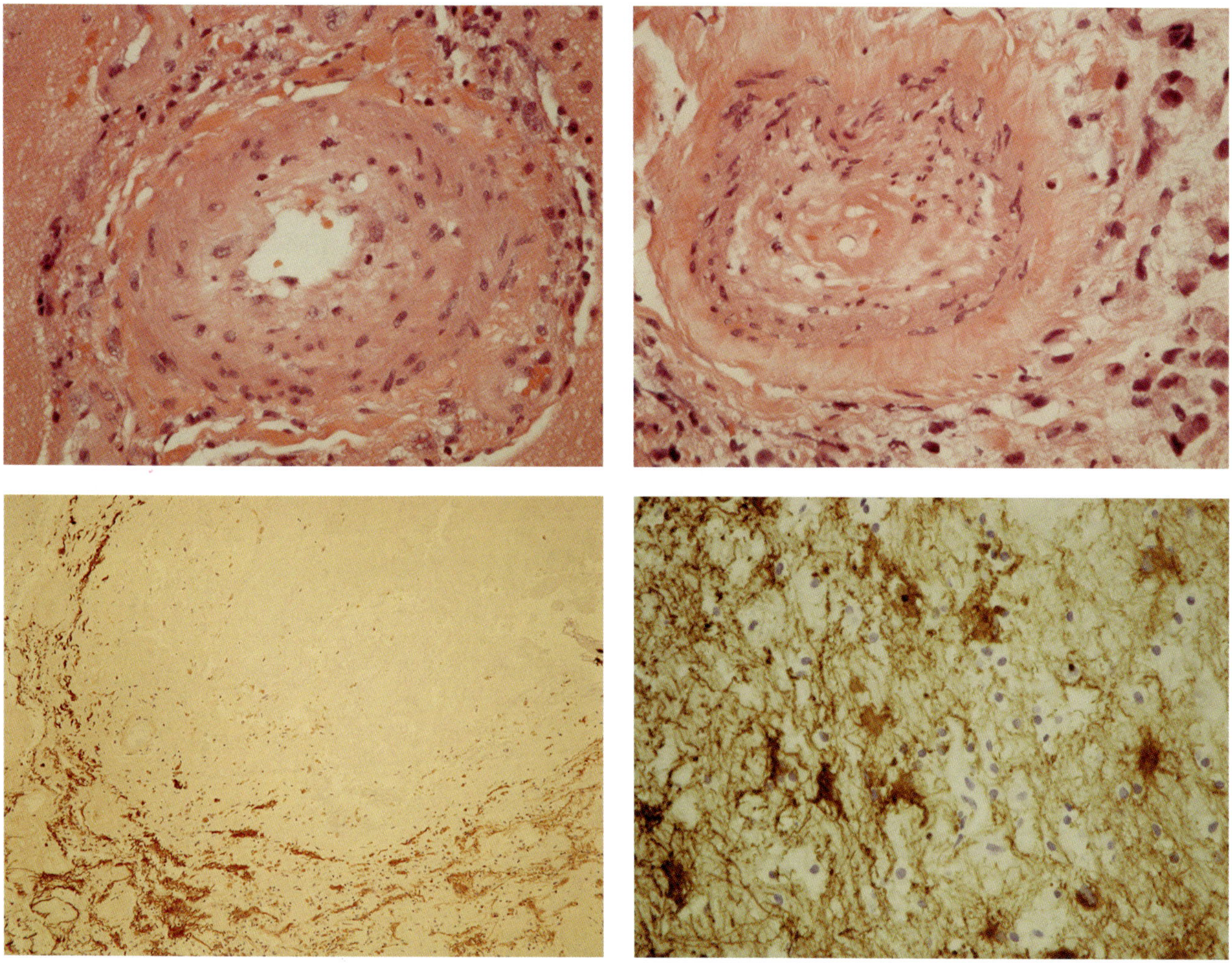

E F G H

Fig. 3.2 *(Continued)* **(E–H)** From a metastatic renal cell carcinoma 7 months following Gamma Knife radiosurgery. **(E)** Proliferative vasculopathy in the stroma (H. & E., ×300). **(F)** Vasculopathy combined with a newly formed fibrin thrombus (H. & E., ×300). **(G)** Reactive gliosis demarcating the radiolesion (glial fibrillary acidic protein [GFAP] immunohistochemistry, ×100). **(H)** Astrocytic cells with processes and fiber production (GFAP, ×300).

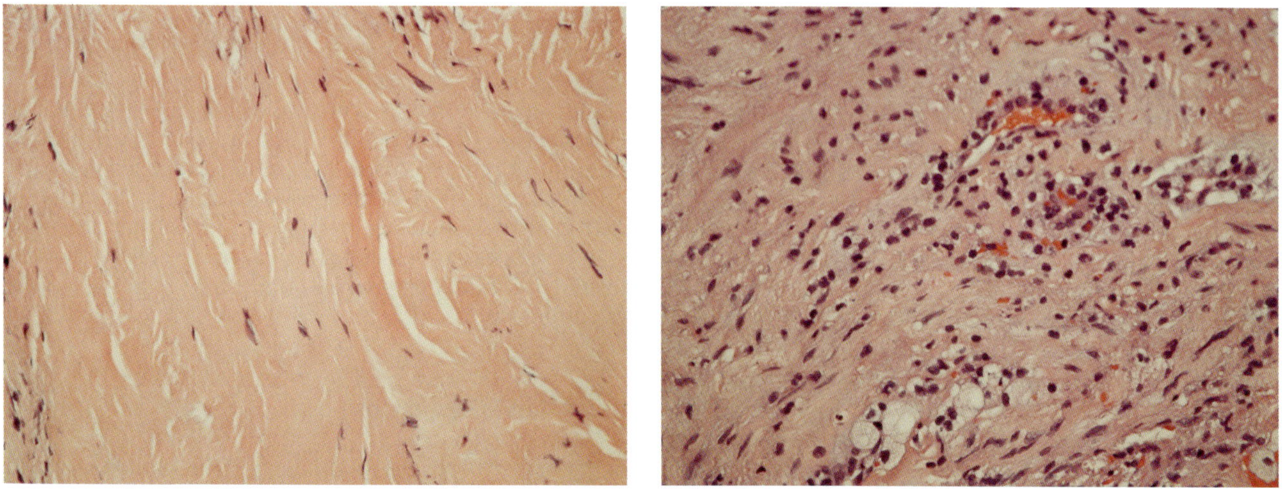

A B

Fig. 3.3 **(A–D)** Chronic-type histological findings in gamma radiolesions from a vestibular schwannoma 18 months after Gamma Knife radiosurgery. **(A)** Hypocellular hyaline degenerated collagen bundles replacing necrotic tissue in the targeted volume (hematoxylin-eosin [H. & E.], ×300). **(B)** Focal lymphocytic infiltration in scar tissue (H. & E., ×300).

(Continued on page 18)

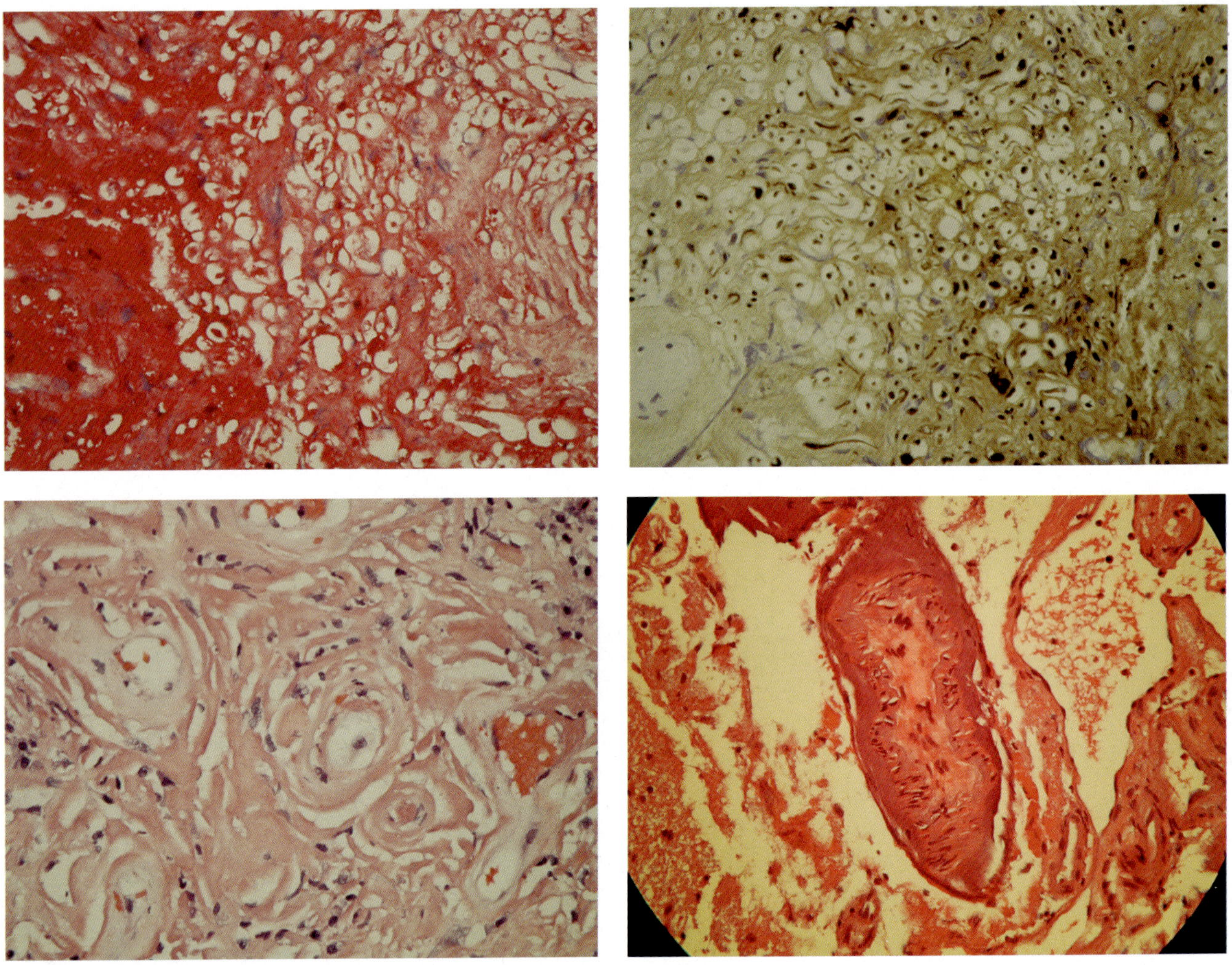

C D E F

Fig. 3.3 *(Continued)* **(C)** S100 immunoreactivity and neurofilament. **(D)** Positivity at the periphery of the treatment volume decreasing toward the center, indicating recurrent or residual tumor tissue at the edge of the lesion (×300). **(E,F)** From an atypical meningioma 33 months following Gamma Knife radiosurgery. **(E)** Fibrotic changes around and in the vessels' wall narrowing the lumina (H. & E., ×300). **(F)** Complete lumen occlusion by spindle cell proliferation in a larger artery (H. & E., ×100).

Discussion

Although a large clinical experience has been accumulated in brain tumor radiosurgery during the past 4 decades, a comprehensive human pathology study has not yet been performed. This is partly due to the high success rate of radiosurgery, but also due to the paucity of postmortem examinations. The term *radiosurgery* signifies the application of ionizing radiation energy, in experimental biology or clinical medicine, aiming at the precise and complete destruction of chosen target structures containing healthy and/or pathological cells, without significant concomitant or late radiation damage to adjacent tissues.[18] Therefore, the goal of radiosurgical pathology and experimental studies should be to investigate short- and long-term effects of high-dose ionizing radiation on neural tissue and its pathologies with histological, tissue culture, and biochemical methods. The experimental basis for brain tumor radiosurgery is well established and provides evidence of the effectiveness of high-dose irradiation.[19–26] Sporadic human pathological case reports[13–17,27–29] and a recent study on vestibular schwannomas have been published.[30] The purpose of the present comprehensive study was to evaluate the effect of Gamma Knife radiosurgery in a series of brain tumors with a variety of histological types and different time intervals after irradiation. It is important to note that these patients had failed radiosurgery in some way, necessitating resection. However, we believe that the histological tumor response would still be indicative of the radiation effect.

Brain Tumor Responses

In the human brain, the morphology of radiolesions appears to be similar to that found in animal models. The temporal development of radiation lesions are divided into three phases in human oncology practice.[31] The immediate response occurs milliseconds to hours after radiation exposure, usually less than 24 hours. Witham et al noted immediate apoptotic responses in brain tumors following radiosurgery.[32] Histologically and clinically, the lesions are regarded as the acute type. The early reaction develops days to weeks after initial exposure, most frequently 24 hours to 2 months. Morphologically and clinically, the lesions may be acute or subacute. The delayed response presents months to years after exposure, often 2 months to many years, and could even occur beyond a decade.[33,34] Pathologically and clinically, the lesions may be acute, subacute, or chronic type.

The morphological appearance of various lesions suggestive of radiation effect in different tumors of this series were not significantly related with the histopathological type of the irradiated neoplasm or with the time interval between radiosurgery and craniotomy.

Three main histopathological types of gamma radiolesions were delineated in the present study (**Table 3.2**). Acute-type gamma radiolesions were characterized mainly with necrotic changes and appeared either early or delayed, and subacute-type gamma radiolesions demonstrated resorptive activity either early or delayed. Chronic-type lesions showed evidence of tissue repair but only at a delayed phase. These changes seemed to follow each other consecutively without any significant relationship between tumor type or time after irradiation and the type of the evoked radiolesion. The only consistent observation was that chronic-type lesions were noted only in delayed fashion, which is in accordance with the idea that these are end-stage alterations. The similar morphological appearance of the target effects in different tumors and different patients suggests that the evoked histopathological reaction is likely related to the biologic effect of radiosurgery. We believe these responses represent both direct cellular effects and vascular mechanisms induced by the radiation energy. The acute effects indicate a direct cellular response, mediated by cytokines released at the time of injury. Subacute and chronic effects appear to be mediated by the inflammatory cascade induced at the time of injury. Research into radiation protection has focused on modulating this inflammation effect.[35,36]

We found that radiation produced effects both in the tumor and in the immediately adjacent tissue. Among degenerative changes, necrosis and apoptosis occurred in the parenchyma of neoplasms contributing to tumor cell destruction, whereas hyaline, fibrinoid, and calcium deposition appeared mostly in the connective tissue stroma and vessel wall. On the other hand, proliferative processes such as granulation tissue formation, inflammatory reaction, macrophage invasion, fibrocyte-fibroblast proliferation, and scar tissue production were found in the stroma and vasculature of the tumor. These effects served a scavenger function, working to remove destroyed neoplastic tissue (necrotic debris) and eventually replace the defect with scar tissue. Scar tissue consists of hyaline degenerated collagen bundles and glial fibrils that have a certain propensity for contraction. This contraction of scar tissue might play a role in the volumetric regression of the tumor, as noted frequently on follow-up imaging studies.

Our human pathological observations are in accordance with the results of recent genetic and pharmacologic studies that revealed the critical role of both radiation-induced microvasculature and tumor cell damage, constituting the fundamental elements of the tumor response to radiation.[37]

Acknowledgment This chapter is dedicated to Professor Pongrác Endes, Department of Pathology, University Medical School of Debrecen, Hungary, for his 100th birthday, recognizing his outstanding character, teaching, and heritage in the field of pathology and ethics.

References

1. Flickinger JC. Radiosurgery of brain metastases from renal cell carcinoma: how can you improve on results like this? Cancer J 2000;6: 360–361
2. Flickinger JC, Kondziolka D, Lunsford LD, et al. A multi-institutional experience with stereotactic radiosurgery for solitary brain metastasis. Int J Radiat Oncol Biol Phys 1994;28:797–802
3. Friedman WA, Foote KD. Linear accelerator radiosurgery in the management of brain tumours. Ann Med 2000;32:64–80
4. Kondziolka D, Lunsford LD, McLaughlin MR, Flickinger JC. Long-term outcomes after radiosurgery for acoustic neuromas. N Engl J Med 1998;339:1426–1433
5. Lunsford LD, Kondziolka D, Flickinger JC. Stereotactic radiosurgery: current spectrum and results. Clin Neurosurg 1992;38:405–444
6. Lunsford LD, Kondziolka D, Flickinger JC. Stereotactic radiosurgery for benign intracranial tumors. Clin Neurosurg 1993;40:475–497
7. Lunsford LD, Maitz A, Lindner G. First United States 201 source cobalt-60 gamma unit for radiosurgery. Appl Neurophysiol 1987;50: 253–256
8. Niranjan A, Lunsford LD. Radiosurgery: where we were, are, and may be in the third millennium. Neurosurgery 2000;46:531–543
9. Niranjan A, Lunsford LD, Gobbel GT, Kondziolka D, Maitz A, Flickinger JC. Brain tumor radiosurgery: current status and strategies to enhance the effect of radiosurgery. Brain Tumor Pathol 2000;17:89–96
10. Payne BR, Prasad D, Szeifert G, Steiner M, Steiner L. Gamma surgery for intracranial metastases from renal cell carcinoma. J Neurosurg 2000;92:760–765
11. Kondziolka D, Lunsford LD, Flickinger JC. The radiobiology of radiosurgery. Neurosurg Clin N Am 1999;10:157–166
12. Yamamoto M. Gamma Knife radiosurgery: technology, applications, and future directions. Neurosurg Clin N Am 1999;10:181–202
13. Hirato M, Hirato J, Zama A, et al. Radiobiological effects of Gamma Knife radiosurgery on brain tumors studied in autopsy and surgical specimens. Stereotact Funct Neurosurg 1996;66(Suppl 1):4–16
14. Szeifert GT, Massager N, Brotchi J, Levivier M. Morphological redifferentiation in a malignant astrocytic tumor after Gamma Knife radiosurgery. J Neurosurg 2002;97:627–630
15. Szeifert GT, Massager N, DeVriendt D, et al. Observations of intracranial neoplasms treated with Gamma Knife radiosurgery. J Neurosurg 2002;97:623–626
16. Szeifert GT, Salmon I, David P, et al. Tumor control and growth in a patient with two cerebral metastases treated with the Leksell Gamma Knife. In: Kondziolka D, ed. Radiosurgery. Basel: Karger; 2002:152–161
17. Thompson BG, Coffey RJ, Flickinger JC, Lunsford LD. Stereotactic radiosurgery of small intracranial tumors: neuropathological correlation in three patients. Surg Neurol 1990;33:96–104
18. Larsson B. Radiobiological fundamentals in radiosurgery. In: Steiner L, ed. Radiosurgery: Baseline and Trends. New York: Raven Press; 1992:3–15
19. Blatt DR, Friedman WA, Bova FJ, Theele DP, Mickle JP. Temporal characteristics of radiosurgical lesions in an animal model. J Neurosurg 1994;80:1046–1055
20. Inoue HK, Kohga H, Hirato M, Nakamura M, Ohye C. Neurobiologic effects of radiosurgery: histologic, immunohistochemical and electron-microscopic studies of a rat model. Stereotact Funct Neurosurg 1994; 63:280–285

21. Kondziolka D, Lunsford LD, Claassen D, Pandalai S, Maitz AH, Flickinger JC. Radiobiology of radiosurgery, II: The rat C6 glioma model. Neurosurgery 1992;31:280–287, discussion 287–288
22. Linskey ME, Martinez AJ, Kondziolka D, et al. The radiobiology of human acoustic schwannoma xenografts after stereotactic radiosurgery evaluated in the subrenal capsule of athymic mice. J Neurosurg 1993; 78:645–653
23. Lunsford LD, Altschuler EM, Flickinger JC, Wu A, Martinez AJ. In vivo biological effects of stereotactic radiosurgery: a primate model. Neurosurgery 1990;27:373–382
24. Niranjan A, Moriuchi S, Lunsford LD, et al. Effective treatment of experimental glioblastoma by HSV vector-mediated TNF alpha and HSV-tk gene transfer in combination with radiosurgery and ganciclovir administration. Mol Ther 2000;2:114–120
25. Niranjan A, Wolfe D, Fellows W, et al. Gene transfer to glial tumors using herpes simplex virus. Methods Mol Biol 2004;246:323–337
26. Niranjan A, Wolfe D, Tamura M, et al. Treatment of rat gliosarcoma brain tumors by HSV-based multigene therapy combined with radiosurgery. Mol Ther 2003;8:530–542
27. Kwon Y, Khang SK, Kim CJ, Lee DJ, Lee JK, Kwun BD. Radiologic and histopathologic changes after Gamma Knife radiosurgery for acoustic schwannoma. Stereotact Funct Neurosurg 1999;72(Suppl 1):2–10
28. Nielsen SL, Kjellberg RN, Asbury AK, Koehler AM. Neuropathologic effect of proton-beam irradiation in man, I: Dose–response relationship after treatment of intracranial neoplasms. Acta Neuropathol 1972;20:348–356
29. Noren G, Arndt J, Hindmarsh T. Stereotactic radiosurgery in cases of acoustic neurinoma: further experiences. Neurosurgery 1983; 13:12–22
30. Szeifert GT, Figarella-Branger D, Roche PH, Régis J. Histopathological observations on vestibular schwannomas after gamma knife radiosurgery: the Marseille experience. Neurochirurgie 2004;50: 327–337
31. Fajardo L-GLF, Berthrong M, Anderson RE. Radiation Pathology. New York: Oxford University Press; 2001
32. Witham TF, Okada H, Fellows W, et al. The characterization of tumor apoptosis after experimental radiosurgery. Stereotact Funct Neurosurg 2005;83:17–24
33. Adams RD. The neuropathology of radiosurgery. Stereotact Funct Neurosurg 1991;57:82–86
34. Julow J, Slowik F, Kelemen J. Late post-irradiation necrosis of the brain. Acta Neurochir (Wien) 1979;46:135–150
35. Kondziolka D, Mori Y, Martinez AJ, McLaughlin M, Flickinger JC, Lunsford LD. Beneficial effects of the radioprotectant 21-aminosteroid U-74389G in a radiosurgery rat malignant glioma model. Int J Radiat Oncol Biol Phys 1999;44(1):179–184
36. Kondziolka D, Somaza S, Martinez AJ, et al. Radioprotective effects of the 21-aminosteroid U-74389G for stereotactic radiosurgery. Neurosurgery 1997;41:203–208
37. Fuks Z, Kolesnick R. Engaging the vascular component of the tumor response. Cancer Cell 2005;8:89–91

4

Image-Guided Stereotactic Radiosurgery

Jasvinder Nangiana, John R. Adler Jr., and Steven D. Chang

Stereotactic radiosurgery combines stereotactic localization with multiple cross-fired beams from a highly collimated high-energy radiation source. This method of noninvasive ablation has proven to be an effective alternative to conventional neurosurgery, cranial irradiation, and brachytherapy for selected small cranial tumors and arteriovenous malformations (AVMs). Most current and historical stereotactic techniques rely on a rigid frame fixed to a patient's skull for head immobilization and target localization. Despite being an effective alternative to invasive neurosurgery and irradiation, frame-based radiosurgery is not ideal for all patient populations. Because they require immobilization, invasive and noninvasive frames are particularly challenging for pediatric patients. Children often require general anesthesia during application of the stereotactic frame and subsequent treatment. Additionally, infants cannot be suitably treated with radiosurgery due to the malleable nature of their skull.

Furthermore, the usefulness of frame-based radiosurgery is largely limited to intracranial tumors. Extracranial lesions beyond the highest cervical level typically cannot be adequately targeted. Although body stereotactic frames have been previously used in a small number of cases, frame-based technologies offer little practicality for spinal lesions, as patients were subjected to lengthy procedures involving placement of metal clamps on spinous processes, exposing them to general anesthesia and the possibility of wound infections.[1] Finally, a fixed frame limits the treatment degrees of freedom, and the metal components of current frames produce imaging artifacts on computed tomography (CT) and magnetic resonance imaging (MRI) scans.

The standard radiosurgery instruments such as the Gamma Knife and conventional linear accelerators are designed to deliver radiation based on a fixed isocenter. This works well with spherical targets but is not ideal for complex or irregular shapes. To treat complex shaped tumors, radiosurgery relies on overlapping spherical dose volumes, a method that results in intralesional dose heterogeneity. A system that achieves shape matching without significantly compromising dose homogeneity could be particularly advantageous for treating many intracranial lesions.

◆ Image-Guided Radiosurgery

Image-guided radiosurgery in the form of the CyberKnife (Accuray Inc., Sunnyvale, CA; **Fig. 4.1**) was developed as a frameless alternative to conventional intracranial radiosurgery.[2] Similar to other stereotactic methods, the system presumes a fixed relationship between the target and the skull. However, the CyberKnife uses real-time image guidance to direct therapy, eliminating the need for skeletal immobilization. Along with noninvasive image-guided localization, a lightweight, high-energy radiation source and

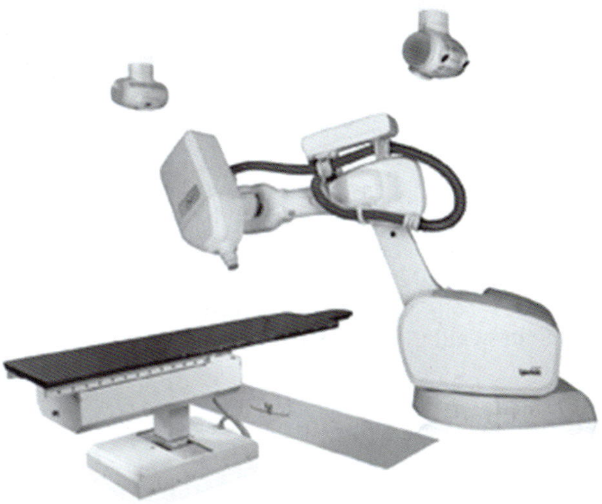

Fig. 4.1 The CyberKnife. From Accuray, Inc. Reprinted with permission.

a robotic delivery system enable the CyberKnife to overcome the limitations of previous modalities. This noninvasive method has proven to be effective for the treatment of intracranial tumors and AVMs, as well as extracranial targets within the spine.

The CyberKnife consists of several distinct parts. The first component is a 130 kg, 6 MV x-ray linear accelerator (linac). This linac is sufficiently light enough to be mounted to a commercially available robotic arm (the second component) that allows it to be pointed with six degrees of freedom and achieve an average treatment precision of 0.3 mm.[3] Compared with a gantry-mounted linac that moves in a planar arc and points to a fixed isocenter, the CyberKnife's unique maneuverability enables it to be positioned to any point in space, thus providing for much greater flexibility and allowing nonisocentric treatment delivery. Furthermore, over the last several years, the dose output of the CyberKnife linac has increased, resulting in reduction of overall patient treatment times.

High-speed computers represent the third component of the CyberKnife. By calculating the location of the treatment site before administering each dose of radiation, the CyberKnife is able to adjust and compensate for the movements of the patient. The fourth distinct feature of the CyberKnife is an x-ray imaging device (amorphous silicon detectors) placed in the floor of the treatment room on both sides of the patient.[4] Initial alignment radiographs are taken to determine the location of the target within the robotic coordinate system prior to treatment. These real-time digital radiographs are registered to digitally reconstructed radiographs (DRRs) from the treatment planning CT study, enabling the skull or spine (and thus treatment) position to be translated to the coordinate frame of the linac. The robotic arm receives information about the target position and compensates for any patient movement by aligning the linac with the treatment site. After the beam is adjusted and realigned with the target, a preplanned radiation dose is administered. Real-time digital radiographs are captured at repeated intervals as the robotic arm moves the linac to ~100 preset points, called nodes, surrounding the patient. Anatomical position can be evaluated at each node, enabling recalibration of the target position before administering each dose of radiation.

This imaging system also allows spinal lesions to be treated with the CyberKnife.[5] The spine is located in the imaging system's coordinating frame in a manner analogous to that used to locate intracranial targets; by comparing the DRRs from the treatment planning study to the current spine location acquired via real-time images, the CyberKnife is able to determine the current position of the patient's spine. The robotic arm adjusts the linac, and treatment doses are administered.

Precision of CyberKnife Treatment Planning

The principal innovation of the CyberKnife is the use of radiographic images of internal anatomical features to align the treatment beam with the target volume.

To achieve this, the position of a patient's anatomy within the camera field of view must be communicated to the robot. By establishing a fixed reference point in both the robot and the camera coordinate frames, the two systems can be aligned with a precision of approximately ± 0.5 mm along each axis.[6]

However, eliminating the need for a stereotactic frame inevitably raises issues about the spatial accuracy of dose placement when compared with existing frame-based systems. The requirement of CT or CT/MR coregistration for the generation of DRRs introduces a level of uncertainty in the treatment planning of the CyberKnife. Standard CyberKnife treatment planning CT slice thickness is 1.25 mm, resulting in the uncertainty in the inferior/superior coordinate of the treatment volume of ~0.63 mm. Furthermore, radiographic technical limitations—edge softening from attenuation of the diagnostic x-rays, blurring from the reconstruction technique, and other ambiguities in the delineation of structure within an image—introduce an uncertainty of ~0.5 to 1.0 mm in the other two planning coordinates. These errors introduced by imaging are comparable to the imaging errors in frame-based systems.[7]

A second component of total clinical error is that introduced by the robot itself (mechanical accuracy of the robot). The linac beam is pointed by the robotic arm at an isocenter from ~75 to 150 different beam positions. The individual beams miss the theoretical targets with errors that are randomly distributed around a zero mean for each coordinate axis, with a net root mean square (rms) radial error of 0.7 mm.[8] For a treatment that uses all beams, the effect of this source of error is to blur rather than offset the dose distribution. The rms radial pointing error of the CyberKnife is comparable to the deviation in the arc motion of a linac moving along a gantry path, which has been reported in one instance to be ≤ 0.6 mm.[9]

Another variable affecting dose precision is patient movement during frameless radiosurgery. In the present CyberKnife system, patient position is measured at select intervals prior to delivering each dose. Any movement during radiation delivery itself will lead to misdirection of that portion of the dose. The patient's changed position is detected and compensated for at the beginning of the next cycle to preserve the pattern in which the beams traverse patient anatomy and intersect within the target. Given that there are typically over 100 nodes, a single patient movement affects no more than about 1% of the total administered dose in a single-fraction treatment. Furthermore, rotational changes in the patient's position can be minimized by using head restraints, such as a molded AquaPlast mask (WFR/Aquaplast Corp., Wyckoff, NJ), during cranial treatments or a custom alpha cradle mold (Smithers Medical Products, Inc., Akron, OH) during spinal treatments. The noninvasive restraints also serve to confine the treatment site to a small region (± 10 mm) within which the imaging system is calibrated to measure translations. More recent advancements in image registration allow for measurement of all six degrees of freedom in the position and orientation of patient anatomy, thus compensating for rotational changes by the patient during the procedure.

CyberKnife Treatment Protocol

The initial steps of patient treatment consist of treatment imaging. Thin-slice CT and/or MR imaging is obtained and loaded onto the treatment planning computer. The treatment planning system (TPS) of the CyberKnife is designed to allow planning based on the geometry of the lesion and surrounding structures, the maximum number of allowable beams, and the dose distribution. Geometry is outlined on CT or MR images, and the amount of radiation each structure can tolerate is specified. A three-dimensional map of the lesion is created using contour data. The system then organizes beams in a manner that allows equal coverage of the tumor, with beams originating from different orientations and nodes. To accommodate dose constraints due to critical structures near the lesion, dose weighting is calculated for different beams. If initial beam configuration does not satisfy dose constraints, information from optimization will aid selection of a new beam; this process continues until a favorable set of beams and doses is obtained. This flexibility enables critical structures adjacent to the lesion to be spared and optimally directs radiation for irregularly shaped tumors. This is accomplished by exploiting the robot's six-degree-of-freedom maneuverability to deliver a homogeneous dose that closely conforms to the irregular volumes.[10,11] Once the inverse treatment planning is complete, the final plan is then reviewed by the treating team prior to delivery. During the actual treatment, the CyberKnife treatment algorithm places the linac at a determined position, uses real-time imaging to locate the target and adjust for movements, delivers radiation, and repeats the process at various nodes surrounding the patient.

◆ CyberKnife Results

Benign Brain Lesions

Acoustic Neuromas

Acoustic neuroma control rates with CyberKnife radiosurgery are comparable to frame-based radiosurgery series, with tumor control rates above 98% and facial and trigeminal nerve complication rates of 1% or less.[12] Multisession radiosurgery can be performed for acoustic neuromas (**Fig. 4.2**) under the hypothesis that multiple smaller sessions of treatment may reduce risk to cranial nerves,[13–15] and several recent clinical studies have investigated the advantages of multisession radiosurgery for treating acoustic neuroma compared with single-session radiosurgery.[16–28] Although the optimal number of sessions or time interval between sessions is not known, our CyberKnife experience with a three-session regimen of radiosurgery has produced hearing preservation rates of 74% at a mean follow-up of 4 years.[7]

Meningiomas

CyberKnife radiosurgical control rates for meningiomas are also comparable to Gamma Knife or frame-based linac radiosurgery, and all meningiomas treatable with frame-based techniques can be treated with image-guided radiosurgery. The CyberKnife does have the flexibility to treat meningiomas that otherwise could not be easily treated with single-session frame-based radiosurgery. One group of such tumors consists of meningiomas immediately adjacent

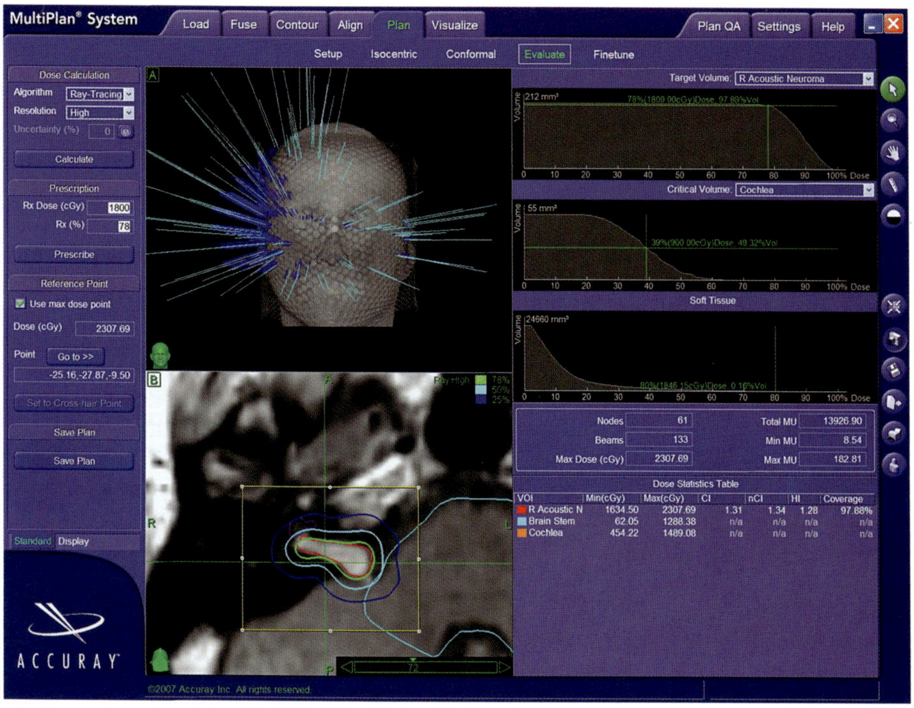

Fig. 4.2 A typical treatment plan for an acoustic neuroma.

to the anterior visual pathways in which single-session radiosurgery is thought to have increased risk. Our experience in using multisession radiosurgery for these lesions has shown excellent control rates (93%).[29] Only two patients suffered visual deterioration, and in both of these patients, the visual deterioration appeared to be from tumor progression, indicating that the tumors may have been undertreated with respect to treatment dose.

Another group of meningiomas that may benefit from multisession radiosurgery are those adjacent to the midline venous sinuses. Reports have suggested that these tumors are more likely to develop posttreatment radiation edema, perhaps due to inflammation and obstruction of cortical veins leading to the sinuses.[30,31] Our experience has been similar to these other reports, with parasagittal and midline meningiomas having a 29% rate of posttreatment edema, whereas nonmidline meningiomas had only a 7.5% rate of posttreatment edema.[32] Multisession radiosurgery using the CyberKnife for these midline meningiomas may be associated with reduced rates of posttreatment edema compared with single-session radiosurgery, and we are currently investigating this hypothesis at Stanford.

Pituitary Tumors

Similar to perioptic meningiomas, pituitary tumors are in close proximity to the optic pathways. Those adenomas that are more than several millimeters from the optic chiasm can be treated with single-session radiosurgery with doses comparable to the Gamma Knife. Pituitary tumors abutting the optic chiasm can be treated with multisession image-guided radiosurgery with good tumor control rates and low risk of visual loss.[29] Our experience with perioptic adenomas reveals that only 1 of 19 patients with treated adenoma 2 mm or closer to the anterior visual pathways suffered visual deterioration; this patient had been treated with prior external beam radiotherapy and two prior courses of frame-based radiosurgery for a multiply recurrent adrenocorticotropic hormone (ACTH)–secreting pituitary tumor.

Glomus Jugulare Tumors

Whether located at the skull base or in the neck, glomus jugulare tumors are excellent targets for radiosurgery due to their well-demarcated borders. Our experience in treating 16 tumors with image-guided radiosurgery has shown 100% tumor control rate to date, with no new permanent neurologic symptoms.[33] For larger tumors, multiple sessions may reduce treatment risk to surrounding structures.

Craniopharyngioma

Craniopharyngiomas represent only a small percentage of brain tumors, but their propensity to recur remains problematic. As such, using radiosurgery to treat residual or recurrent craniopharyngiomas has been performed in select cases. As with perioptic meningiomas or pituitary tumors, the ability to deliver multisession radiosurgery may reduce complications from anterior visual field pathway injury. Our CyberKnife experience to date has been limited to 16 patients, all of whom were treated with multisession radiosurgery.[34] Ninety-one percent of the patients with follow-up imaging and clinical evaluation achieved tumor control or shrinkage without any neuroendocrine or visual complications.

Trigeminal Neuralgia

Trigeminal neuralgia radiosurgery with the CyberKnife has the same basic concept as Gamma Knife radiosurgery in that a small high-dose lesion is created within the prepontine segment of the trigeminal nerve. The only significant difference is that the CyberKnife uses nonisocentric planning, and thus the lesion volume is typically an ellipse instead of a round isocenter (**Fig. 4.3**). A recent multicenter publication of nonisocentric CyberKnife radiosurgery for trigeminal neuralgia revealed an initial pain relief rate of 67% with median time to pain relief of 14 days.[35]

Malignant Brain Lesions

Brain Metastases

Brain metastases remain one of the most common indications for the CyberKnife, but results of single-session radiosurgery for solid metastases are comparable to published linac and Gamma Knife series.[2,36] Recent efforts at our institution to expand the use of radiosurgery for brain metastases have focused on the use of adjuvant stereotactic radiosurgery targeted at the resection cavities of brain metastases without whole-brain radiation irradiation.[37] In this group of 76 patients, the metastasis resection cavity was treated with radiosurgery using one to five sessions, depending on cavity size. The most common histology was lung (42%), melanoma (18%), and breast (16%). Treatment was given in a single session in 78% of patients, with two to five sessions used in the remainder. Radiosurgery was delivered to a median marginal dose of 18.6 Gy (range 15–30 Gy), mean maximum dose of 23.8 Gy (range 17.8–40.5 Gy), to an average tumor volume of 9.8 cm^3 (range 0.1–66.8 cm^3) and a 79% median isodose line. With a median follow-up of 8.1 months (0.1–80.5 months), 69 patients had follow-up imaging evaluable for control analyses. Crude overall local and distant failure rates were 14% (10/69 patients) and 51% (35/69), respectively. Actuarial local control rates at 6 and 12 months were 88% and 79%, respectively. On univariate analysis, the conformality and modified conformality indices were the only treatment variables that significantly correlated with improved local control. Target volume, dose, and number of sessions were not statistically significant. Median overall survival was 16.2 months. The crude local failure rate of 14% compares favorably to historical results with observation alone (46%) and for postoperative whole-brain radiation (10–20%). Given the improved local control seen with less conformal plans, we now use a 2 mm margin around the resection cavity when using this technique.

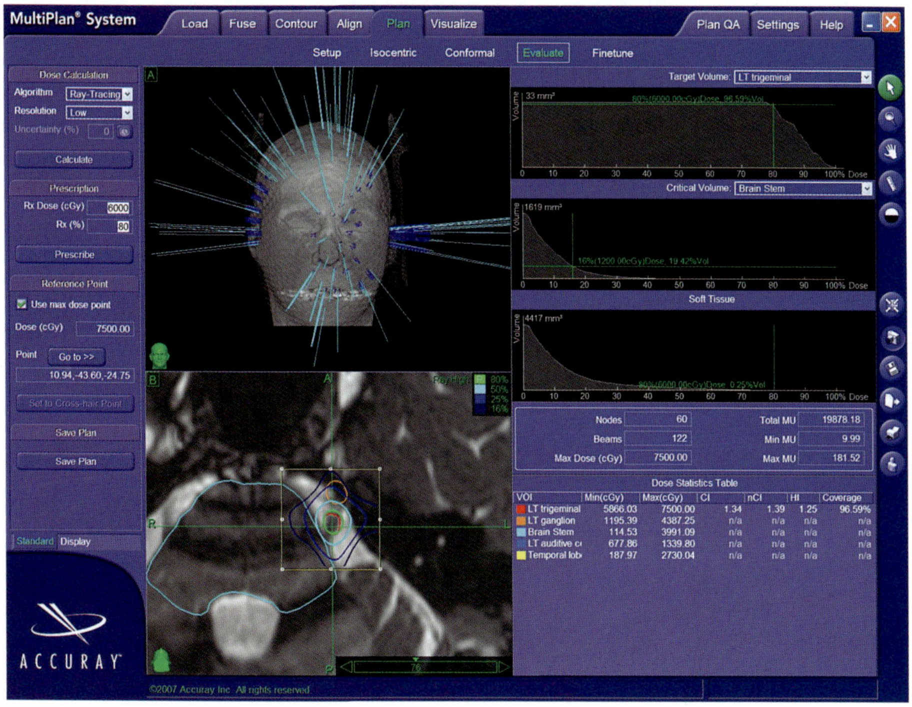

Fig. 4.3 A typical treatment plan for trigeminal neuralgia.

Nasopharynx Carcinoma

The use of a stereotactic radiosurgical boost after external beam radiotherapy has become a common treatment for nasopharyngeal carcinoma. Over a 14-year period at our institution, 82 patients received a radiosurgical boost after radiotherapy.[38] Patients received 66 Gy of radiotherapy followed by a single fraction radiosurgical boost of 7 to 15 Gy, delivered 2 to 6 weeks after radiotherapy completion (70 patients also received cisplatin-based chemotherapy delivered concurrently with and adjuvant to radiotherapy) (**Fig. 4.4**). At median follow-up of 40.7 months (6.5–144.2 months) for

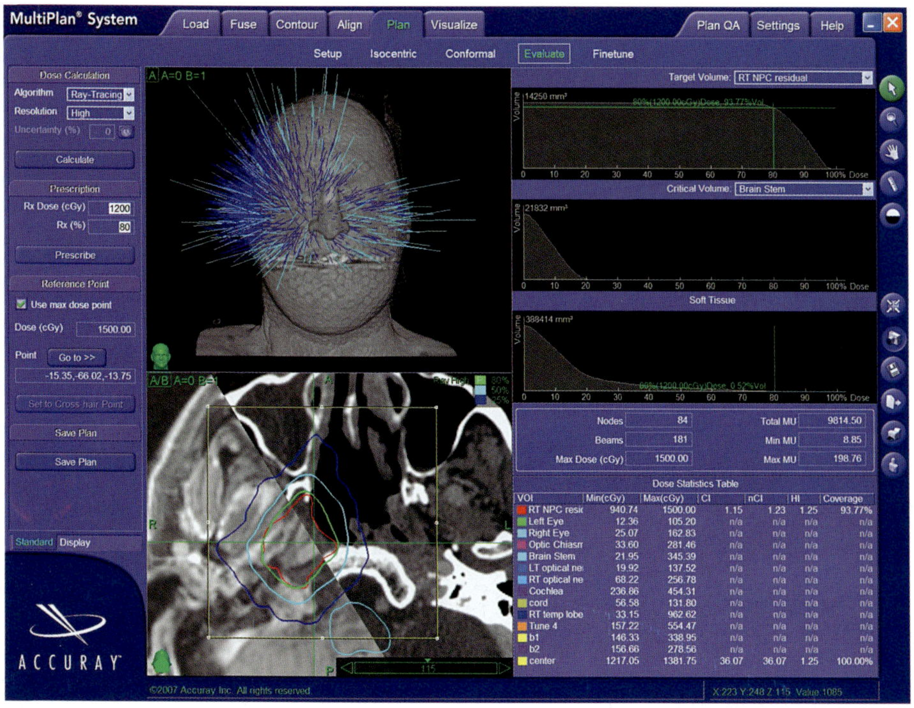

Fig. 4.4 A typical treatment plan for a nasopharynx cavity radiosurgery boost.

living patients, there was only one local failure. At 5 years, the freedom from local relapse rate was 98%, freedom from nodal relapse was 83%, freedom from distant metastasis was 68%, freedom from any relapse was 67%, and overall survival was 69%. Late toxicity included unresolved V2 or V3 numbness in 3, radiation-related retinopathy in 3, carotid aneurysm in 1, and radiographic temporal lobe necrosis in 10 patients, of whom 2 were symptomatic with seizures.

Spinal Lesions

Benign Spine Tumors

Since 1999, CyberKnife radiosurgery was used to manage 71 patients (median age 46 years; range 12–86 years) with 78 benign spinal tumors (36 schwannomas, 16 neurofibromas, 26 meningiomas) at our institution.[39] Total treatment doses for spinal cord tumors ranged from 14 to 30 Gy (mean 20 Gy) delivered in consecutive daily sessions[2,4,16,17,29] to tumor volumes that varied from 0.14 to 54.5 cm^3. Mean follow-up for the benign spinal tumor patient was 2.5 years posttreatment. Two patients had tumor progression (one at 6 months posttreatment and the second at 1 year posttreatment). Both of these patients underwent tumor progression. Three other patients (one meningioma, one schwannoma, and one neurofibroma) underwent surgery for progression of symptoms, even though the tumor size was stable following radiosurgery treatment. In total, 76 of the 78 tumors were controlled after radiosurgery and were either stable (59%) or smaller (39%) in size (**Fig. 4.5**). Two patients died during the follow-up period from causes unrelated to their spine tumor. Radiation-induced myelopathy appeared 8 months postradiosurgery in one patient. These preliminary results are supported by similar results from the University of Pittsburgh.[40]

Spine Metastases

The treatment of spinal metastases has been one of the fastest-growing indications for extracranial radiosurgery. From 1996 to 2005, 74 patients with 102 spinal metastases were treated using the CyberKnife at our institution.[41] Sixty-two (84%) patients were symptomatic. Seventy-four percent (50/68) of previously treated patients had prior radiation. Using the CyberKnife, 16 to 25 Gy in one to five fractions was delivered. Patients were followed clinically and radiographically for at least 3 months or until death. With mean follow-up of 9 months (range 0–33 months), 36 patients were alive, and 38 were dead at the last follow-up. No death was treatment related. Eighty-four percent of symptomatic patients experienced improvement or resolution of symptoms after treatment. Three patients developed treatment-related spinal injury. Analysis of dose–volume parameters and clinical parameters failed to identify predictors of spinal cord injury. Others have reported similar control rates for spine metastases.[42–46]

Spinal Arteriovenous Malformations

To date, 23 patients with spinal cord AVMs have been treated with CyberKnife radiosurgery, with our initial experience of the first 15 patients previously published.[47] Seventeen spinal AVMs were located in the cervical region, three in the thoracic spine, and three in the lumbar spine. Radiosurgery was delivered in two to five sessions with a mean dose of 20.5 Gy. For the spinal AVM patients, mean follow-up was also 2.5 years. Ten patients were more than 3 years following radiosurgery treatment, and 4 of these 10 patients showed complete obliteration of their spinal AVMs (**Fig. 4.6**). Of the remaining six patients who were more than 3 years posttreatment, five showed significant reduction of AVM

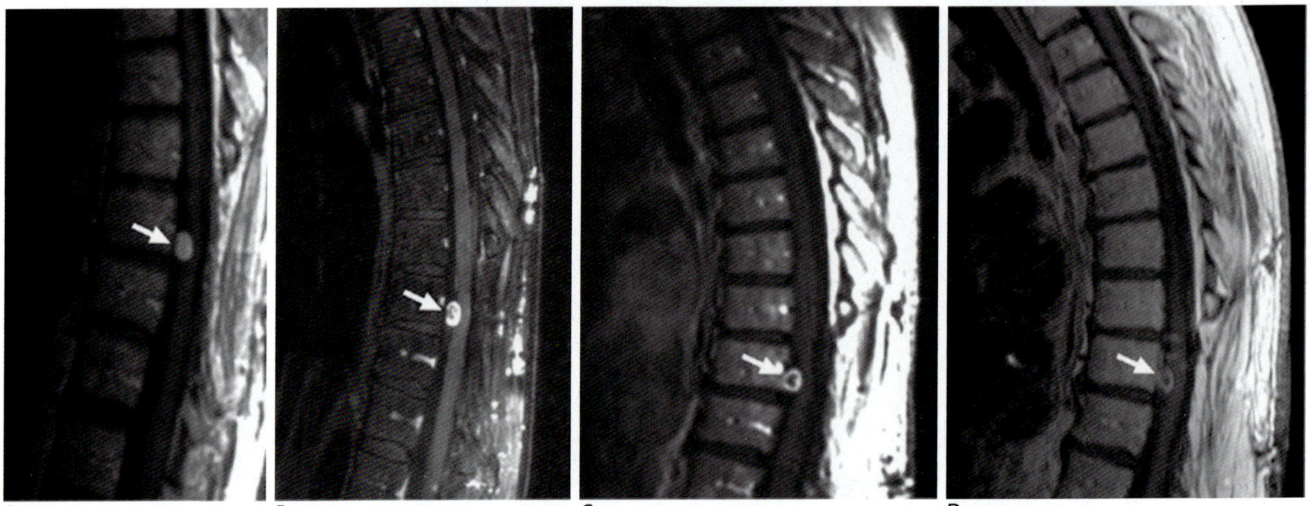
A B C D

Fig. 4.5 Magnetic resonance imaging (MRI) scans showing temporal response to radiosurgery in a patient with recurrent T9 schwannoma treated with 22 Gy in three sessions. **(A)** Pretreatment sagittal T1 postcontrast MRI scan. **(B)** Six-month sagittal postcontrast MRI scan illustrating a slight change in the enhancement pattern. **(C)** Twenty-four- and **(D)** 73-month sagittal postcontrast MRI scans illustrating size reduction and further loss of central enhancement. (From Dodd RL, Ryu M, Kamnerdsupaphon P, Gibbs IC, Chang SD, Adler JR Jr. CyberKnife radiosurgery treatment of benign intradural extramedullary spinal tumors. Neurosurgery 2006;58(4):674–685. Reprinted with permission.)

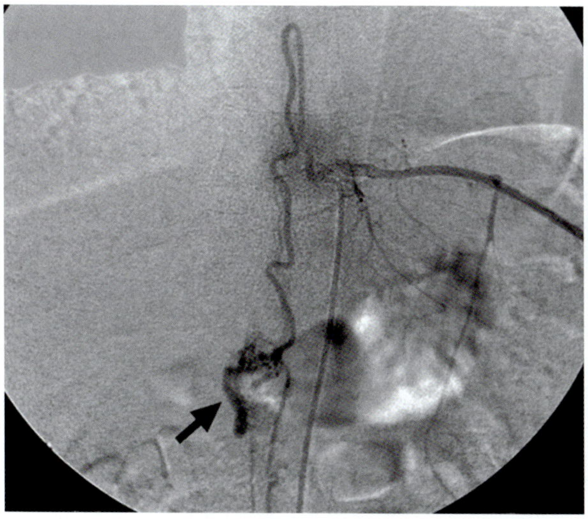
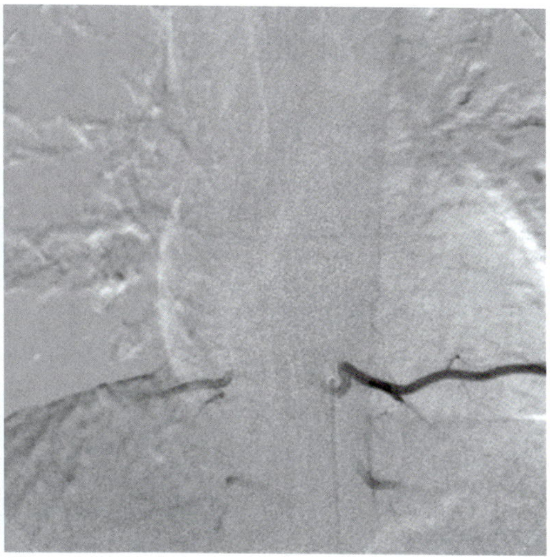

A B

Fig. 4.6 Pre- and postoperative stereotactic radiosurgery angiograms demonstrating angiographic obliteration of the conus medullaris type II (glomus) spinal cord arteriovenous malformation (AVM). **(A)** Selective intercostal angiogram pretreatment demonstrating an enlarged anterior spinal artery feeding an AVM (*arrow*) of the conus medullaris. **(B)** Frontal projection from a selective injection of the feeding intercostal artery posttreatment demonstrating no residual AVM. (From Sinclair J, Chang SD, Gibbs IC, Adler JR Jr. Multisession CyberKnife radisosurgery for intramedullary spinal cord arteriovenous malformations. Neurosurgery 2006;58(6):1081–1089. Reprinted with permission.)

volume on posttreatment angiography. Two patients developed radiation edema after treatment. One of these patients had complete AVM obliteration 9 months posttreatment and had resolution of the spinal edema. The second patient is 24 months posttreatment and has persistent spinal cord edema associated with worsening neurologic function. No patients developed a hemorrhage from their spinal cord AVMs after radiosurgery treatment.

◆ Summary

Image-guided radiosurgery has several advantages, and it is more flexible than conventional stereotactic radiosurgery. By removing the constraints of invasive stereotactic frames, the CyberKnife is more amenable to multisession radiosurgery, targeting of lesions outside the cranium, and delivery of homogeneous conformal dose distribution to targets of irregular shape. Furthermore, patient comfort is improved, eliminating the need for general anesthesia in pediatric populations. To date worldwide, more than 40,000 patients have been treated with CyberKnife radiosurgery. For lesions in the brain, clinical and radiographical outcomes are comparable to those achieved with conventional linac and Gamma Knife systems.

Because the CyberKnife introduces new flexibility to radiosurgery, its usefulness can be extended beyond intracranial to spinal (and other extracranial) lesions. With the introduction of advanced amorphic silicon detectors, radiographic imaging of the spine has improved significantly. Processing of the high-quality images by the six-dimensional registration software can further achieve significant improvements in spatial resolution. As such, the CyberKnife has been used to treat spinal lesions with promising results, including AVMs, and benign and malignant spinal neoplasms.

References

1. Takacs I, Hamilton AJ, Lulu B, et al. Frame based stereotactic spinal radiosurgery: experience from the first 19 patients. Paper presented at: Quadrennial Meeting of the American Society for Stereotactic and Functional Neurosurgery; Snowbird, UT, July 7–10, 1999
2. Adler JR Jr, Murphy MJ, Chang SD, Hancock SL. Image-guided robotic radiosurgery. Neurosurgery 1999;44:1299–1306
3. Yu C, Main W, Taylor D, Kuduvalli G, Apuzzo ML, Adler JR Jr. An anthropomorphic phantom study of the accuracy of CyberKnife spinal radiosurgery. Neurosurgery 2004;55:1138–1149
4. Antonuk LE, Yorkston J, Huang W, et al. A real time, flat panel, amorphous silicon, digital x-ray imager. Radiographics 1995;15:993–1000
5. Ryu SI, Chang SD, Kim DH, et al. Image-guided hypo-fractionated stereotactic radiosurgery to spinal lesions. Neurosurgery 2001;49:838–846
6. Murphy MJ, Cox RS. Frameless radiosurgery using real-time image correlation for beam targeting. Med Phys 1996;23:1052–1053
7. Lemieux L, Kitchen ND, Hughes SW, Thomas DG. Voxel-based localization in frame-based and frameless stereotaxy and its accuracy. Med Phys 1994;21:1301–1310
8. Murphy MJ, Cox RS. The accuracy of dose localization for an image-guided frameless radiosurgery system. Med Phys 1996;23:2043–2049
9. Winston KR, Lutz W. Linear accelerator as a neurosurgical tool for stereotactic radiosurgery. Neurosurgery 1988;22:454–464
10. Schweikard A, Adler JR, Latombe JC. Motion planning in stereotaxic radiosurgery. Proc IEEE Int Conf Robotics and Automation 1993: 1909–1916
11. Schweikard A, Tombropoulos RZ, Adler JR, Latombe JC. Treatment planning for a radiosurgical system with general kinematics. Proc IEEE Conf Robotics and Automation 1994:1720–1727
12. Chang SD, Gibbs IC, Sakamoto GT, Lee E, Oyelese A, Adler JR Jr. Staged stereotactic irradiation for acoustic neuroma. Neurosurgery 2005;56: 1254–1261
13. Flickinger JC. An integrated logistic formula for prediction of complications from radiosurgery. Int J Radiat Oncol Biol Phys 1989;17:879–885
14. Lederman G, Lowry J, Wertheim S, et al. Acoustic neuroma: potential benefits of fractionated stereotactic radiosurgery. Stereotact Funct Neurosurg 1997;69:175–182

15. Lo YC, Ling CC, Larson DA. The effect of setup uncertainties on the radiobiological advantage of fractionation in stereotaxic radiotherapy. Int J Radiat Oncol Biol Phys 1996;34:1113–1119
16. Andrews DW, Silverman CL, Glass J, et al. Preservation of cranial nerve function after treatment of acoustic neurinomas with fractionated stereotactic radiotherapy: preliminary observations in 26 patients. Stereotact Funct Neurosurg 1995;64:165–182
17. Andrews DW, Suarez O, Goldman HW, et al. Stereotactic radiosurgery and fractionated stereotactic radiotherapy for the treatment of acoustic schwannomas: comparative observations of 125 patients treated at one institution. Int J Radiat Oncol Biol Phys 2001;50:1265–1278
18. Bush DA, McAllister CJ, Loredo LN, Johnson WD, Slater JM, Slater JD. Fractionated proton beam radiotherapy for acoustic neuroma. Neurosurgery 2002;50:270–275
19. Fuss M, Debus J, Lohr F, et al. Conventionally fractionated stereotactic radiotherapy (FSRT) for acoustic neuromas. Int J Radiat Oncol Biol Phys 2000;48:1381–1387
20. Fuss M, Salter BJ, Sadeghi A, Vollmer DG, Hevezi JM, Herman TS. Fractionated stereotactic intensity-modulated radiotherapy (FS-IMRT) for small acoustic neuromas. Med Dosim 2002;27:147–154
21. Meijer OW, Wolbers JG, Baayen JC, Slotman BJ. Fractionated stereotactic radiation therapy and single high-dose radiosurgery for acoustic neuroma: early results of a prospective clinical study. Int J Radiat Oncol Biol Phys 2000;46:45–49
22. Poen JC, Golby AJ, Forster KM, et al. Fractionated stereotactic radiosurgery and preservation of hearing in patients with vestibular schwannoma: a preliminary report. Neurosurgery 1999;45:1299–1305
23. Suh JH, Barnett GH, Sohn JW, Kupelian PA, Cohen BH. Results of linear accelerator-based stereotactic radiosurgery for recurrent and newly diagnosed acoustic neuromas. Int J Cancer 2000;90:145–151
24. Varlotto JM, Shrieve DC, Alexander E III, Kooy HM, Black PM, Loeffler JS. Fractionated stereotactic radiotherapy for the treatment of acoustic neuromas: preliminary results. Int J Radiat Oncol Biol Phys 1996;36:141–145
25. Williams JA. Fractionated stereotactic radiotherapy for acoustic neuromas. Stereotact Funct Neurosurg 2002;78:17–28
26. Williams JA. Fractionated stereotactic radiotherapy for acoustic neuromas. Int J Radiat Oncol Biol Phys 2002;54:500–504
27. Williams JA. Fractionated stereotactic radiotherapy for acoustic neuromas. Acta Neurochir (Wien) 2002;144:1249–1254
28. Williams JA. Fractionated stereotactic radiotherapy for acoustic neuromas: preservation of function versus size. J Clin Neurosci 2003;10:48–52
29. Adler JR Jr, Gibbs IC, Puataweepong P, Chang SD. Visual field preservation after multisession CyberKnife radiosurgery for perioptic lesions. Neurosurgery 2006;59:244–254
30. Kalapurakal JA, Silverman CL, Akhtar N, et al. Intracranial meningiomas: factors that influence the development of cerebral edema after stereotactic radiosurgery and radiation therapy. Radiology 1997;204:461–465
31. Kan P, Liu JK, Wendland MM, Shrieve D, Jensen RL. Peritumoral edema after stereotactic radiosurgery for intracranial meningiomas and molecular factors that predict its development. J Neurooncol 2007;83:33–38
32. Patil CG, Hoang S, Borchers J, et al. Predictors of peritumoral edema following stereotactic radiosurgery for supratentorial meningiomas. Neurosurgery 2008;63(3):435–442
33. Lim M, Bower R, Nangiana JS, Adler JR, Chang SD. Radiosurgery for glomus jugulare tumors. Technol Cancer Res Treat 2007;6:419–423
34. Lee M, Gibbs IC, Adler JR, Chang SD. Radiation therapy and CyberKnife radiosurgery in the management of craniopharyngiomas. Neurosurg Focus 2007;24: In press
35. Villavicencio AT, Lim M, Burneikiene S, et al. CyberKnife radiosurgery for trigeminal neuralgia treatment: a prelimiary multicenter experience. Neurosurgery 2008;62(3):647–655
36. Chang SD, Murphy M, Geis P, et al. Clinical experience with image-guided robotic radiosurgery (the CyberKnife) in the treatment of brain and spinal cord tumors. Neurol Med Chir (Tokyo) 1998;38:780–783
37. Soltys SG, Adler JR, Lipani JD, et al. Stereotactic radiosurgery of the postoperative resection cavity for brain metastases. Int J Radiat Oncol Biol Phys 2008;70:187–193
38. Hara W, Loo BW Jr, Goffinet DR, et al. Excellent local control with stereotactic radiotherapy boost after external beam radiotherapy in patients with nasopharyngeal carcinoma. Int J Radiat Oncol Biol Phys 2008;71(2):393–400
39. Dodd RL, Ryu MR, Kamnerdsupaphon P, Gibbs IC, Chang SD Jr, Adler JR Jr. CyberKnife radiosurgery for benign intradural extramedullary spinal tumors. Neurosurgery 2006;58:674–685
40. Gerszten PC, Burton SA, Ozhasoglu C, McCue KJ, Quinn AE. Radiosurgery for benign intradural spinal tumors. Neurosurgery 2008;62(4):887–896
41. Gibbs IC, Kamnerdsupaphon P, Ryu MR, et al. Image-guided robotic radiosurgery for spinal metastases. Radiother Oncol 2007;82:185–190
42. Gagnon GJ, Henderson FC, Gehan EA, et al. CyberKnife radiosurgery for breast cancer spine metastases: a matched-pair analysis. Cancer 2007;110:1796–1802
43. Gerszten PC, Burton SA, Belani CP, et al. Radiosurgery for the treatment of spinal lung metastases. Cancer 2006;107:2653–2661
44. Gerszten PC, Burton SA, Ozhasoglu C, et al. Stereotactic radiosurgery for spinal metastases from renal cell carcinoma. J Neurosurg Spine 2005;3:288–295
45. Gerszten PC, Burton SA, Ozhasoglu C, Welch WC. Radiosurgery for spinal metastases: clinical experience in 500 cases from a single institution. Spine 2007;32:193–199
46. Gerszten PC, Burton SA, Quinn AE, Agarwala SS, Kirkwood JM. Radiosurgery for the treatment of spinal melanoma metastases. Stereotact Funct Neurosurg 2005;83:213–221
47. Sinclair J, Chang SD, Gibbs IC, Adler JR Jr. Multisession CyberKnife radiosurgery for intramedullary spinal cord arteriovenous malformations. Neurosurgery 2006;58:1081–1089

5

Stereotactic Radiosurgery for Arteriovenous Malformations

L. Dade Lunsford, Ajay Niranjan, Hideyuki Kano, John C. Flickinger, and Douglas Kondziolka

Arteriovenous malformations (AVMs) are congenital vascular anomalies comprised of an abnormal number of blood vessels that are abnormally constructed. The blood vessels directly shunt blood from arterial input to the venous system without an intervening capillary network to dampen pressure. Both abnormal blood vessel construction and abnormal blood flow lead to a risk of rupture and intracranial hemorrhage. In addition, patients with lobar vascular malformations may suffer from intractable vascular headaches or develop seizure disorders. The annual incidence of AVM recognition is thought to be ~10,000 patients per year in the United States. However, the reliance on magnetic resonance imaging (MRI) has led to an increasing recognition of these vascular anomalies even in patients with minimal symptoms. The decision making relative to management of an AVM must be carefully evaluated based on several risk factors. The options for management include observation, endovascular embolization alone or in preparation for other adjuvant management, craniotomy and surgical removal, and stereotactic radiosurgery (SRS).[1] All treatments may be done in one or more stages.

In general, the following factors are evaluated when a patient is seen with an AVM: the patient's age, associated medical condition, history of a prior hemorrhagic event, prior management if any, overall volume and morphology, location of the AVM, initial presenting symptoms (headache, seizures, and local neurologic deficits), the AVM angioarchitecture (e.g., compact vs diffuse nidus), estimation of its surgical risks, presence of a proximal or intranidal aneurysm, and prior surgical experience in training. In making a decision for management strategies, we often employ a decision tree algorithm as shown in **Fig. 5.1.**

Optimal care depends on careful weighing of each of the above factors and the estimated risk of subsequent hemorrhage. The patient's clinical presentation and location are important issues as well as symptoms in each patient. Age, prior bleeding event, smaller AVM size, deep venous drainage, and high flow rates have been suggested by some as increasing the potential for subsequent bleeding. For larger volume AVM (average diameter 4–5 cm), observation may be the only reasonable strategy in view of the risks of even multimodality management.[2] This may be especially true for patients who have never bled previously. Endovascular embolization employing a variety of particulate, glue, or coil methods may be used as an adjunct prior to craniotomy and surgical removal.[3,4] It has also been performed in preparation for SRS, although its role prior to radiosurgery has declined with the realization that embolization rarely leads to significant volumetric reduction. Although the flow within the AVM may change after embolization, SRS must include the original volume. In contrast, before surgical removal, embolization may provide major benefit, either by reducing flow or eliminating deep-seated feeders that would otherwise be a significant problem during AVM resection. Recanalization of embolized AVM components over time may require repeat SRS.

Surgical removal is an important option for patients with lobar vascular malformations of suitable size, especially at centers of excellence with extensive AVM experience. Incomplete removal requires adjuvant management, perhaps including radiosurgery. Spetzler and Martin, among others, defined the relationship of AVM volume, pattern of venous drainage, and location within critical areas of the brain as important considerations that help to facilitate outcome prediction at the time of surgical resection at centers of excellence. Outcomes after AVM radiosurgery do not correlate with the same predictions of the Spetzler–Martin scale when microsurgery is used.[5] Outcomes after radiosurgery may be predicted based on volume, location, age, angioarchitecture, and dose delivered.[6] SRS is an excellent management strategy for patients with AVMs < 30 mm in average diameter (for a single procedure). Staged procedures are

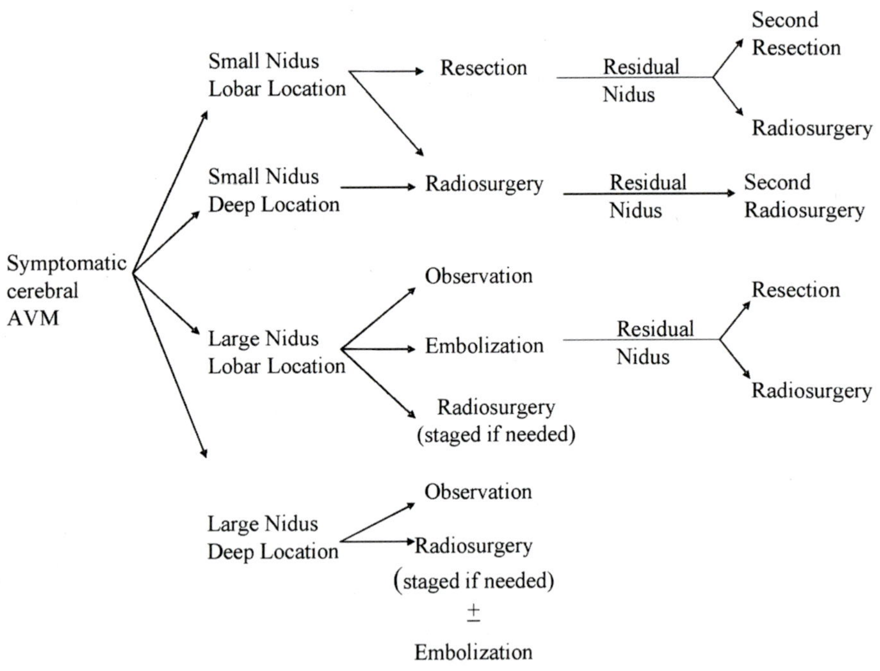

Fig. 5.1 Clinical algorithm for choosing management options for patients with intracranial arteriovenous malformations (AVMs).

used for larger vascular malformations or for those that were incompletely obliterated 3 years or more after an initial procedure.

The chief benefit of radiosurgery management is risk reduction; the chief deficit of radiosurgery is the latency interval that is required to achieve complete obliteration of the AVM.[7,8] The latency interval is generally 2 to 3 years, but in selected patients it may be longer. AVM radiosurgery has been used for children not suitable for other management strategies, as well as for older patients who have significant medical risk factors for surgical removal.

History of Radiosurgery for Arteriovenous Malformations

Radiation to obliterate abnormal blood vessels in the brain is a procedure that was first considered in the late 1960s. Raymond Kjellberg, using the Harvard-affiliated proton facility in Cambridge, Massachusetts, advocated proton Bragg peak stereotactic radiation during the 1970s and early 1980s.[9,10] More than 1000 AVM patients were treated, but the dose-planning technique was quite rudimentary. The technology of the Bragg peak proton facility was designed to provide a low exit dose based on the radiophysiological characteristics of this technology. The doses that were actually used in this series of patients were quite low and do not correspond to doses that we now know may be effective in the obliteration of AVMs. Although Kjellberg maintained that Bragg peak radiation stabilized AVM blood vessel walls and reduced the subsequent risk of hemorrhage (in comparison to age-related survivals from a life insurance table), only 20% of patients had complete obliteration of their AVM over time. Fabrikant et al, working at the Lawrence Livermore National Laboratory, began to use helium ion beam to perform multisession AVM irradiation in the 1980s.[11]

In Stockholm, Lars Leksell and Ladislau Steiner initiated work with the first-generation Leksell Gamma Knife unit.[12] The first patient was treated in March 1970, using the original prototype 179 cobalt source photon beam unit designed by Borje Larsson and Lars Leksell. The target definition was based on biplane angiography done during the procedure itself. Patients were observed for a period of time in preparation for a larger experience that began to emerge in Stockholm using the second-generation unit, which was built in 1975.

Linear accelerator (linac) technologies have been adapted for SRS. O.O. Betti, working in Paris and Buenos Aires,[13] J.L. Barcia-Salorio in Spain,[14,15] and Colombo in Vincenza, Italy,[16–18] were pioneers in the application of photon radiation using newer generation linacs. In addition, surgeons and radiation oncologists working at the Joint Center in Boston[19] and in Gainesville, Florida,[20] used modified linacs to treat a large number of vascular malformations. Most centers continue to evaluate SRS as part of an overall management plan that may include embolization, microsurgical removal, or radiosurgery alone or in combination. We will discuss our current viewpoint relative to the role of embolization subsequently.

Radiosurgery for Arteriovenous Malformations at the University of Pittsburgh

History

Our first AVM patient was treated in August 1987,[21] and we reported our initial experience in 227 patients in 1991.[22] Confirming the work of others, we noted that the 2-year

Table 5.1 Patient Demographics from Radiosurgery Experience at the University of Pittsburgh, 1987–2004

Number of patients	906
Patient age	
Median	36 years
Range	3–80 years
Gender	
Male	474 (52%)
Female	432 (48%)
Presenting symptoms	
Hemorrhage	417 (46%)
Seizures	213 (24%)
Headache	164 (18%)
Sensory motor deficit	74 (8%)
Incidental	38 (4%)
Prior management	
Embolization	194 (21%)
Surgery	63 (7%)

success rate in terms of complete obliteration was related to nidus volume and dose. In high-dose cases (AVM < 1 cc), obliteration rates of 100% were noted, which declined to 85% for volumes of 1 to 4 cc and 58% for AVMs > 4 cc in volume.

Our subsequent 20-year experience in Pittsburgh has now increased to more than 1100 patients who have undergone Gamma Knife radiosurgery for their AVM using one or more radiosurgical procedures. We have more recently analyzed the outcome data of 906 patients who underwent radiosurgery between 1987 and 2004 (**Tables 5.1, 5.2,** and **5.3**). Our median patient age was 36 years, with a range of 3 to 80 years. Typical symptoms at presentation included hemorrhage (46%), seizures (24%), and headache (18%). Eight percent had neurologic deficits (8%). An incidental AVM was detected in 4% of patients. Prior management strategies included surgical removal or clot evaluation in 7%. Twenty-one percent underwent one or more interventional procedures (embolization). The median target volume was 3.4 cc (range 0.065–57.7 cc). The median margin dose was 20 Gy (range 13–32 Gy). A single procedure was performed in 865 (95.5%) of patients, and repeat radiosurgery for incomplete nidus obliteration after 3 years was needed in 113 (12.5%) patients. Prospective volume staged radiosurgery was performed in 41 (4.5%) patients.

Table 5.2 Locations and Grades of Arteriovenous Malformations from Radiosurgery Experience at the University of Pittsburgh, 1987–2004 ($N = 906$)

AVM locations	Percentage
Temporal	18.50
Frontal	18
Parietal	17.50
Thalamus/basal ganglia	16.0
Occipital	11.50
Cerebellar	6.30
Brainstem	5.50
Dural	2.70
Corpus callosal	2.0
Intraventricular	1.0
Pineal	1.0
Spetzler–Martin grade	
Grade I	2.1
Grade II	24.4
Grade III	42.4
Grade IV	15.0
Grade V	2.7
Grade VI	13.4
Coexistence of aneurysm	77 (8.5)

Table 5.3 Radiosurgical Parameters of Arteriovenous Malformations Treated at the University of Pittsburgh, 1987–2004

AVM volume	
Median	3.4 mL
Range	0.065–57.7 mL
Radiosurgery dose	
Median	20 Gy
Range	13–32 Gy
Radiosurgery	
Single session	865/906 (95.5%)
Prospective volume staged	41/906 (4.5%)
Repeat radiosurgery	113/906 (12.5%)

At a median follow-up of 3 years, complete nidus obliteration was achieved in 78% (confirmed by angiography or MRI). In addition, 21% of patients achieved subtotal obliteration of the nidus. During the follow-up interval, 38 bleeds (4.1%) occurred after the procedure. Seizure control was improved in 51% of patients who presented with seizures. Adverse radiation effects (AREs) resulting in neurologic deficits developed in 24 patients (2.6%) and the detection of new T2 signal increase surrounding the AVM target in 108 patients (12%). We noted long-term complications such as delayed cyst formation and encephalomalacia in 16 patients (1.7%). No patient in this AVM series has developed a radiation-related tumor at the time of this writing.

Stereotactic Radiosurgical Procedure

We perform intracranial radiosurgery using the Leksell Gamma Knife (Elekta Instruments AB, Stockholm, Sweden), beginning with the model unit U, and proceeding to the B, C, 4-C, and in recent experience Perfexion model. The patient's clinical studies and imaging are reviewed for suitability for SRS. As noted previously, we evaluate the bleeding history, the age of the patient, existing comorbidities, location, and clinical symptomatology. Patients with lobar AVMs were placed prophylactically on anticonvulsants for a period of 2 to 4 weeks around the time of the procedure. This has reduced the risk of a perioperative seizure event from as high as 5% in year 1 of our 20-year experience to a risk of < 1% at the current time. We require that all women within the child-bearing age have a recent negative pregnancy test, or we perform it on the day of the procedure.

Patients are evaluated preoperatively by the neurosurgeon, the radiation oncologist, and the nursing team. On the morning of the procedure, the patients arrive at 6 o'clock and begin conscious sedation using oral lorazepam followed by intravenous (IV) conscious sedation (fentanyl and midazolam) as needed. Scalp anesthetic injection using a combination of Marcaine and Xylocaine is injected at the sites of pin application. At the current time, we prefer to use titanium pins with plastic inserts, to minimize the risk of MRI artifacts. General anesthesia may be required for frame application in imaging in patients younger than 12 years of age.

Neurodiagnostic imaging follows using both IV paramagnetic contrast-enhanced three-dimensional (3D) volumetric MRI scan and a whole-head T2 fast spin echo imaging sequence. Patients subsequently undergo biplane digital subtraction angiography (DSA) as the next step. In patients where MRI scans are not possible (those with undetermined implants, pacemakers, old aneurysm clips, etc.), we use contrast-enhanced stereotactic computed tomography angiography (CTA). The development of axial imaging as part of the imaging paradigm is critical for AVM management. This has allowed us to make superior 3D conformal plans much more carefully in comparison to using two-plane angiography alone.

Imaging studies are placed in a dose-planning computer system (Elekta Instruments), which currently has both high speed and high resolution. We begin the planning using MRI while the patient is undergoing angiography. Angiography is used to "fine-tune" or idealize the angiographic plan. In both the 4-C and Perfexion models currently used, optimization of the dose planning is achieved by confining the sharpest fall-off isodose (usually the 50%) to the edge of the 3D defined volume. Each slice is looked at serially to confirm excellent conformality (conforming the edge dose to the 3D target volume). High selectivity (rapid fall-off of the radiation dose outside the target) is equally important (**Fig. 5.2**). We also assess the patient for the presence of proximal and intranidal aneurysms. We strive to reduce dose to draining veins when feasible. Typical doses at the margin of the AVM are 18 to 25 Gy and never below 16 Gy. Maximal doses are usually 36 to 50 Gy

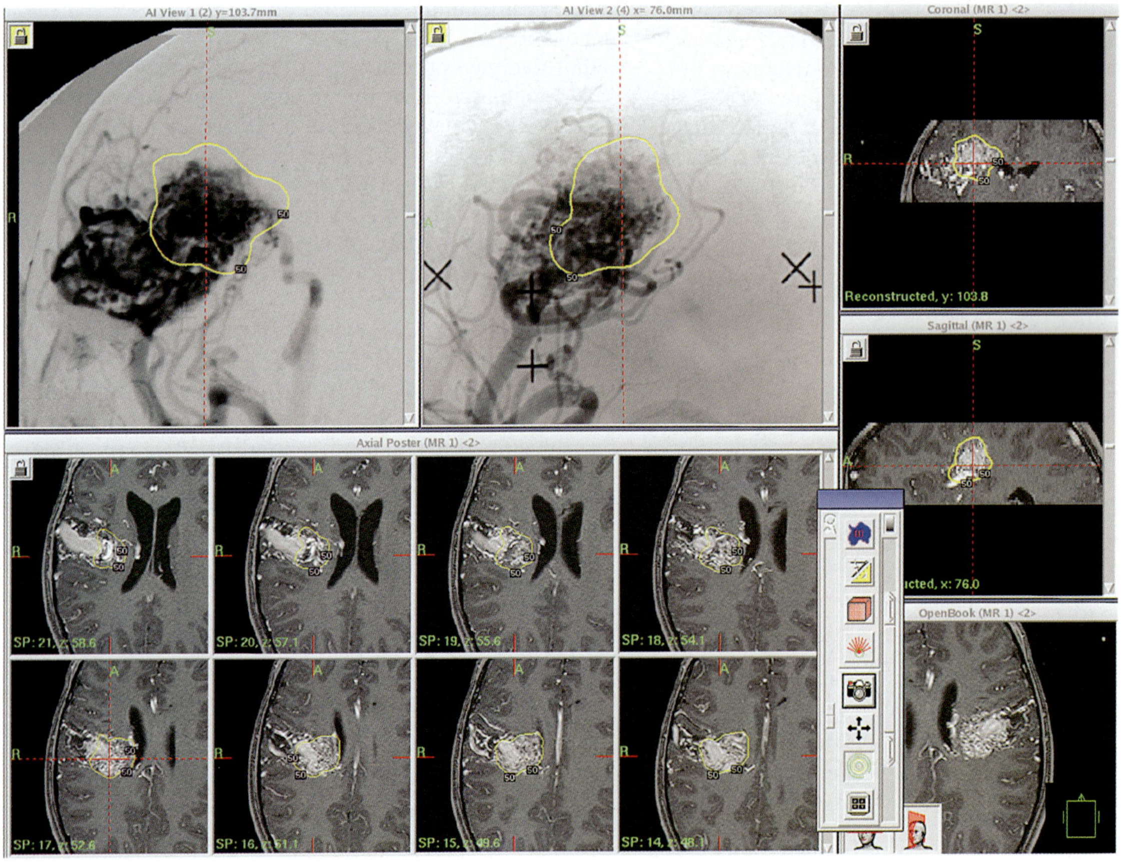

Fig. 5.2 Gamma Knife dose plan for a right hemisphere arteriovenous malformation showing the 50% isodose line projecting on anteroposterior and lateral views of angiograms and axial poster, as well as coronal and sagittal reconstruction of magnetic resonance images. This plan was created using Leksell GammaPlan PFX.

at the margin of the AVM. Final dose selection depends on the volume and location, which also helps to estimate ARE risks. We also consider the presence of preexisting neurologic conditions, the patient's age, and prior bleeding history. Because the dose to the surrounding brain is a critical predictor of ARE, we must maximize conformality and selectivity.

At the conclusion of the procedure, patients receive 20 to 40 mg of methylprednisolone. This coupled with anticonvulsants in lobar AVM patients tends to reduce the risk of perioperative seizures. For those patients who have previously undergone embolization in an attempt to reduce flow or to achieve volumetric reduction of the AVM, or for those who have had intracranial surgery or hematoma evacuation, Gamma Knife radiosurgery may be used as an adjuvant strategy rather than a primary management. We often perform radiosurgery once the patient has achieved stable neurologic improvement but almost never within the first month after an ictal event, such as a bleed or embolization. For patients who have had intracranial hemorrhages, we prefer to wait between 1 and 3 months to see if there will be a regional clot reabsorption. The AVM nidus should not be compressed by clot at the time of the radiosurgery. Failure of radiosurgery can be traced in some ways to inadequate planning, inadequate recognition of the 3D geometry of the AVM, reappearance of a component of the AVM previously embolized, or reappearance of a component of the AVM that was previously compressed by intracerebral hematoma.

Follow-up imaging is recommended at regular intervals. Whenever possible, imaging is done at our center, but if the patient lives a distance, we recommended the images be done at an imaging site closer to home. Communication with the patient's referring physician team is critical. We normally recommend MRI scans at 6 months and then annually to assess the effect of radiosurgery. If at the end of 3 years MRI suggests complete obliteration, then we request that a repeat DSA be performed. If MRI clearly defines residual nidus, angiography is delayed, and the patient is contacted to suggest the possible need for repeat radiosurgery to achieve the final obliteration response. In such cases, repeat stereotactic imaging may include both repeat MRI and angiography.

For those patients who have large AVMs (determined by multiplying the MRI X, Y, and Z dimensions of the AVM and dividing by 2, a rough approximation of an ellipsoid volume), we recommend consideration of prospective staged SRS. Staged radiosurgery, with two stages separated usually by 3 months, is recommended for AVMs > 15 cm^3. We also consider it for those AVMs between 10 and 15 cm^3. For those AVM volumes 10 cm^3 or smaller, we normally perform single-stage radiosurgery. The interval between stages varies from 3 to 6 months based on the goal of some radiobiological repair of surrounding brain during the observation interval. However, we do not want to wait too long, as the goal of protection from bleeding cannot begin until the radiosurgical procedure has been completed for all volumetric components of the AVM.

◆ Current Outcomes of Stereotactic Radiosurgery of Arteriovenous Malformations

In the absence of treatment, the overall risk of a spontaneous bleed from a brain AVM appears to range from 1 to 5% per year, depending on various risk factors.[23] In the Finnish population-based 24-year study, hemorrhage was a relatively constant lifetime risk, with an annual death risk of ~1% and approximately a 4% risk of bleed per year.[23] Recent work reported from the cooperative trial in Canada suggested that an annual bleed rate may be as high as 5% (C Wallace, personal communication). We performed an individualized analysis of the hemorrhage risk of AVM patients before radiosurgery.[24] Our findings demonstrated an overall crude annual hemorrhage rate of 2.4% per year.

There were several factors associated with hemorrhage risk, the primary one being a prior hemorrhage (an identification of a single draining vein on angiography), along with the detection of a diffuse AVM nidus on angiography. Pollock et al constructed an estimation of bleed risks related to these significant factors[24] (**Tables 5.4** and **5.5**). For low-risk AVMs (no prior hemorrhage and no other risk factors, diffuse nidus, or single draining vein), the annual risk rate was ~1% per year. In contrast, the risk of a second hemorrhage for patients with additional risk factors ranged from 2.0 to 3.7% for AVMs with a compact nidus up to 8.94% for those with high-risk features of the angioarchitecture (one draining vein or diffuse morphology).

In talking with families, we often use a "rule of thumb" to estimate the lifetime bleeding risk related to a patient's age. The age at which the risk of a bleed is greater than the risk of morbidity from radiosurgery may well depend on the location and size of the AVM. A simple lifetime analysis risk rate suggests that a patient's age subtracted from 105 will give the total cumulative risk of that patient having a bleeding event.[25,26] Clearly, for a child, the risk is very large, whereas for a senior citizen, the remaining lifetime risk of a bleed for a patient who has never bled before may be reasonably low.

Bleeding Risks after Stereotactic Radiosurgery for Arteriovenous Malformations

We have also analyzed the bleeding rate during the observation interval (latency interval) after radiosurgery and before

Table 5.4 Estimated Annual Risk of First and Second Hemorrhage in AVM Patients

	Estimated Risk of Intracranial Hemorrhage	
AVM Characteristics	**First Bleed**	**Second Bleed**
Low-risk AVM (well-defined nidus and > 1 draining vein)	1.00%	3.70%
High-risk AVM (diffuse nidus or only 1 draining vein)	2.20%	8.90%

Abbreviation: AVM, arteriovenous malformation.

Table 5.5 Estimated Cumulative Lifetime Risk of Hemorrhage According to History of Prior Hemorrhage and Whether Any High-Risk Morphologic Risk Features* Are Absent or Present

Patient Age at Diagnosis (years)	Expected Survival (years)	Lifetime Risk of Intracranial Bleed			
		Low Hemorrhage Risk AVMs		High Hemorrhage Risk AVMs	
		No Prior Bleed	Prior Bleed	No Prior Bleed	Prior Bleed
15	77	46.0	90.5	75.1	99.7
25	67	40.4	86.1	68.9	99.2
35	78	34.8	80.4	61.9	98.2
45	79	28.7	72.4	53.4	95.9
55	80	22.0	61.2	43.0	90.4
65	83	16.4	49.5	33.2	81.5
75	86	10.4	34.1	21.9	64.3
85	91	5.8	20.3	12.6	43.0

* Increased risk diffuse morphology or one draining vein.
Abbreviation: AVM, arteriovenous malformation.

complete AVM obliteration.[27] For this study, we evaluated 312 patients with clinical angiographic outcomes followed for an average of 4 years. Twenty-one patients suffered AVM bleeds at a median of 8 months after radiosurgery. The overall total risk of postradiosurgery hemorrhage per patient was 7.4%, after exclusion of additional bleeding risk factors such as untreated aneurysms. The actual hemorrhage rate from a patent AVM before complete obliteration was 4.8% per year during the first 2 years after radiosurgery, and 5% per year for the third to fifth years after radiosurgery, if the AVM continued to be unobliterated. Our data have not provided strong evidence to date that there is a protective benefit of radiosurgery that gradually emerges during the observation years, even before complete obliteration has occurred. In contrast, studies from the University of Tokyo experience reported by Maruyama et al[28] as well as reinterpretation of the outcome data from the Karolinska experience[29] of Steiner have suggested that there may be some protective benefit to AVMs even before complete obliteration of their nidus occurs.

Patients who have a proximal unsecured aneurysm have an increased risk of postradiosurgical hemorrhage. If the aneurysm is immediately proximal to the AVM, it will likely close as the AVM obliterates. We have not found that intranidal aneurysms increase the risk of bleeding during the latency interval. For those patients with aneurysms more than one arterial branch proximal to their AVM, we believe that the aneurysm requires a different management algorithm that should be determined based on those characteristics that guide whether surgery or endovascular is the best management. Such aneurysms generally do not go away at the time that the AVM is obliterated.

To date, in our experience, no patient has suffered a hemorrhage after definitive high-resolution angiography has confirmed complete obliteration of their AVM. We have a single patient with more than 50 aneurysm clips who has undergone multiple surgical procedures. The AVM was thought to be obliterated after radiosurgery, but the patient suffered a subsequent hemorrhage. A new AVM was identified on follow-up angiography (neither CT nor MRI scan was feasible in this patient). The possibility of recanalization of a previously treated AVM requiring additional treatment and monitoring is important. For this reason, even in those patients who have angiographic complete closure of their AVM, we recommend MRI scans at 2-year intervals to assess the overall brain response to detect late ARE or delayed cyst development.

Although the studies of both Maruyama et al and Karlsson et al[28,29] provide some evidence of an overall reduction in bleeding rates during the latency interval, this hypothesis remains largely unproven at the present time. In addition, both ours and other outcome studies have shown that even with complete obliteration, the hemorrhage rate is not zero. For patients who have defined angiographic obliteration, we may safely estimate that the lifetime risk of a bleed is now < 1%.

Arteriovenous Malformation Obliteration after Stereotactic Radiosurgery

In our study of 351 patients followed for 3 to 11 years by imaging, and using dosages at the margin of 20 Gy (median), we documented AVM obliteration (**Fig. 5.3**) in 73% of those patients studied by angiography and in 86% of those patients studied by MRI alone.[30] Furthermore, we believe that there is approximately a 95% accuracy that MRI-detected obliteration will be confirmed by follow-up angiography.[31] There are some patients who are unwilling to undergo repeat angiography even though this remains the gold standard for detection of response. Even the presence of an early draining vein, without discernible nidus, is a sign of satisfactory response. To our knowledge, no patient has subsequently bled when only an early draining vein is seen. Follow-up angiography afterwards at 6 months to 1 year in such cases invariably shows loss of the early draining vein as well.

Failure of obliteration is multifactorial and as noted earlier may be related to dose, volume, inadequate recognition of the 3D geometry, recanalization of the previously embolized component, or clot-compressed AVM that was

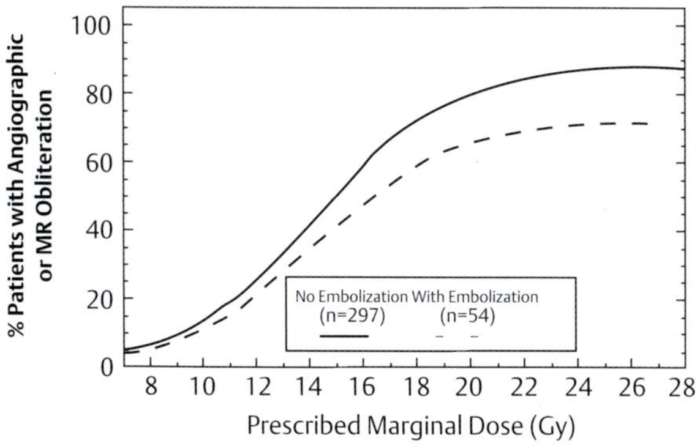

Fig. 5.3 Graph showing a higher percentage of arteriovenous malformation obliteration rates with higher margin doses. MR, magnetic resonance.

subtotally treated. In our studies designed to detect the reasons for marginal failure, we noted that such persistence of out-of-field residual AVM was seen in 18% of previously embolized patients but only 5% of nonembolized patients. We have also noted that the successful obliteration for the same-volume AVMs may be slightly lower in women, is higher in children, and occurs more completely and at a faster rate in children than in adults.

Adverse Effects of Radiosurgery

Early adverse effects are relatively rare and include headache from the frame application, nausea from conscious sedation medications, and the relatively small risk of developing seizures in patients with subcortical lobar AVMs.[31–34] It is for this reason that prophylactic anticonvulsants are used in these patients but not in patients with deep-seated AVMs. Late AREs of radiosurgery are relatively rare. We evaluated data from 85 AVM patients who developed symptomatic complications after Gamma Knife radiosurgery and compared them with 337 patients who had no complications and were evaluated as part of another multiinstitutional study.[35] Thirty-five of 85 patients were classified as having a permanent symptomatic sequela. We constructed various models to study the effects of AVM location and the volume of tissue receiving 12 Gy or more (the 12 Gy volume) with the risk of developing permanent postradiosurgery ARE. AVM locations in increasing order of risk as might be expected were frontal, temporal, interventricular, parietal, cerebellar, corpus callosum, occipital, medulla, thalamus, basal ganglia, and pons and midbrain. We were able to construct statistical models predicting the risk of permanent radiation sequelae with a 12 Gy volume. Such data are very important for subsequent planning of additional patients relative to a risk/benefit analysis. This database, though useful, was constructed with a relatively small number of complications, considering the large number of patients and the relatively large number of variables. It is likely that the risk predictions for some brainstem locations are significantly overestimated. Certainly, the risk of complications is expected to be high for large-volume AVMs in critical locations of the brain (**Table 5.6**). It is for this reason that for larger volume AVMs, 15 cc or more, we clearly recommend staging. The goal of this is to increase the eventual obliteration rate while maintaining safety. We generally divide the AVM into two volumes of approximately equal proportion. At the time of the first procedure (which is done with angiography and MRI), we devise a plan for the

Table 5.6 Estimated Percentage Risk of Symptomatic Adverse Radiation Effects for Arteriovenous Malformations Measuring 1, 2, 3, and 4 cm in Average Diameter According to Location

	Risk of Symptomatic Radiosurgery-Related Complication by AVM Diameter			
AVM Location	**1 cm**	**2 cm**	**3 cm**	**4 cm**
Low-risk brain regions				
Frontal lobe	0.04	0.07	0.11	1.48
Temporal lobe	0.59	0.94	1.45	16.95
Mild-risk brain regions				
Intraventricular	1.32	2.11	3.22	31.63
Cerebellum	1.65	2.62	4.00	36.68
Parietal lobe	2.61	2.55	3.88	35.99
Moderate-risk brain regions				
Corpus callosum	3.73	5.88	8.80	57.32
Occipital lobe	3.87	6.09	9.11	58.20
High-risk brain regions				
Medulla	7.43	11.46	16.66	73.55
Thalamus	12.36	18.51	25.98	83.00
Basal ganglia	15.01	22.15	30.54	85.95
Pons/midbrain	44.02	55.89	66.19	96.46

Abbreviation: AVM, arteriovenous malformation.
*Marginal doses were chosen according to 3% guidelines from the integrated logistic formula.[32] Because of limited experience, estimated brainstem risks are probably less than predicted in this table.

entire AVM and then gradually subtract isocenters from the plan until we develop a 50% volume that corresponds to the initial stage. The second-stage volume is then done to reproduce the original plan at an interval of 3 to 6 months. This strategy increases the brain's ability to repair normal tissue and to prevent AREs.

Other complications of AVM radiosurgery are relatively rare. Such complications have taken many years to fully understand or even develop. These include the risk of hemorrhage despite obliteration (1% lifetime), the risk of temporary or permanent radiation injury, the risk of late cyst formation at the site of the obliterated nidus, and the long-term risk for radiation-induced tumor. Cyst formation after AVM radiosurgery was first reported by Japanese investigators who had sent patients to receive Gamma Knife radiosurgery in Sweden in the early years of radiosurgery.[36] Cyst formation has also been reported in other long-term follow-up studies.[37,38] In our 20 years of experience, we have detected 16 patients (1.7%) with delayed cyst formation. We also observed that patients who developed delayed cyst formation were more likely to have had prior bleeds. This raises the intriguing possibility that residual iron deposition in the brain tissue may serve as a radiation sensitizer that could potentiate the effects of radiosurgery on a long-term basis. Such cysts have been managed with observation, simple drainage, cyst shunting, or surgical fenestration. Patients with perioperative T2 signal change without additional neurologic problems do not require additional treatment.

In our experience of almost 9000 Gamma Knife procedures, we have not identified a patient who fits the Cahan requirements for a radiation-related tumor. Recently, Sheehan et al reported two patients who have had radiosurgery for their AVM and developed delayed meningiomas.[39] As a relatively common tumor in older patients, it is not clear from a population basis that this represents a significant increased risk compared with the natural history of meningioma development. There are, however, two additional cases of a glioblastoma reported after AVM radiosurgery.[40,41] With more than a half million patients having undergone Gamma Knife radiosurgery over the last 40 years, the denominator (number treated) is relatively known, but the numerator (the incidence of radiation-related tumors) remains largely an estimate. We provide an estimate to patients that the gross risk of developing a radiation-related tumor is ~4 in 50,000, a 1 in 12,500 risk. We do, nonetheless, warn our patients the risk of a radiation-related tumor may be as high as 1 in 1000, although neither our personal experience nor data recently published from Sheffield, England, can confirm this incidence.[42]

Repeat Radiosurgery

For those patients who have a residual nidus identified by imaging 3 or more years after radiosurgery, we recommend repeat radiosurgery. For such patients, we are occasionally able to increase the dose slightly to the residual smaller volume AVM. Permanent neurologic injury was slightly higher than would be expected with those patients who had no prior radiation injury.[43] However, it should be recalled that most patients had relatively larger AVMs to begin with and received relatively lower radiation margin doses. If we are unable to give in a single procedure 16 Gy or more, we believe that staged radiosurgery must be considered to try to increase the chances of the obliteration rate. We know that the successful obliteration response declines rapidly below a 15 Gy edge dose.

◆ The Management of Large Arteriovenous Malformations

Large AVMs pose a major challenge for both surgical resection embolization and radiosurgery. Multimodality management is probably going to be critical for such AVMs that have any hope of treatment. AVM embolization has been performed using a variety of agents over the course of time, including isobutyl cyanoacrylate glue, coils, silk threads, polyvinyl alcohol, and, more recently, Onyx (ev3 Neurovascular, Irvine, CA). Prior studies have shown the recanalization rates of 14 to 15% of patients who had prior AVM embolization. Because we cannot use a single-staged radiosurgical procedure for such large-volume AVMs, we have recommended a staged prospective approach. Although fractionated radiation therapy (2–4 Gy per fraction to a total dose of 50 Gy) has virtually no significant benefit[44] in terms of AVM obliteration and at the same time has significant long-term side effect risks, radiosurgery divided into two sessions seems to have an acceptable risk prediction. Kjellberg et al, using stereotactic Bragg peak radiation therapy, achieved obliteration rates < 20%, although they postulated that such radiation-stabilized blood vessel walls reduced the risk of a subsequent bleed.[10] Most of the AVMs treated by this technique had large-volume AVMs. In a group of 48 patients treated by Pan et al,[45] an obliteration rate of only 25% was noted after 14 months in a single radiosurgical strategy when relatively larger doses were given to the edge (16.5–17.7 Gy). Approximately 37% of patients had moderate and 12% severe adverse radiation effects when the AVM volume was > 10 cc. We noted the rather narrow window between dose response and complication, as well as the minimal chance of receiving a total obliteration with low dose. We switched to prospective volume staging (**Fig. 5.4**) as an option to manage larger AVMs unsuitable for primary single-session radiosurgery.

◆ The Role of Preradiosurgical Embolization

Embolization has a major benefit in preparation for craniotomy and microsurgical removal.[46] Its primary benefit is reducing the flow through the AVM or removal of deep-seated feeders that may be problematic for subsequent surgical removal. We used embolization early in our experience for larger volume AVMs.[47] The goal was to decrease the volume of the AVM to make it more effective for radiosurgery.

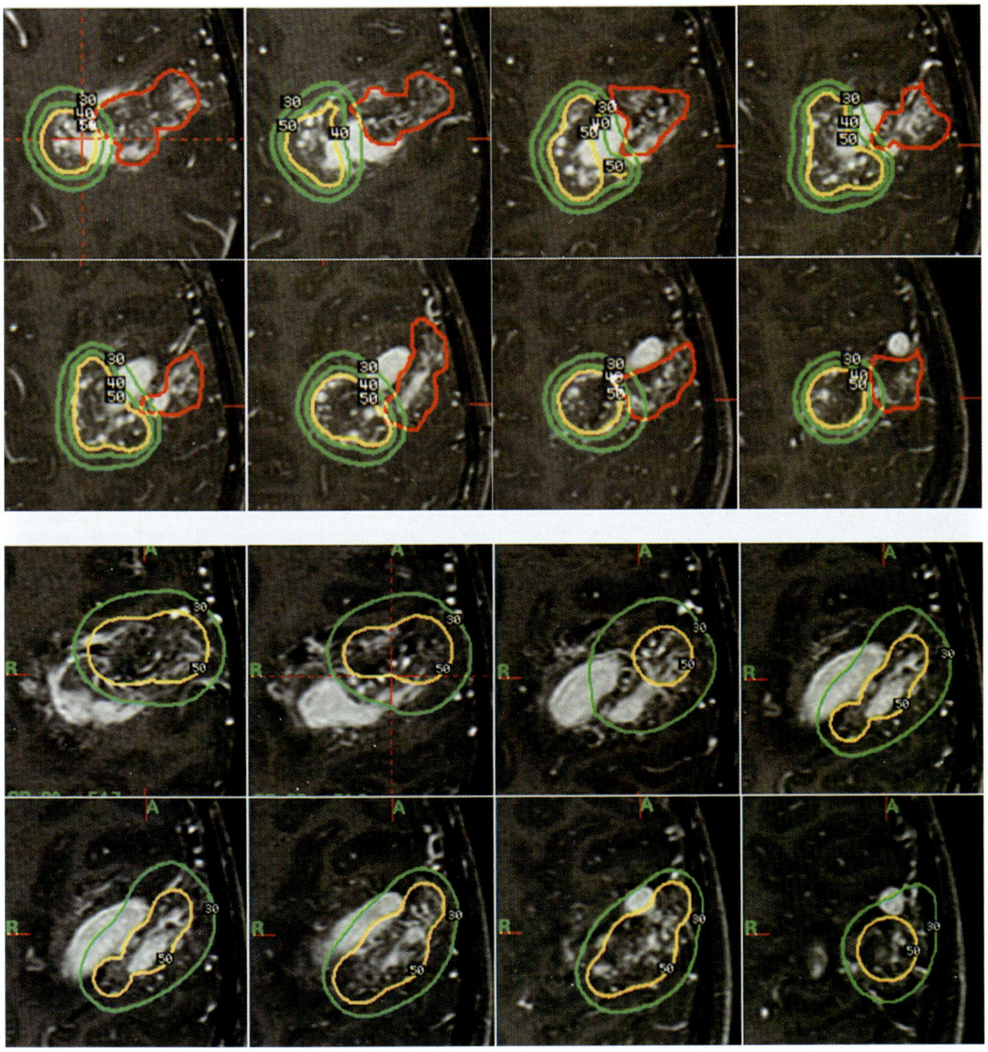

Fig. 5.4 Radiosurgery dose plans of staged radiosurgery for a large-volume arteriovenous malformation (AVM). **(A)** The medial part of the nidus was selected for stage 1 treatment. A margin dose of 18 Gy was prescribed to this target (*yellow line*). The nidus volume for stage 2 radiosurgery (*outlined in red*) was also defined at the time of first radiosurgery. **(B)** Dose plan of second-stage radiosurgery showing complete coverage of the remaining AVM nidus.

However, embolization can be effective only if it permanently reduces the nidus volume. Reduction in flow from an AVM does not provide improvement in radiosurgical outcome data. Our most recent analysis suggests that radiosurgical embolization had a negative effect on AVM obliteration rates.[48] Others have reported that up to 30% of patients who had AVM embolization subsequently had an increase in the nidus volume when a subsequent angiogram was performed at the time of radiosurgical targeting.[49] Twelve percent of embolized AVMs showed recanalization within a year.[50] Unlike surgery that removes an AVM nidus within a few weeks of embolization, radiosurgery takes several years to be fully effective. This latency interval, unfortunately, allows sufficient time for embolized AVM components to recanalize, remodel, or even recruit new feeding blood vessels. In a recent report using both embolization and radiosurgery, permanent neurologic deficits ranged from 5 to 12% of patients, with a mortality rate of 1.5 to 2.7% of patients.[49–51] Complete obliteration rates varied from 47 to 55%.[49–51] In a study of 47 patients who had radiosurgery and embolization in comparison to 47 matched patients who were treated with radiosurgery alone, nidus obliteration was achieved in 47% of the embolization group but in 70% of the radiosurgery group.[52] The experience using adhesive agents such as Onyx is too early yet to define whether radiosurgery will have a significant improvement in patients who have previously undergo liquid adhesive embolization.

Treatment of Dural Arteriovenous Malformations

In contrast to the experience with intracranial AVMs, dural vascular malformations or dural arteriovenous fistulas (DAVFs, **Fig. 5.5**) may indeed benefit from embolization and radiosurgery.[53] The timing of the individual procedures

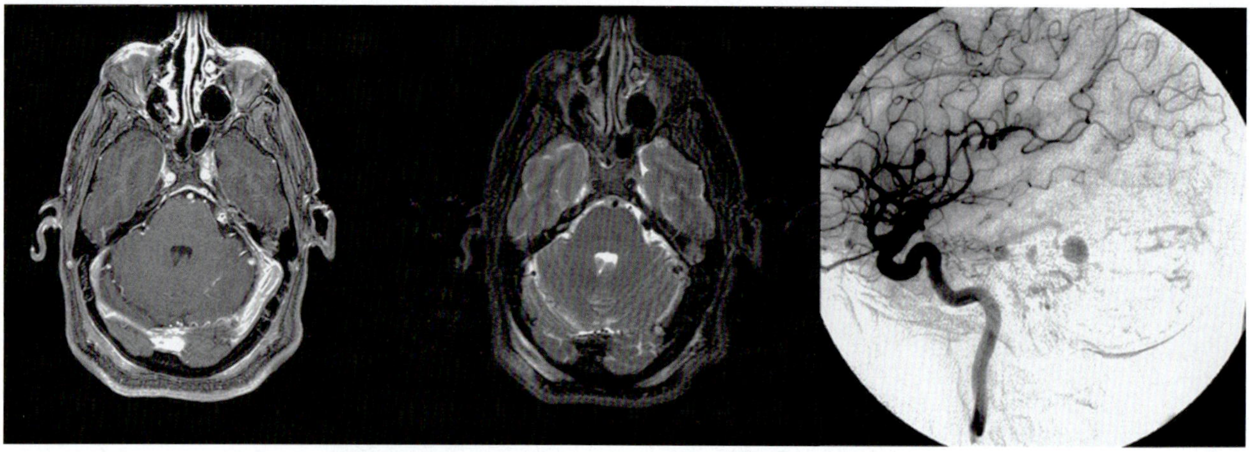

Fig. 5.5 (A) Axial T1-weighted contrast-enhanced and (B) T2-weighted magnetic resonance images showing a left cerebellopontine (CP) angle dural arteriovenous malformation (AVM). (C) Digital subtraction angiography showing the left meningohypophyseal trunk feed into the left CP angle dural AVM.

is critical. In general, we prefer to do radiosurgery first in a newly diagnosed patient, at a time when the entire connection of the fistula can be defined. Most of these lesions occur in the region of the transverse or sigmoid sinus and may be associated with pulsatile tinnitus.[54] Others may occur in the cavernous sinus and are associated with diplopia, impaired vision, or exophthalmos. Lesions of the superior sagittal sinus may cause papilledema, vision loss, and hydrocephalus. Those lesions that have cortical venous drainage are prone to have intracranial hemorrhages, progressive deficits, or seizures. Because such patients have an overall intracranial hemorrhage rate of ~2% per year, management of these lesions may be very important.[54] We generally recommend early radiosurgery followed the same day by embolization. Patients have their frame placed and undergo MRI, followed by initial angiography, and are transferred to Gamma Knife for radiosurgery with a femoral sheath catheter left in position. After completion of the radiosurgical component of the procedure, they are transferred back to the interventional radiology suite, where they undergo embolization. The combination of radiosurgery and embolization provides both early symptom relief of the DAVF and long-term relief of the condition by radiosurgery.

◆ Summary

AVM radiosurgery is a well-established management strategy for AVMs at the present time. With more than 25 years of experience using Gamma Knife technique, and with thousands of patients worldwide who have undergone this procedure, we understand the overall success rate, the complication rate, and the various alternative strategies. We believe that at the present time embolization has an important role prior to microsurgery, an important role after radiosurgery for the management of DAVFs, and a relatively limited role in the prospective management of AVMs within the brain. Although outcome studies continue to be looked at both in Canada and in the United States, we suspect that most patients with an intracranial AVM require strong consideration for intervention, providing the management strategy has an acceptable risk to the patient. It seems unlikely that higher doses will be feasible. The ability to conform dose and to restrict dose (selectivity) seemed to be maximized with the current imaging techniques as well as radiation delivery systems, including the new Perfexion Gamma Knife. We may be able to increase the chance of obliteration by developing specific radiation sensitizers delivered by microcatheters immediately before radiosurgery. To date, brain protection technologies and drugs have been disappointing. The greatest remaining issue for AVM radiosurgery is the risk of a latency interval hemorrhage, so efforts to reduce the latency interval would be important. The recognition of late long-term side effects, including the possible risk of radiation-related tumors or late cyst development, continues to be evaluated. Within the context of a disease that has a 1% annual mortality left untreated, the current data have shown that SRS is a safe and effective management strategy that can be applied to both lobar and deep-seated AVMs. Many patients with AVMs were never treatable by any technique prior to the development of radiosurgery.

Acknowledgments Drs. Lunsford and Kondziolka are consultants with Elekta Instruments AB. Dr. Lunsford is a stockholder with Elekta.

References

1. Deruty R, Pelissou-Guyotat I, Morel C, Bascoulergue Y, Turjman F. Reflections on the management of cerebral arteriovenous malformations. Surg Neurol 1998;50(3):245–255, discussion 55–56
2. Han PP, Ponce FA, Spetzler RF. Intention-to-treat analysis of Spetzler–Martin grades IV and V arteriovenous malformations: natural history and treatment paradigm. J Neurosurg 2003;98(1):3–7

3. Ledezma CJ, Hoh BL, Carter BS, Pryor JC, Putman CM, Ogilvy CS. Complications of cerebral arteriovenous malformation embolization: multivariate analysis of predictive factors. Neurosurgery 2006;58(4): 602–611
4. Raymond J, Iancu D, Weill A, et al. Embolization as one modality in a combined strategy for the management of cerebral arteriovenous malformations. Interventional Neuroradiol 2005;11(Suppl):57–62
5. Spetzler RF, Martin NA. A proposed grading system for arteriovenous malformations. J Neurosurg 1986;65(4):476–483
6. Pollock BE, Flickinger JC. A proposed radiosurgery-based grading system for arteriovenous malformations. J Neurosurg 2002;96(1):79–85
7. Liscak R, Vladyka V, Simonova G, et al. Arteriovenous malformations after Leksell Gamma Knife radiosurgery: rate of obliteration and complications. Neurosurgery 2007;60(6):1005–1014, discussion 1015–1016
8. Pollock BE, Gorman DA, Coffey RJ. Patient outcomes after arteriovenous malformation radiosurgical management: results based on a 5- to 14-year follow-up study. Neurosurgery 2003;52(6):1291–1296, discussion 1296–1297
9. Kjellberg RN. Stereotactic Bragg peak proton beam radiosurgery for cerebral arteriovenous malformations. Ann Clin Res 1986;18(Suppl 47):17–19
10. Kjellberg RN, Hanamura T, Davis KR, Lyons SL, Adams RD. Bragg-peak proton-beam therapy for arteriovenous malformations of the brain. N Engl J Med 1983;309(5):269–274
11. Fabrikant JI, Levy RP, Steinberg GK, et al. Heavy-charged-particle radiosurgery for intracranial arteriovenous malformations. Stereotact Funct Neurosurg 1991;57(1–2):50–63
12. Steiner L, Leksell L, Greitz T, Forster DM, Backlund EO. Stereotaxic radiosurgery for cerebral arteriovenous malformations: report of a case. Acta Chir Scand 1972;138(5):459–464
13. Betti OO, Munari C, Rosler R. Stereotactic radiosurgery with the linear accelerator: treatment of arteriovenous malformations. Neurosurgery 1989;24(3):311–321
14. Barcia-Salorio JL, Barcia JA, Soler F, Hernandez G, Genoves JM. Stereotactic radiotherapy plus radiosurgical boost in the treatment of large cerebral arteriovenous malformations. Acta Neurochir Suppl (Wien) 1993;58:98–100
15. Barcia-Salorio JL, Soler F, Hernandez G, Barcia JA. Radiosurgical treatment of low flow carotid-cavernous fistulae. Acta Neurochir Suppl (Wien) 1991;52:93–95
16. Colombo F, Benedetti A, Pozza F, Marchetti C, Chierego G. Linear accelerator radiosurgery of cerebral arteriovenous malformations. Neurosurgery 1989;24(6):833–840
17. Colombo F, Cavedon C, Francescon P, et al. Three-dimensional angiography for radiosurgical treatment planning for arteriovenous malformations. J Neurosurg 2003;98(3):536–543
18. Colombo F, Pozza F, Chierego G, Casentini L, De Luca G, Francescon P. Linear accelerator radiosurgery of cerebral arteriovenous malformations: an update. Neurosurgery 1994;34(1):14–20
19. Loeffler JS, Alexander E III, Siddon RL, Saunders WM, Coleman CN, Winston KR. Stereotactic radiosurgery for intracranial arteriovenous malformations using a standard linear accelerator. Int J Radiat Oncol Biol Phys 1989;17(3):673–677
20. Friedman WA, Bova FJ, Mendenhall WM. Linear accelerator radiosurgery for arteriovenous malformations: the relationship of size to outcome. J Neurosurg 1995;82(2):180–189
21. Altschuler EM, Lunsford LD, Coffey RJ, Bissonette DJ, Flickinger JC. Gamma Knife radiosurgery for intracranial arteriovenous malformations in childhood and adolescence. Pediatr Neurosci 1989;15(2):53–61
22. Lunsford LD, Kondziolka D, Flickinger JC, et al. Stereotactic radiosurgery for arteriovenous malformations of the brain. J Neurosurg 1991;75(4):512–524
23. Ondra SL, Troupp H, George ED, Schwab K. The natural history of symptomatic arteriovenous malformations of the brain: a 24-year follow-up assessment. J Neurosurg 1990;73(3):387–391
24. Pollock BE, Flickinger JC, Lunsford LD, Bissonette DJ, Kondziolka D. Factors that predict the bleeding risk of cerebral arteriovenous malformations. Stroke 1996;27(1):1–6
25. Brown RD Jr. Simple risk predictions for arteriovenous malformation hemorrhage. Neurosurgery 2000;46(4):1024
26. Kondziolka D, McLaughlin MR, Kestle JR. Simple risk predictions for arteriovenous malformation hemorrhage. Neurosurgery 1995;37(5): 851–855
27. Pollock BE, Flickinger JC, Lunsford LD, Bissonette DJ, Kondziolka D. Hemorrhage risk after stereotactic radiosurgery of cerebral arteriovenous malformations. Neurosurgery 1996;38(4):652–659, discussion 9–61
28. Maruyama K, Shin M, Tago M, Kishimoto J, Morita A, Kawahara N. Radiosurgery to reduce the risk of first hemorrhage from brain arteriovenous malformations. Neurosurgery 2007;60(3):453–458, discussion 458–459
29. Karlsson B, Lax I, Soderman M. Risk for hemorrhage during the 2-year latency period following Gamma Knife radiosurgery for arteriovenous malformations. Int J Radiat Oncol Biol Phys 2001;49(4):1045–1051
30. Flickinger JC, Kondziolka D, Maitz AH, Lunsford LD. An analysis of the dose-response for arteriovenous malformation radiosurgery and other factors affecting obliteration. Radiother Oncol 2002;63(3):347–354
31. Pollock BE, Kondziolka D, Flickinger JC, Patel AK, Bissonette DJ, Lunsford LD. Magnetic resonance imaging: an accurate method to evaluate arteriovenous malformations after stereotactic radiosurgery. J Neurosurg 1996;85(6):1044–1049
32. Flickinger JC, Kondziolka D, Lunsford LD, et al. Development of a model to predict permanent symptomatic postradiosurgery injury for arteriovenous malformation patients. Arteriovenous Malformation Radiosurgery Study Group. Int J Radiat Oncol Biol Phys 2000;46(5): 1143–1148
33. Flickinger JC, Kondziolka D, Maitz AH, Lunsford LD. Analysis of neurological sequelae from radiosurgery of arteriovenous malformations: how location affects outcome. Int J Radiat Oncol Biol Phys 1998;40(2): 273–278
34. Flickinger JC, Kondziolka D, Pollock BE, Maitz AH, Lunsford LD. Complications from arteriovenous malformation radiosurgery: multivariate analysis and risk modeling. Int J Radiat Oncol Biol Phys 1997; 38(3):485–490
35. Flickinger JC, Kondziolka D, Lunsford LD, et al. A multi-institutional analysis of complication outcomes after arteriovenous malformation radiosurgery. Int J Radiat Oncol Biol Phys 1999;44(1):67–74
36. Hara M, Nakamura M, Shiokawa Y, et al. Delayed cyst formation after radiosurgery for cerebral arteriovenous malformation: two case reports. Minim Invasive Neurosurg 1998;41(1):40–45
37. Izawa M, Hayashi M, Chernov M, et al. Long-term complications after gamma knife surgery for arteriovenous malformations. J Neurosurg 2005;102(Suppl):34–37
38. Pan HC, Sheehan J, Stroila M, Steiner M, Steiner L. Late cyst formation following gamma knife surgery of arteriovenous malformations. J Neurosurg 2005;102(Suppl):124–127
39. Sheehan J, Yen CP, Steiner L. Gamma Knife surgery-induced meningioma: report of two cases and review of the literature. J Neurosurg 2006;105(2):325–329
40. Berman EL, Eade TN, Brown D, et al. Radiation-induced tumor after stereotactic radiosurgery for an arteriovenous malformation: case report. Neurosurgery 2007;61(5):E1099
41. Kaido T, Hoshida T, Uranishi R, et al. Radiosurgery-induced brain tumor: case report. J Neurosurg 2001;95(4):710–713
42. Rowe J, Grainger A, Walton L, Silcocks P, Radatz M, Kemeny A. Risk of malignancy after Gamma Knife stereotactic radiosurgery. Neurosurgery 2007;60(1):60–65, discussion 65–66
43. Maesawa S, Flickinger JC, Kondziolka D, Lunsford LD. Repeated radiosurgery for incompletely obliterated arteriovenous malformations. J Neurosurg 2000;92(6):961–970
44. Karlsson B, Lindqvist M, Blomgren H, et al. Long-term results after fractionated radiation therapy for large brain arteriovenous malformations. Neurosurgery 2005;57(1):42–49
45. Pan DH, Guo WY, Chung WY, Shiau CY, Chang YC, Wang LW. Gamma Knife radiosurgery as a single treatment modality for large cerebral arteriovenous malformations. J Neurosurg 2000;93(Suppl 3):113–119
46. Mathis JA, Barr JD, Horton JA, et al. The efficacy of particulate embolization combined with stereotactic radiosurgery for treatment of large arteriovenous malformations of the brain. AJNR Am J Neuroradiol 1995;16(2):299–306
47. Dawson RC III, Tarr RW, Hecht ST, et al. Treatment of arteriovenous malformations of the brain with combined embolization and stereotactic radiosurgery: results after 1 and 2 years. AJNR Am J Neuroradiol 1990;11(5):857–864
48. Pollock BE, Flickinger JC, Lunsford LD, Maitz A, Kondziolka D. Factors associated with successful arteriovenous malformation radiosurgery. Neurosurgery 1998;42(6):1239–1244, discussion 1244–1247
49. Miyachi S, Negoro M, Okamoto T, et al. Embolisation of cerebral arteriovenous malformations to assure successful subsequent radiosurgery. J Clin Neurosci 2000;7(Suppl 1):82–85
50. Gobin YP, Laurent A, Merienne L, et al. Treatment of brain arteriovenous malformations by embolization and radiosurgery. J Neurosurg 1996;85(1):19–28

51. Henkes H, Nahser HC, Berg-Dammer E, Weber W, Lange S, Kuhne D. Endovascular therapy of brain AVMs prior to radiosurgery. Neurol Res 1998;20(6):479–492

52. Andrade-Souza YM, Ramani M, Scora D, Tsao MN, terBrugge K, Schwartz ML. Embolization before radiosurgery reduces the obliteration rate of arteriovenous malformations. Neurosurgery 2007;60(3):443–451, discussion 451–452

53. Houser OW, Campbell JK, Campbell RJ, Sundt TM Jr. Arteriovenous malformation affecting the transverse dural venous sinus—an acquired lesion. Mayo Clin Proc 1979;54(10):651–661

54. Awad IA, Little JR, Akarawi WP, Ahl J. Intracranial dural arteriovenous malformations: factors predisposing to an aggressive neurological course. J Neurosurg 1990;72(6):839–850

6

Stereotactic Radiosurgery for Dural Arteriovenous Fistulas

Michael Söderman, Bengt Karlsson, Bodo Lippitz, and Tommy Andersson

In the adult population, intracranial dural arteriovenous fistulas (DAVFs), also called dural arteriovenous shunts or malformations, are about 10 times less frequent than brain arteriovenous malformations (AVMs).[1] DAVFs are lesions in the dura mater, acquired in relation to a thrombotic process in the intracranial venous system, most often in a dural sinus.[2–5] The symptoms at presentation and the prognosis depend on the location of the arteriovenous fistula, particularly on the venous drainage pattern.[6] A DAVF that drains, directly or indirectly, into the cortical venous system may cause venous congestion, leading to intradural hemorrhage or, less commonly, to increased intracranial pressure. The elevated intracranial pressure can cause nonfocal neurologic symptoms such as dementia.

Patients at risk for bleeding or other adverse events are usually offered treatment.[7–10] Intolerable bruit or significant exophthalmos or chemosis related to increased pressure in the superior ophthalmic vein may also prompt treatment.

Microsurgery and embolization are established treatment options for DAVFs, and the indications and methods have been well described elsewhere.[10,11]

Irradiation as a means of DAVF treatment has been proposed by several groups. There are several reports on the use of fractionated irradiation (i.e., various forms of radiotherapy).[12–16] However, radiosurgery, initially with a single cobalt 60 source and subsequently with the Gamma Knife (Elekta Instruments AB, Stockholm, Sweden), seems to have emerged as the preferred method.[17–22] There are very few reports on linear accelerator radiosurgery of DAVFs.[23–25]

◆ Pathophysiology of DAVFs

DAVFs are acquired abnormal arteriovenous connections within the dura mater.[26] The blood supply is from meningeal arteries, albeit a minor contribution from pial arteries is not uncommon. The venous exit is directly to a dural sinus, to a leptomeningeal vein contiguous with the dura mater, or both. DAVFs in the cavernous sinus most often empty into the superior ophthalmic vein.

The pathophysiology of spontaneous DAVFs seems to be related to venous thrombosis and venous hypertension, both prior to and after the emergence of the shunt.[27,28]

In this disease there is upregulation of vascular endothelial growth factor as well as basic fibroblast growth factor, epinephrine B2, and hypoxia-inducible factor 1 in rat models with induced intracranial venous hypertension.[29–32] A similar pattern of growth factor upregulation has been found in operative specimens and blood samples from patients with DAVFs.[33–36]

◆ Clinical Presentation and Natural History of DAVF

The presentation and relevance of a DAVF depend on the location of the shunt and on the venous drainage pattern.[6,37–42] Widely used classification systems mix anatomical location and venous drainage but can be useful for descriptive purposes.[43–45] However, it is principally the venous drainage pattern that determines the prognosis.[3,46]

Thus, a DAVF without cortical venous drainage or reflux may present with externally audible pulse-synchronous bruit or symptoms related to orbital venous congestion, but it will not cause a hemorrhage or elevated intracranial pressure. Not infrequently it is an incidental finding during a neuroradiological investigation performed for an unrelated reason.[8,47]

Lesions localized in the wall of the cavernous sinus regularly drain through the superior ophthalmic vein, causing orbital venous congestion visible as chemosis and exophthalmos.

The risk for intracranial hemorrhage is elevated if the blood is not redirected into the cortical venous system, directly or indirectly. In this context it should be noted that some patients use several venous pathways to drain a DAVF and that drainage through a dural sinus or the superior orbital vein may coexist with leptomeningeal drainage; consequently, the patient is at risk for intracranial hemorrhage. Also, a change in symptoms in a fistula without cortical venous reflux, including disappearance of a symptom like bruit, may indicate rerouting of the venous drainage, potentially into cortical veins, converting a "benign" fistula into a dangerous one. Such changes, therefore, should always warrant an angiographic investigation. A DAVF with cortical venous reflux may present with bruit or chemosis, but also with neurologic deficits, frequently because of intracranial hemorrhage.

The data on the natural course of DAVFs are limited and ambiguous, to say the least. Brown et al found an annual incidence of hemorrhage of 1.8% in all patients with DAVFs and 3% among those with drainage into leptomeningeal veins.[47] In this series, all the patients that bled had leptomeningeal drainage with a venous varix. Duffau et al analyzed the early outcome of 20 consecutive patients and found a 35% rebleeding rate within 2 weeks of the first hemorrhage.[7] In 2002 van Dijk et al reported an annual hemorrhage rate of 8% and an annual mortality rate of 10%[9] from DAVFs with long-standing cortical venous drainage. In the most recent and largest series, the annual risk of hemorrhage was 7.4% in patients who presented with intracranial hemorrhage and 1.5% in those who did not. There was no mortality.[8]

To summarize, it may very well be that the annual risk of hemorrhage from a nonruptured DAVF is $< 2\%$, whereas it is $\sim 7\%$ if it presents with bleeding. In this context, the angioarchitecture of the lesion should probably also be taken into consideration, but more data are needed.

◆ Indications for Radiosurgery

In a patient with limited symptoms and without cortical venous drainage from a DAVF, abstention from treatment is clearly a management option, particularly in view of the relatively high likelihood of spontaneous occlusion or symptom regress.[6,9,47,48] However, these patients should be monitored both clinically and radiologically, as a benign DAVF may in rare instances develop leptomeningeal venous drainage.[49] A change in symptoms, even an improvement (e.g., a reduced bruit), should arouse suspicion of conversion that warrants an angiographical investigation.

Patients harboring a DAVF with cortical venous drainage, and therefore at risk for intracranial hemorrhage or nonfocal neurologic deficits, are usually offered treatment.[7–10,46] In this patient group, radiosurgery is a treatment alternative if embolization or surgery is considered unacceptably dangerous or impossible. Patients with hemorrhage as the presenting event and those with a focal leptomeningeal venous dilatation may be at considerable risk for bleeding during the time before the DAVF obliterates and should be subjected to radiosurgery only if there is no other realistic alternative.[8,47]

Patients with intolerable bruit from a DAVF without cortical venous drainage can be treated with radiosurgery if they accept the latency period and the fact that not all patients will be cured.

Significant exophthalmos or chemosis secondary to a DAVF in the cavernous sinus should also prompt an active approach, particularly because visual impairment secondary to the increased intraorbital pressure has been reported.[47] These patients can usually be cured with transvenous embolization, mostly with detachable coils, of the cavernous sinus through a skull base sinus or occasionally through the superior ophthalmic vein. Transarterial embolization with liquid adhesive in this region requires precise knowledge of the individual patient's anatomy, and in view of the possible complications, it should not be taken on lightly.[50] Transarterial particle embolization with the aim to alleviate symptoms and speed up the obliteration process has been attempted.[51] However, some patients have severe symptoms from a cavernous sinus DAVF that is inaccessible for embolization and not amenable to surgery, whereas others have relatively little orbital congestion. Both of these patient groups could be offered treatment with radiosurgery.

◆ Radiosurgical Technique

Prior to radiosurgery, stereotactic angiography is required to define the target, that is, the arteriovenous shunting zone, because this zone can seldom be adequately located using magnetic resonance imaging (MRI) or computed tomography (CT) alone (**Fig. 6.1A**). The angiographic technique is very similar to that previously described for radiosurgery for brain AVMs.[52]

The initial target volume is projected onto cross-sectional stereotactic imaging, usually MRI, so that radiation doses to sensitive tissue such as the skin, the brainstem, and the cranial nerves can be calculated and kept acceptably low (**Fig. 6.1B**).[20] In DAVFs of the cavernous sinus, the optic apparatus is of particular concern because of its low tolerance for ionizing radiation. Traditionally, the maximum radiation dose to the optic pathways has been 8 Gy; however, recent data indicate that the optic nerve can probably tolerate higher radiation doses, up to 11 Gy, over a short distance with a low risk of radiation-induced optic neuritis.[53,54]

The arteriovenous shunt is located in the dura, most often in the wall of a dural sinus, but it may extend into the previous lumen in the presence of a neovascularization within an old thrombosis. Gadolinium-enhanced T1-weighted images in axial and coronal planes are helpful to identify the dura mater and the sinus.

DAVFs are treated with radiation doses similar to those in radiosurgery for brain AVMs.[22] Thus, lesions remote from cranial nerves and other radiation-sensitive tissue are irradiated with 25 Gy to the 40 to 60% isodose. Dose plans are adjusted according to the radiation sensitivity of adjacent structures (**Fig. 6.2**). Using the Gamma Knife, collimator plugging with the aim to reduce skin radiation doses is frequent in these often superficial targets.

The treatment volume is usually below 2 mL, and radiation doses therefore do not have to be reduced below 25 Gy to decrease the risk for an adverse radiation reaction in the

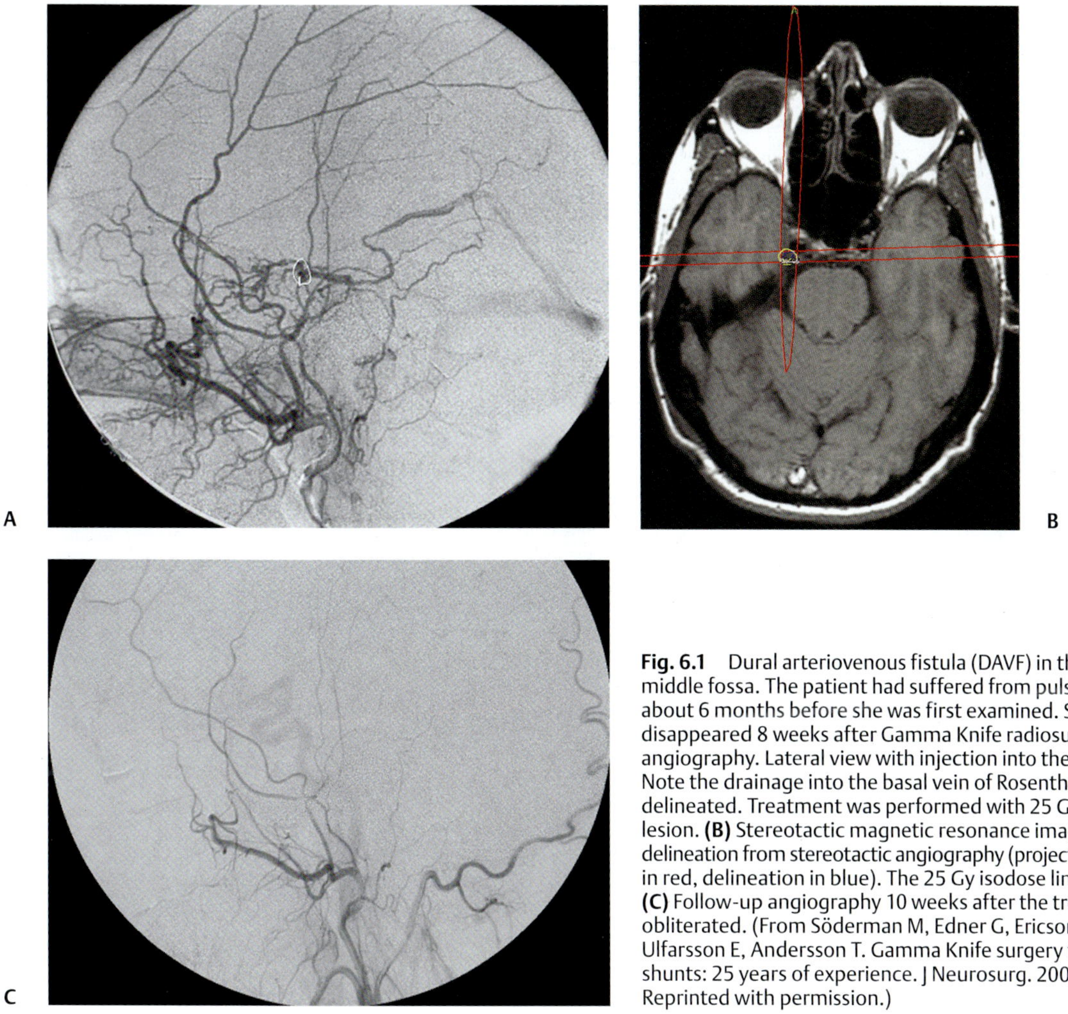

Fig. 6.1 Dural arteriovenous fistula (DAVF) in the medial wall of the middle fossa. The patient had suffered from pulse-synchronous bruit for about 6 months before she was first examined. She had not bled. The bruit disappeared 8 weeks after Gamma Knife radiosurgery. **(A)** Stereotactic angiography. Lateral view with injection into the external carotid artery. Note the drainage into the basal vein of Rosenthal. The target volume is delineated. Treatment was performed with 25 Gy to the periphery of the lesion. **(B)** Stereotactic magnetic resonance imaging with superimposed delineation from stereotactic angiography (projection lines from angiography in red, delineation in blue). The 25 Gy isodose line is shown in yellow. **(C)** Follow-up angiography 10 weeks after the treatment. The DAVF had obliterated. (From Söderman M, Edner G, Ericson K, Karlsson B, Rähn T, Ulfarsson E, Andersson T. Gamma Knife surgery for dural arteriovenous shunts: 25 years of experience. J Neurosurg. 2006 Jun;104(6):867–875. Reprinted with permission.)

adjacent brain. Thus, volume is generally not a limiting factor, particularly because some of the structures in the periphery of the target are often relatively insensitive to radiation, such as bone and dural sinus.

Guo et al reported relatively heterogeneous dose plans in Gamma Knife radiosurgery for DAVFs of the cavernous sinus; maximum doses ranged from 22 to 38 Gy, and target coverage was within the 50 to 90% isodose.[20] Their results were excellent, with an 80% cure rate and no complications.

Endovascular Treatment and Radiosurgery

In 1996 Link et al reported obliteration in 72% of their cases and regression in 28% of 29 patients with DAVFs in various locations treated either with radiosurgery alone or with a combination of particle embolization and radiosurgery. Twelve of 14 patients with cortical venous drainage were embolized in conjunction with the radiosurgical treatment. No patient bled during the follow-up period.[19] Similar results were reported by Pollock et al in their 20 patients with cavernous sinus DAVFs treated with the same technique.[51] They also noted rapid improvement of symptoms in most cases. Favorable symptomatic outcomes were also noted by Friedman et al using the same technique in the treatment of DAVFs without cortical venous reflux in the transverse and sigmoid sinus.[55]

Koebbe et al reported on 18 patients with 23 DAVFs who underwent radiosurgery alone ($N = 8$) or in combination with embolization ($N = 10$).[21] Prescription doses ranged from 15 to 25 Gy and maximum doses from 30 to 50 Gy. All patients were treated to the 50% isodose. In five patients, symptoms resolved after the irradiation, and five noted improvement but still had residual cranial nerve deficit secondary to the DAVF or the endovascular treatment. Two of these patients had complications from the embolization. No complications related to the radiosurgery were observed. Only 2 of the 10 patients with cavernous sinus DAVFs had radiological follow-up with conventional angiography. Both were cured.

Hasuo et al reported on nine patients with DAVFs in the cavernous sinus who were subjected to particle embolization followed by radiosurgery with a prescription dose of

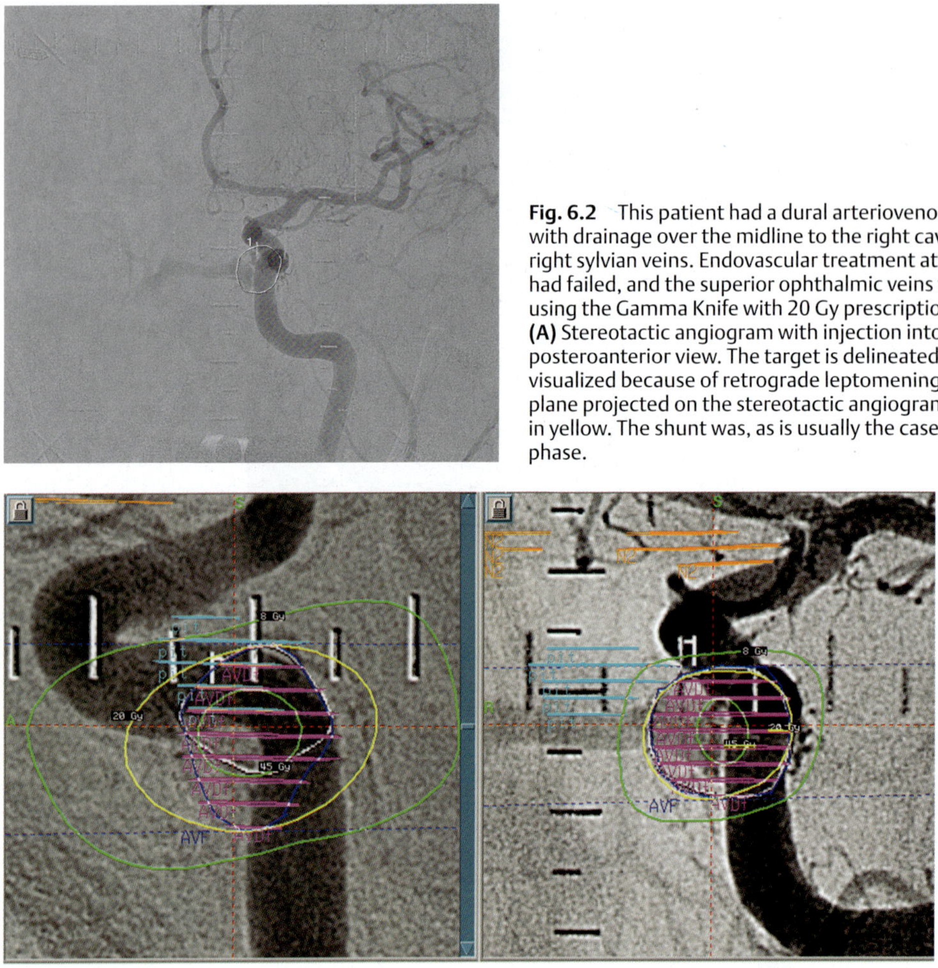

A

B

Fig. 6.2 This patient had a dural arteriovenous fistula in the left cavernous sinus with drainage over the midline to the right cavernous sinus and secondarily to the right sylvian veins. Endovascular treatment attempts through the petrosal sinuses had failed, and the superior ophthalmic veins were thrombosed. He was treated using the Gamma Knife with 20 Gy prescription dose to the 50% isodose. **(A)** Stereotactic angiogram with injection into the internal carotid artery, posteroanterior view. The target is delineated in white. The sylvian veins are visualized because of retrograde leptomeningeal blood flow. **(B)** The final dose plane projected on the stereotactic angiogram. The 20 Gy isodose line is depicted in yellow. The shunt was, as is usually the case, best seen in the early arterial phase.

30 Gy.[56] In seven patients, rapid clinical improvement and resolution of symptoms could be seen over the following 4 to 19 months. One patient was irradiated a second time with the same treatment parameters, and the DAVF subsequently obliterated. In one patient the shunt persisted, but the flow and the clinical symptoms were markedly reduced.

Results of Radiosurgery

The 2-year obliteration rate in the series reported by Söderman et al, proven by angiography, was 68%, and significant flow regression was seen in 24% of the patients.[22] This is very close to the 70% obliteration rate predicted by the Karlsson obliteration model for brain AVMS treated with the same radiation doses.[57]

Other studies have reported similar figures, regardless of the location of the DAVF and whether radiosurgery had been used as a single treatment or in combination with embolization.[18–22,24,51,55,58–60]

Several authors have noted the sometimes remarkably short time span between radiosurgery and symptomatic cure of DAVFs, in some cases also obliteration proven by angiography (**Fig. 6.1**).[18,20,22,51] The location within the dura mater and the usually narrow blood vessels that these transdural shunting zones represent may be factors underlying this rapid obliteration process, with subsequent reduction of the time at risk for hemorrhage.

One might assume that there is a dose–effect relationship similar to what has been established in radiosurgery of brain AVMs.[57] If so, it would be expected that the higher the radiation dose, the higher the obliteration rate. However, in the only study where this aspect was investigated,[22] no such dose–effect relationship was seen, perhaps because of the limited number of patients. The data may also have been skewed because of spontaneous cures among the patients with slow flow lesions, most of which were in the cavernous sinus and were treated with low radiation doses. Both Davies et al and van Dijk et al showed that symptoms often improve or resolve without treatment.[9,49,61] Brown et al also found that spontaneous obliteration was not unusual.[47]

In most cases where the DAVF has not obliterated, flow regression or regression of clinical symptoms has been obvious.[20,22,51] Some of these patients have been retreated with subsequent obliteration. To our knowledge, there is no

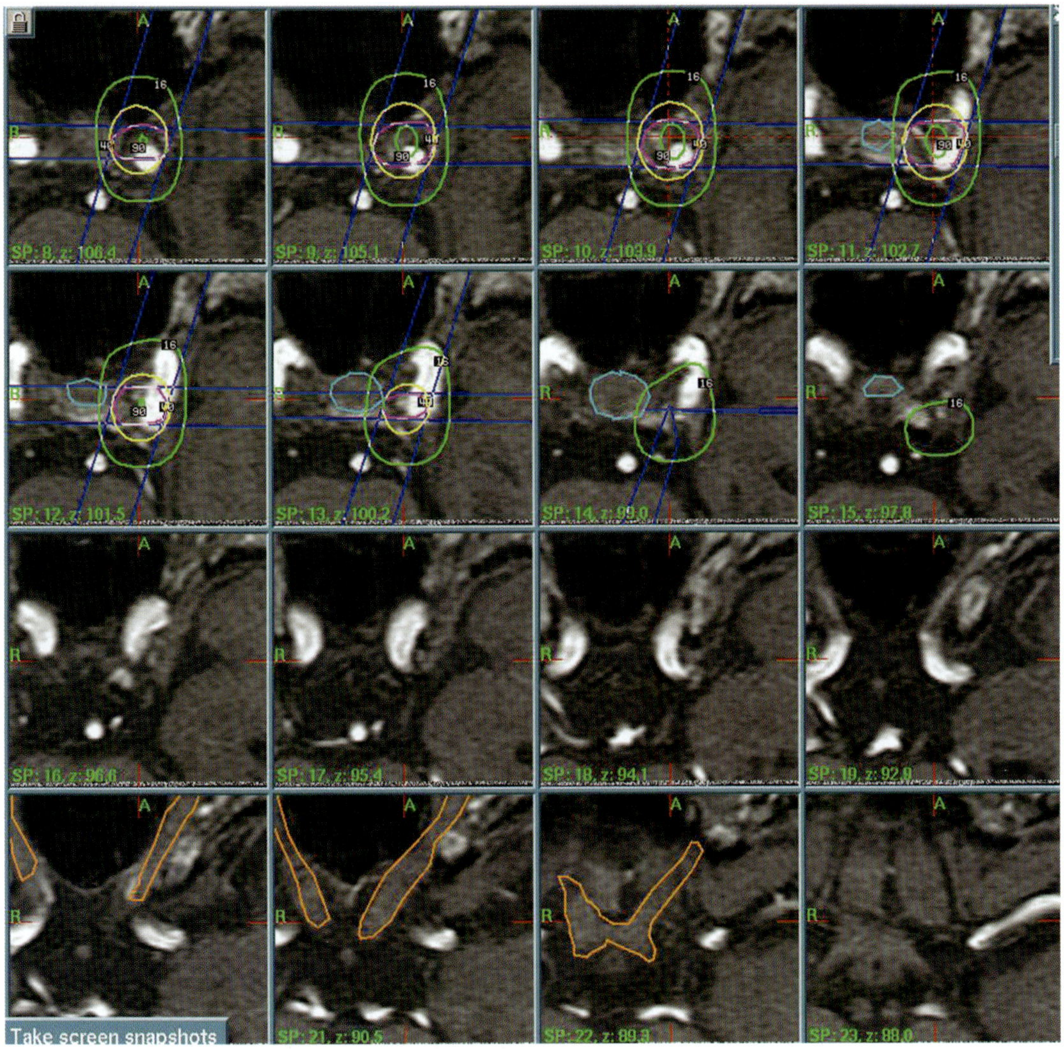

C

Fig. 6.2 *(Continued)* **(C)** The final dose plan projected onto axial gradient echo magnetic resonance images (time-of-flight technique). The pituitary has been delineated in turquoise, the optic apparatus in orange, and the target volume in violet. The DAVF was obliterated at the two-year follow-up angiography.

report that a DAVF treated solely with radiosurgery has recurred after it has been proven by angiography to be obliterated.

Complications of Radiosurgery

Hemorrhage and Thrombosis

The risk of intracranial hemorrhage after radiosurgery for a DAVF with cortical venous drainage persists until such leptomeningeal reflux has ceased, which is equivalent to the closure of the arteriovenous shunt. However, this hemorrhagic risk in the latency period before occlusion may be quite low. Söderman et al reported an annual incidence of hemorrhage after radiosurgery of ~2.6%.[22]

Thrombosis of the superior ophthalmic vein has been reported after radiosurgery for a cavernous sinus DAVF.[62] Barcia-Solario et al reported that 2 of their 25 patients experienced temporary worsening of the symptoms as the shunt occluded.[18]

Adverse Radiation Effects

There is one report of a late cystic hemorrhagic complication, similar to those seen after brain AVM radiosurgery.[22,63] It healed without clinical consequences. In several series of radiosurgery for cavernous sinus DAVF, there were no postradiation injuries to the optical or oculomotor nerves, nor any other adverse radiation effect.[18,20,64] Transient cranial nerve damage has been reported, but it seems to be unusual.[22] Transient alopecia has been noted.

Effects of Angiography

Cerebral angiography carries a low but not negligible risk for complications.[65,66] The reported complications, which were related to the stereotactic or follow-up angiograms, resolved without sequel.[22,51]

◆ Mechanism of Radiosurgery

In brain AVMs, the gradual occlusion of the nidus after treatment by radiosurgery has been attributed to endothelial damage in pathological arteries inducing the proliferation of smooth muscle cells and the elaboration of extracellular collagen by these cells, which in turn leads to progressive stenosis and obliteration of the AVM.[67] Even though the "nidus" in a DAVF basically consists of normal vessels, the occlusion process may be similar and thus comprise thrombosis, neovascularization, and medial hyperplasia.

The mechanism of the sometimes very rapid effect of radiosurgery on the DAVF is not known. It could be speculated to be the effect of direct damage to the endothelium with subsequent thrombosis.

◆ Comparison of Radiosurgery to the Natural History of DAVF

The natural history of DAVF is not very well understood except that cortical venous drainage entails a risk of intracranial hemorrhage; the magnitude of the risk varies considerably between studies.[7–9,47] It is not clear whether the location of the shunt has any impact on the risk. The cortical venous drainage pattern may influence the risk for bleeding, but this aspect has not been analyzed in any of the studies on radiosurgery of DAVFs.[47]

As has been stated, several reports have noted that the time span between radiosurgery for DAVF and symptomatic cure, in some cases also proven obliteration, can be remarkably short.[18,20,22,56,64] DAVFs have a high rate of spontaneous thrombosis and occlusion.[6,9,47,48] It is not entirely clear to what extent obliteration after radiosurgery can be attributed to the treatment, the natural course of the disease, or even the angiography. Nevertheless, a rapid closure of the arteriovenous shunt will reduce the time that the patient suffers from orbital or other symptoms and also, in cases with cortical venous reflux, reduce the time at risk for intracranial hemorrhage.

◆ Limitations of Radiosurgery of DAVFs

Some authors have noted that high-flow arteriovenous shunts respond less favorably to irradiation.[18,22] We speculate that this may be for simple geometrical reasons; that is, the vessel diameters were too large for the thrombus formation and wall thickening to have the desired occlusive effect. This concurs with the observation in a single-center series that brain AVMs with plexiform nidi may respond better to radiosurgery than lesions with high-flow arteriovenous shunts.[68]

Another limitation is the fact that all DAVFs do not obliterate after the irradiation and thus can remain symptomatic or put the patient at risk for hemorrhage for a considerable time.

◆ Summary

Radiosurgery is an effective treatment for dural arteriovenous fistulas, with a low risk of complications. In DAVFs with cortical venous drainage, there is a risk for hemorrhage before obliteration of the shunt.

Radiosurgery can be used in the treatment of DAVFs with subjectively intolerable symptoms and in the treatment of DAVFs not amenable to embolization or surgery, even in the presence of cortical venous drainage or reflux.

References

1. Newton TH, Cronqvist S. Involvement of dural arteries in intracranial arteriovenous malformations. Radiology 1969;93:1071–1078
2. Chaudhary MY, Sachdev VP, Cho SH, Weitzner I Jr, Puljic S, Huang YP. Dural arteriovenous malformation of the major venous sinuses: an acquired lesion. AJNR Am J Neuroradiol 1982;3:13–19
3. Houser OW, Baker HL Jr, Rhoton AL Jr, Okazaki H. Intracranial dural arteriovenous malformations. Radiology 1972;105:55–64
4. Houser OW, Campbell JK, Campbell RJ, Sundt TM Jr. Arteriovenous malformation affecting the transverse dural venous sinus—an acquired lesion. Mayo Clin Proc 1979;54:651–661
5. Mironov A. Pathogenetical consideration of spontaneous dural arteriovenous fistulas (DAVFs). Acta Neurochir (Wien) 1994;131:45–58
6. Lasjaunias P. Angioarchitecture and natural history of dural arteriovenous shunts. Interv Neurorad 1997;3:313–317
7. Duffau H, Lopes M, Janosevic V, et al. Early rebleeding from intracranial dural arteriovenous fistulas: report of 20 cases and review of the literature. J Neurosurg 1999;90:78–84
8. Söderman M, Pavic L, Edner G, Holmin S, Andersson T. Natural history of dural arteriovenous shunts. Stroke 2008;39(6):1735–1739
9. van Dijk JM, terBrugge KG, Willinsky RA, Wallace MC. Clinical course of cranial dural arteriovenous fistulas with long-term persistent cortical venous reflux. Stroke 2002;33:1233–1236
10. Sarma D, terBrugge K. Management of intracranial dural arteriovenous shunts in adults. Eur J Radiol 2003;46:206–220
11. van Dijk JM, terBrugge KG, Willinsky RA, Wallace MC. Selective disconnection of cortical venous reflux as treatment for cranial dural arteriovenous fistulas. J Neurosurg 2004;101:31–35
12. Bitoh S, Hasegawa H, Fujiwara M, Nakao K. Irradiation of spontaneous carotid-cavernous fistulas. Surg Neurol 1982;17:282–286
13. Yamada F, Fukuda S, Matsumoto K, Yoshii N. Effect of radiotherapy on dural arteriovenous malformation: long-term follow-up study and clinical evaluation. Neurol Med Chir (Tokyo) 1984;24:591–599
14. Yasunaga T, Takada C, Uozumi H, et al. Radiotherapy of spontaneous carotid-cavernous sinus fistulas. Int J Radiat Oncol Biol Phys 1987;13:1909–1913
15. Hidaka H, Terashima H, Tsukamoto Y, Nakata H, Matsuoka S. Radiotherapy of dural arteriovenous malformation in the cavernous sinus. Radiat Med 1989;7:160–164
16. Pierot L, Poisson M, Jason M, Pontvert D, Chiras J. Treatment of type D dural carotid-cavernous fistula by embolization followed by irradiation. Neuroradiology 1992;34:77–80
17. Barcia-Salorio JL, Herandez G, Broseta J, Gonzalez-Darder J, Ciudad J. Radiosurgical treatment of carotid-cavernous fistula. Appl Neurophysiol 1982;45:520–522
18. Barcia-Salorio JL, Soler F, Barcia JA, Hernandez G. Stereotactic radiosurgery for the treatment of low-flow carotid-cavernous fistulae: results in a series of 25 cases. Stereotact Funct Neurosurg 1994;63:266–270
19. Link MJ, Coffey RJ, Nichols DA, Gorman DA. The role of radiosurgery and particulate embolization in the treatment of dural arteriovenous fistulas. J Neurosurg 1996;84:804–809
20. Guo WY, Pan DH, Wu HM, et al. Radiosurgery as a treatment alternative for dural arteriovenous fistulas of the cavernous sinus. AJNR Am J Neuroradiol 1998;19:1081–1087

21. Koebbe CJ, Singhal D, Sheehan J, et al. Radiosurgery for dural arteriovenous fistulas. Surg Neurol 2005;64:392–398, discussion 398–399
22. Söderman M, Edner G, Ericson K, et al. Gamma Knife surgery for dural arteriovenous shunts: 25 years of experience. J Neurosurg 2006;104: 867–875
23. Kobayashi H, Hayashi M, Noguchi Y, Tsuji T, Handa Y, Caner HH. Dural arteriovenous malformations in the anterior cranial fossa. Surg Neurol 1988;30:396–401
24. Chandler HC Jr, Friedman WA. Successful radiosurgical treatment of a dural arteriovenous malformation: case report. Neurosurgery 1993; 33:139–141, discussion 141–132
25. Lewis AI, Tomsick TA, Tew JM Jr. Management of tentorial dural arteriovenous malformations: transarterial embolization combined with stereotactic radiation or surgery. J Neurosurg 1994;81:851–859
26. Lasjaunias P, terBrugge K, Chiu M. Dural AVM. Neurosurgery 1985;16: 435–436
27. Herman JM, Spetzler RF, Bederson JB, Kurbat JM, Zabramski JM. Genesis of a dural arteriovenous malformation in a rat model. J Neurosurg 1995;83:539–545
28. Terada T, Higashida RT, Halbach VV, et al. Development of acquired arteriovenous fistulas in rats due to venous hypertension. J Neurosurg 1994;80:884–889
29. Shin Y, Uranishi R, Nakase H, Sakaki T. Vascular endothelial growth factor expression in the rat dural arteriovenous fistula model. No To Shinkei 2003;55:946–952
30. Zhu Y, Lawton MT, Du R, et al. Expression of hypoxia-inducible factor-1 and vascular endothelial growth factor in response to venous hypertension. Neurosurgery 2006;59:687–696, discussion 687–696
31. Kojima T, Miyachi S, Sahara Y, et al. The relationship between venous hypertension and expression of vascular endothelial growth factor: hemodynamic and immunohistochemical examinations in a rat venous hypertension model. Surg Neurol 2007;68:277–284, discussion 284
32. Shin Y, Nakase H, Nakamura M, Shimada K, Konishi N, Sakaki T. Expression of angiogenic growth factor in the rat DAVF model. Neurol Res 2007;29(7):727–733
33. Terada T, Tsuura M, Komai N, et al. The role of angiogenic factor bFGF in the development of dural AVFs. Acta Neurochir (Wien) 1996;138: 877–883
34. Uranishi R, Nakase H, Sakaki T. Expression of angiogenic growth factors in dural arteriovenous fistula. J Neurosurg 1999;91:781–786
35. Klisch J, Kubalek R, Scheufler KM, Zirrgiebel U, Drevs J, Schumacher M. Plasma vascular endothelial growth factor and serum soluble angiopoietin receptor sTIE-2 in patients with dural arteriovenous fistulas: a pilot study. Neuroradiology 2005;47:10–17
36. Tirakotai W, Bertalanffy H, Liu-Guan B, Farhoud A, Sure U. Immunohistochemical study in dural arteriovenous fistulas and possible role of local hypoxia for the de novo formation of dural arteriovenous fistulas. Clin Neurol Neurosurg 2005;107:455–460
37. Castaigne P, Laplane D, Djindjian R, Bories J, Augustin P. Spontaneous arteriovenous communication between the external carotid and the cavernous sinus. Rev Neurol (Paris) 1966;114:5–14
38. Castaigne P, Bories J, Brunet P, Cassan JL, Meininger V, Merland JJ. Arteriovenous fistulae of the dura mater: clinical and radiological study of 13 cases. Ann Med Interne (Paris) 1975;126:813–817
39. Castaigne P, Bories J, Brunet P, Merland JJ, Meininger V. Meningeal arterio-venous fistulas with cortical venous drainage. Rev Neurol (Paris) 1976;132:169–181
40. Djindjian R, Cophignon J, Comoy J, Rey J, Houdart R. Polymorphisme neuroradiologique des fistules carotico.caverneuses. Neurochirurgie 1968;14:881–890
41. Djindjian R, Merland JJ. Superselective Angiography of the External Carotid Artery. Berlin/Heidelberg/New York: Springer Verlag; 1978
42. Lasjaunias P, Halimi P, Lopez-Ibor L, Sichez JP, Hurth M, De Tribolet N. Endovascular treatment of pure spontaneous dural vascular malformations: review of 23 cases studied and treated between May 1980 and October 1983. Neurochirurgie 1984;30:207–223
43. Barrow DL, Spector RH, Braun IF, Landman JA, Tindall SC, Tindall GT. Classification and treatment of spontaneous carotid-cavernous sinus fistulas. J Neurosurg 1985;62:248–256
44. Borden JA, Wu JK, Shucart WA. A proposed classification for spinal and cranial dural arteriovenous fistulous malformations and implications for treatment. J Neurosurg 1995;82:166–179
45. Cognard C, Gobin YP, Pierot L, et al. Cerebral dural arteriovenous fistulas: clinical and angiographic correlation with a revised classification of venous drainage. Radiology 1995;194:671–680
46. Awad IA, Little JR, Akarawi WP, Ahl J. Intracranial dural arteriovenous malformations: factors predisposing to an aggressive neurological course. J Neurosurg 1990;72:839–850
47. Brown RD Jr, Wiebers DO, Nichols DA. Intracranial dural arteriovenous fistulae: angiographic predictors of intracranial hemorrhage and clinical outcome in nonsurgical patients. J Neurosurg 1994;81:531–538
48. Luciani A, Houdart E, Mounayer C, Saint Maurice JP, Merland JJ. Spontaneous closure of dural arteriovenous fistulas: report of three cases and review of the literature. AJNR Am J Neuroradiol 2001;22:992–996
49. Davies MA, Saleh J, ter Brugge K, Willinsky R, Wallace MC. The natural history and management of intracranial dural arteriovenous fistulae, I: Benign lesions. Interv Neurorad 1997;3:295–302
50. Lasjaunias P, Lopez-Ibor L, Abanou A, Halimi P. Radiological anatomy of the vascularization of cranial dural arteriovenous malformations. Anat Clin 1984;6:87–99
51. Pollock BE, Nichols DA, Garrity JA, Gorman DA, Stafford SL. Stereotactic radiosurgery and particulate embolization for cavernous sinus dural arteriovenous fistulae. Neurosurgery 1999;45:459–466, discussion 466–457
52. Guo WY, Lindqvist M, Lindqvist C, et al. Stereotaxic angiography in Gamma Knife radiosurgery of intracranial arteriovenous malformations. AJNR Am J Neuroradiol 1992;13:1107–1114
53. Mehta MP, Kinsella TJ. Cavernous sinus cranial neuropathies: is there a dose-response relationship following radiosurgery? Int J Radiat Oncol Biol Phys 1993;27:477–480
54. Stafford SL, Pollock BE, Leavitt JA, et al. A study on the radiation tolerance of the optic nerves and chiasm after stereotactic radiosurgery. Int J Radiat Oncol Biol Phys 2003;55:1177–1181
55. Friedman JA, Pollock BE, Nichols DA, Gorman DA, Foote RL, Stafford SL. Results of combined stereotactic radiosurgery and transarterial embolization for dural arteriovenous fistulas of the transverse and sigmoid sinuses. J Neurosurg 2001;94:886–891
56. Hasuo K, Mizushima A, Matsumoto S, et al. Type D dural carotid-cavernous fistula: results of combined treatment with irradiation and particulate embolization. Acta Radiol 1996;37:294–298
57. Karlsson B, Lax I, Söderman M. Can the probability for obliteration after radiosurgery for arteriovenous malformations be accurately predicted? Int J Radiat Oncol Biol Phys 1999;43:313–319
58. Shin M, Kurita H, Tago M, Kirino T. Stereotactic radiosurgery for tentorial dural arteriovenous fistulae draining into the vein of Galen: report of two cases. Neurosurgery 2000;46:730–733, discussion 733–734
59. Pan DH, Chung WY, Guo WY, et al. Stereotactic radiosurgery for the treatment of dural arteriovenous fistulas involving the transverse-sigmoid sinus. J Neurosurg 2002;96:823–829
60. Maruyama K, Shin M, Kurita H, Tago M, Kirino T. Stereotactic radiosurgery for dural arteriovenous fistula involving the superior sagittal sinus: case report. J Neurosurg 2002;97:481–483
61. Davies MA, terBrugge K, Willinsky R, Wallace C. The natural history and management of intracranial dural arteriovenous fistulae, II: Aggressive lesions. Interv Neurorad 1997;3:303–311
62. Lau LI, Wu HM, Wang AG, Yen MY, Hsu WM. Paradoxical worsening with superior ophthalmic vein thrombosis after Gamma Knife radiosurgery for dural arteriovenous fistula of cavernous sinus: a case report suggesting the mechanism of the phenomenon. Eye 2006;20:1426–1428
63. Kihlstrom L, Guo WY, Karlsson B, Lindquist C, Lindqvist M. Magnetic resonance imaging of obliterated arteriovenous malformations up to 23 years after radiosurgery [see comments]. J Neurosurg 1997;86: 589–593
64. Onizuka M, Mori K, Takahashi N, et al. Gamma Knife surgery for the treatment of spontaneous dural carotid-cavernous fistulas. Neurol Med Chir (Tokyo) 2003;43:477–482, discussion 482–473
65. Dawkins AA, Evans AL, Wattam J, et al. Complications of cerebral angiography: a prospective analysis of 2,924 consecutive procedures. Neuroradiology 2007;49:753–759
66. Willinsky RA, Taylor SM, terBrugge K, Farb RI, Tomlinson G, Montanera W. Neurologic complications of cerebral angiography: prospective analysis of 2,899 procedures and review of the literature. Radiology 2003;227:522–528
67. Schneider BF, Eberhard DA, Steiner LE. Histopathology of arteriovenous malformations after Gamma Knife radiosurgery. J Neurosurg 1997;87:352–357
68. Meder JF, Oppenheim C, Blustajn J, et al. Cerebral arteriovenous malformations: the value of radiologic parameters in predicting response to radiosurgery. AJNR Am J Neuroradiol 1997;18:1473–1483

7

Stereotactic Radiosurgery for Cavernomas

Bengt Karlsson and Michael Söderman

There is a consensus that radiosurgery has an important role to play in the management of vascular lesions. Its importance in the management of arteriovenous malformations (AVMs) is well established and discussed elsewhere in this book. It is therefore remarkable that the use of radiosurgery in the management of the other clinically important vascular malformations, namely, cavernoma, is still controversial. Some experts claim that cavernomas respond to radiosurgery just like AVMs, some that radiosurgery can be used as a salvage treatment only, and others that radiosurgery should not be used at all. In general, such diverse opinions are caused by anecdotal reports and limited experience, which leads to extrapolation of results from an insignificant number of cases. It is therefore to be expected that the literature reporting cavernomas responding to radiosurgery is sparse, which is certainly true as compared with the number of publications reporting results following AVM radiosurgery. Another thing to be noticed is that few, if any, experts recommend radiosurgery for cavernomas that have not hemorrhaged, whereas prior hemorrhage has little or no influence on AVM management.

If knowledge is limited in regard to how cavernomas respond to radiosurgery, the situation is even less satisfactory following fractionated radiation treatment. For comparison, there are few publications addressing AVM response to fractionated radiation, and the reported experience varies from article to article, making it difficult to draw any definite conclusions. We therefore performed a meta-analysis recently, suggesting that fractionation as compared with radiosurgery offers no or very limited benefit in the management of AVMs.[1] It is to be noted that no published information is available on how cavernomas respond to fractionated radiation treatments. One possible conclusion is that the absence of such articles reflects the lack of favorable treatment results, but it is also possible that no group has treated a sufficiently large enough number of patients to allow the researchers to publish their experience.

One may argue that cavernomas were difficult to visualize in the era prior to magnetic resonance imaging (MRI) and, consequently, that AVMs, which have been treated with radiosurgery since the 1960s, have had at least a 20-year head start in terms of treatment results. However, cavernomas have been treated based on MR images from the late 1980s, and thus a sufficient number of patients should have been treated to allow conclusions to be drawn about the efficacy of the treatment. In addition, with the increased use of MR scanners, there are more and more cavernomas diagnosed, significantly more than AVMs, making them the most commonly diagnosed vascular malformation. It is therefore not surprising that the interest in managing cavernomas in general, and the role of radiosurgery in particular, has increased. To address that issue, we will summarize, assess, and interpret the published results and also relate them to our own very limited experience.

◆ Characteristics and Incidence of Cavernomas

Cavernomas are one of four classically described types of vascular malformations, the others being AVMs, venous malformations, and capillary telangiectasias. A cavernoma is also referred to as a capillary hemangioma, cavernous angioma, cavernous hemangioma, and cavernous malformation, although some researchers suggest that cavernous hemangiomas are a different entity.[2] Some believe that the old term *angiograpically occult vascular malformation* (AOVM), which described an intracerebral hemorrhage where the source of the hemorrhage could not be identified on angiography, equals a cavernoma, but this is not entirely true, as spontaneously obliterated small AVMs were included in this category as well.

Cavernomas are discrete, lobulated, and well-circumscribed lesions. They are composed of dilated, thin-walled capillaries that have a simple endothelial lining with variably thin fibrous adventitia indistinguishable from the lining of capillary telangiectasia. They consist of cavernous spaces lined by endothelial cells and collagen. They have no brain parenchyma between the centrally placed vascular channels, and elastic fibers in the walls of the vascular spaces are absent. The arterial supply is rarely visualized.[3]

The incidence of cavernomas is unknown. Articles from the pre-MRI era suggest a 0.5 to 4.0% incidence.[3] With the growing use of MRI, an increasing number of cavernomas are diagnosed, and an incidence of three central cavernomas per million per year was recently suggested.[4] There is a hereditary component, and up to 50% of patients with cavernomas have a strong family history that is usually autosomal dominant with incomplete penetration. They may occur throughout the central nervous system, including the spinal cord and cauda equina. Although usually solitary, multiple lesions also occur, especially in the familial cases.

It has been suggested that intraparenchymal cavernomas are a different identity as compared with cavernous sinus cavernomas,[2] and we will thus address the two types separately.

Cavernomas versus Cavernous sinus Cavernomas

Gonzales et al described a multitude of differences between cavernomas and cavernous sinus hemangiomas (CSHs).[2] CSHs are more common in women, whereas cavernomas are not. There is no hereditary component in CSH. Cavernomas are vascular malformations, whereas CSHs grow over time, a behavior consistent with a neoplastic lesion. CSHs do not manifest with acute bleedings, but cause compression symptoms from the cranial nerves. They are high-flow lesions, whereas cavernomas are low flow. They have a capsule or pseudocapsule and show no evidence of previous hemorrhage. They tend to hemorrhage profusely at surgery, and a 36% surgery related morbidity has been reported.[5]

From a radiosurgical perspective, the above would suggest that CSHs respond to radiosurgery like meningiomas and hemangiopericytomas. Although sparse, the published reports are consistent with this assumption. Shibata and Mori were the first to publish results on the radiation response of a CSH.[6] They reported three cases treated with fractionated radiotherapy; all lesions responded favorably and decreased, but the follow-up time was short. Maryishi et al[7] confirmed the findings, reporting a decrease in the tumor 8 months after radiotherapy. Other authors have reported similar results following radiosurgery.[8–13] The number of cases are few, with each article reporting between 1 and 5 patients, for a total of 16 patients. The observation time varies between 0.5 and 5 years, with a mean time of 2.5 years. The prescription doses vary between 12 and 19 Gy, with a mean value of 15 Gy. Nine patients improved clinically after the treatment, mostly with an improved cranial nerve function. One tumor decreased slightly, 11 significantly, and 4 almost disappeared. No complications were reported. It is interesting to note that all lesions responded in a similar way despite the different doses given; thus, it seems preferable to use lower treatment doses. The only caveat is the relatively short follow-up times, and later tumor recurrence is a possibility that may change the preceding results. Still, CSHs seem to respond favorably to radiosurgery, so well that radiosurgery is probably the treatment of choice for such hemangiomas.

◆ Indications for Radiosurgery

There are three reasons to treat cavernomas: for the mass effect in CHSs (as reported above), for the propensity to cause clinically symptomatic hemorrhages, and/or seizures for the intracerebral lesions. This means that the results following CSH radiosurgery are best assessed by MRI. For intracerebral lesions, the aim is to affect the impact of the cavernoma on surrounding brain tissue for patients suffering from epilepsy and to change the natural course of the malformation for the other patients. A very important consequence of the above is that the treatment results in patients with intracerebral cavernomas that cannot be assessed by imaging. Unlike for AVMs, imaging, whether angiography, MRI, or MR angiography (MRA), is therefore of very limited value in evaluating the response to the treatment.

For patients with epilepsy, a successful treatment will result in a significant decrease or a cessation of seizures. In regard to a change in the risk for cavernoma rupture, it can only be judged by a comparison to the natural cause of the cavernoma or by histological verification that the cavernoma has been obliterated.

◆ Cavernomas, Epilepsy, and Radiosurgery

Seizures are one of the most common clinical presentations of cavernomas. It is assumed that the epileptic activity from a cavernoma arises not from the lesion itself, but from the surrounding hemosiderin deposit as well as from other degradation products from hemoglobin. Thus, it seems illogical to treat the cavernoma with radiation to affect the surrounding neural tissue. In addition, seizure is one of the complications following radiosurgery, which raises some concern regarding treating epilepsy with radiation. Finally, the dose given to the cavernoma must be low to avoid complications, resulting in low doses to the surrounding neural tissue as well. One can argue that it could be possible to affect the epileptogenic activity without causing tissue necrosis, but our very limited experience at the Karolinska Institute contradicts this assumption.

By analyzing the literature, one must conclude that the clinical results published contradict the speculations above. We have found three articles in which the results following radiosurgery for epilepsy associated with cavernomas are presented.[14–16] Because two of them reported experiences from the same patient material,[14,15] we will focus on the more recent of the two.[15]

Regis et al and Hsu et al reported results following radiosurgery for cavernomas associated with seizures.[15,16] We will concentrate on the patients with intractable epilepsy, here defined as uncontrolled for at least 1 year as well as having a follow-up for at least 1 year after radiosurgery.

Regis et al reported on 49 patients, all with intractable epilepsy and all followed for at least 1 year after radiosurgery.[15] The prescription doses varied between 15 and 24 Gy, and the follow-up time varied between 11 and 37 months (which contradicts the 1-year minimum follow-up time, although the difference is insignificant). Regis et al found that 26 patients (53%) were seizure free or having an aura only (Engel I), 12 (24%) were almost seizure free (Engel II), two (4%) experienced worthwhile improvement (Engel III), and 11 (22%) showed no worthwhile improvement (Engel IV). They also noticed that the results were inferior for mesiotemporal epilepsy, which makes sense, as the microsurgical results are better if the hippocampus is removed. A caveat from this study is that the complication rate is not reported, and we cannot exclude the possibility that some of the short-term beneficial effects from the radiosurgical treatments are mediated through radiation-induced edema. Thus, follow-up studies over a longer period of time would have been valuable.

Hsu et al reported the results from 14 patients in whom the cavernomas causing seizures were treated with radiosurgery.[16] In eight patients, the history of seizures was 1 year or less, leaving six patients with intractable epilepsy. The follow-up time was over 1 year for all patients. All six patients improved, three to Engel I, two to Engel II, and one to Engel III. One patient developed an asymptomatic radiation-induced edema. The antiepileptic medication was increased in one patient, making it difficult to assess if the medication or the radiation was responsible for the improvement, but the medication was either unchanged (four patients) or decreased (one patient) for the other five patients.

The details of the seizure disorders are usually not included in the publications reporting general treatment results. Some report the time between the onset of seizures and the radiosurgical treatment, and others only note that the patients had pretreatment seizures. We are not informed if the epilepsy is intractable or not for patients with long-lasting seizure problems. Thus, the results from these articles are more nonspecific, as factors other than radiation may contribute to a change in seizure activity. Amin-Hanjani et al reported that 18 patients had seizures before the treatment, 8 with fair and 10 with poor seizure control.[17] After the treatment, 1 had no seizures, 13 had fair, and 4 had poor seizure control. Chang et al reported that seizures resolved in two of the four patients with this problem.[18] Huang et al[19] reported 13 patients with seizures, 5 of whom suffered from seizures for more than a year before the treatment. Three of these patients improved to Engel I and two to Engel III. Among the other patients, five improved to Engel I and three to Engel II. Kida et al[20] reported that seven patients had seizures before treatment and that the seizures disappeared in three patients, improved in three cases, and deteriorated in one. Kim et al did not report details about pretreatment seizures but they concluded that 9 of 12 patients were seizure free without medication after the treatment and that the seizures persisted in the other 3 patients.[21] Liscak et al reported that 44 patients had seizures before treatment and that improvement occurred in 20 of them.[22] They also observed transient seizure deterioration caused by radiation-induced edema in two patients. Liu et al defined patients with a seizure history of longer than 6 months as having chronic epilepsy.[22] In the 17 with chronic epilepsy, 4 improved to Engel I, and 13 were reported as Engel III or IV. Stea et al reported that two of the treated patients had experienced seizures.[23] One of the patients became seizure free, and one improved after the radiosurgical treatment. However, the latter improved with change in his medication. Tsien et al reported that one patient who had seizures before the treatment became seizure free and remained so 4.5 years later.[24] Finally, Zhang et al reported that 33 patients had seizures before the treatment and that follow-up information is available from 31 of them.[25] Twenty-two patients improved, and the other nine were unchanged. Zhang et al make an important observation and write that "Six patients whose cavernous hemangiomas were located in the temporal lobe had seizure control when there was manifest brain edema. However, the seizure control deteriorated when the edema resolved."

The conclusion from analyzing the studies above must be that radiosurgery does decrease the epileptic activity from a cavernoma and its surrounding hemoglobin degradation products.

◆ Cavernomas, Hemorrhage, and Radiosurgery

In the rest of the chapter we will analyze and assess the risk for hemorrhage of a cavernoma and how it responds to radiosurgical treatment.

Histopathological Analysis of Radiation Response

One way to assess the response to radiation is to analyze the irradiated lesion histopathologically. For AVMs, several reports have shown how they respond to radiation.[26–33] In contrast, only two publications have been found analyzing histological postradiation changes in cavernomas.

Gewirtz et al analyzed 8 cavernomas that were surgically excised after radiation treatment, radiation being fractionated radiation, Gamma Knife Surgery® (Elekta Instruments AB, Stockholm, Sweden) surgery, or helium ion particle beam.[34] These 8 were compared to 10 nonirradiated cavernomas. The mean time between radiation and surgical extirpation was 28 months. Seven of the irradiated lesions showed marked fibrosis of the vascular channels, fibrinoid necrosis, and ferrugination. The fibrinoid necrosis was the only finding unique to the irradiated lesions as compared with the controls. Gewirtz et al conclude: "Our present results suggest that there is little pathological changes that can be ascribed to radiation in these AOVMs. Clearly, the vascular channels remain patent, unlike high-flow arteriovenous malformations, which often sclerose and thrombose close with radiosurgery." They continue: "Perhaps the lack of an elastic lamina or a muscular layer prevents AOVMs from sclerosing like the high-flow AVMs."

Nyáry et al reported the histopathological analysis of a cavernoma that was excised after having been irradiated with fractionated radiation to a total dose of 40 Gy and removed 1 year later.[35] Dose per fraction is not reported. The specimen was compared to nonirradiated cavernoma. The comparison "indicated that there was endothelial cell destruction and marked fibrosis with hyaline degeneration and scar tissue formation in the connective tissue stroma" of the irradiated cavernoma. In addition, most of the vessels were obliterated in the irradiated tissue sampling." As seen, the two articles contradict each other. One possible explanation for this may be found in the paper by Seo et al.[36] They treated 9 cavernomas with radiosurgery, and one of the patients was operated on after the treatment. They write in the abstract that "Histological findings revealed an arteriovenous malformation [AVM] and a cavernous angioma. There was hypertrophy of the internal membrane of the AVM, but no effect on the cavernous malformation." It seems possible that the case reported by Nyáry et al is similar to this, and thus it is fair to conclude that histopathological verification fails to show that radiosurgery changes the natural course of a cavernoma. To define the efficacy of radiosurgery, we must therefore compare the pre- and posttreatment risk for hemorrhage. Consequently, we must define the risk for hemorrhage from an untreated cavernoma, in other words, the natural course of the disease, before the impact of radiosurgery can be assessed.

Risk for Hemorrhage from an Untreated Cavernoma

The common way to assess the risk for hemorrhage is to follow a number of untreated patients, register the number of hemorrhages and the number of years that the patients have been observed, and divide by two. This seems straightforward, but there are several pitfalls with such a study. First, we must assume that the patients studied are representative of the whole patient population. This may not be the case, as the cases studied are a selected group of patients referred to an MRI examination for a reason; thus, an asymptomatic cavernoma is far less likely to be diagnosed. Consequently, we do not know how many patients have undiagnosed cavernomas, which certainly will affect the statistics. In addition, the patients followed are those who were not surgically treated, and we cannot assume a priori that the natural course is identical in the two groups of patients. A study like this is also sensitive for lack of information: the more patients that are underreported, the lower the estimated risk for hemorrhage. All hemorrhages that occur must thus be reported to avoid this flaw. This raises the need to define a hemorrhage, as we can be sure that some subclinical hemorrhages will not be reported, and we can be equally sure to detect several subclinical hemorrhages on MRI. The most accurate way to follow patients would be to conduct regular clinical and MRI follow-up examinations and to report subclinical and clinical hemorrhages separately, a study that, unfortunately, has yet to be published. Awaiting for this study to be published, we have to critically analyze the available articles reporting the annual risk of hemorrhage from cavernomas. There are only a few, and they are summarized in the following discussion. We have, if necessary, recalculated the hemorrhage rates from per patient to per cavernoma if the information allowing us to do so was available. Most authors have defined a hemorrhage as a clinical event, and if not, we have tried to recalculate the numbers to include clinical hemorrhages only. We have also studied the pretreatment hemorrhage rates in the studies reporting treatment results, and the studies are summarized here.

The only purely retrospective article found was the one by Del Curling et al, who studied 8131 MR images and found 32 patients having a total of 76 cavernomas.[37] Fifty lesions were found in the six patients having multiple lesions. Only three patients had radiographically identifiable hemorrhages, resulting in a 0.25% annual incidence of hemorrhage per patient and a 0.1% annual incidence per cavernoma. Peripheral hemosiderin deposition was identifiable around all lesions. The criticism of the article is obvious. The authors have defined a hemorrhage as when the imaging and hemorrhage occur simultaneously, in other words, when a suspicion of a stroke was the indication for performing the MRI examination. It is questionable how this is related to the natural course of the disease. It is not mentioned but assumed that the three patients with fresh hemorrhages were symptomatic. However, it is mentioned that another 10 patients had a history of present or prior focal neurologic deficits; if these symptoms are assumed to be related to earlier hemorrhages, the risk for hemorrhages will be higher, and thus the 0.1% annual risk is most likely an underestimation of the natural course of a cavernoma.

In the next two articles, the patient material was studied in both a retrospective and a prospective manner. Kim et al studied images from 9954 MR examinations and found 62 patients having a total of 108 cavernomas.[38] The risk for hemorrhage was defined as the number of years at risk, assuming that the patient was born with the cavernoma, divided by the number of hemorrhages. The number of risk years given in the article is 2510, and the resulting annual incidence of hemorrhages was found to be 2.3% per patient and 1.4% per lesion. Here, a hemorrhage was defined as an acute event; thus, the old hemorrhages, the evidence of which can be seen as hemosiderin deposits, were not included, which presents an obvious flaw in the statistics. Kim et al also analyzed the prospective annual risk for hemorrhage, which was found to be 3.8% per patient and 2.6% per lesion.

The study by Kondziolka et al analyzed the largest patient material.[39] Of the 235 patients referred to them, no treatment was recommended for 162 patients, and data were obtained from 122 of them. The number of cavernomas was not reported, and the risk of hemorrhage was calculated per patient, but as we know that 25 had multiple lesions, we can conclude that the number of cavernomas was at least 147. A hemorrhage was defined as a clinically detectable event. The mean age was 37.3 years, and 50% of patients in the study had never experienced a clinically detectable hemorrhage. The pretreatment hemorrhage rate was calculated as 1.3% per year and per patient, assuming a constant risk per year and that the cavernoma has been present since birth. However, the 1.3% found also reflects the mean age at diagnosis and the relative number of patients who have not hemorrhaged, which does not necessarily equal the natural course of cavernomas. The pretreatment hemorrhage rate can be calculated by dividing the median age by 100 and multiplying the result by the relative number of bleeders, here $(37.3/100) \times 0.5 = 1.3\%$. If we assume that it is relatively more common to refer cavernomas to a neurosurgical department when the cavernoma has hemorrhaged, the 1.3% will be too high. The only way to avoid this potential flaw is to analyze the age distribution at the first hemorrhage per cavernoma, and based on this to calculate the annual risk for hemorrhage, which is insensitive to the potential bias mentioned earlier.[40] It should be noted that the numbers above express the annual risk for hemorrhage per patient. The risk will be 1.1% or lower if we calculate the incidence of hemorrhage per cavernoma instead.

In the prospective part of the study, a 2.6% annual incidence of hemorrhage per patient is given, which equals a risk per lesion of $\leq 2.2\%$. Because it is prospective, it should equal the annual risk for hemorrhage, assuming that all hemorrhages have been reported. Thus, the prospective risk is twice the retrospective risk. As no treatment was given, and as the true risk for hemorrhage is unrelated to being studied retro- or prospectively (if not, we could decrease the risk for hemorrhages just by studying them retrospectively only), the results contradict the assumptions that the patient is born with the cavernoma and/or that the risk for hemorrhage is age independent. Another possible explanation for this difference is that a cavernoma hemorrhage has a higher likelihood to be symptomatic if it hemorrhaged earlier. An increased hemorrhage risk for earlier ruptured cavernomas is also concluded in the study. A 0.6% annual risk for a clinical hemorrhage was found among patients with an earlier nonruptured cavernoma, which should be compared with a 4.5% ($\leq 3.7\%$ per lesion) annual risk for patients who had suffered from a prior hemorrhage. However, as all cavernomas have imaging evidence of prior hemorrhage, the 3.7% risk is applicable to the recently hemorrhaged cavernomas only. The very important question is: how long does this increased hemorrhage rate persist after a prior hemorrhage?

We found three purely prospective studies. Moriarity et al[43] analyzed 68 patients, with a mean number of 3.4 cavernomas per patient. They followed the patients prospectively and found 11 symptomatic hemorrhages in a median follow-up time of 5.2 years. They reported a 3.1% annual risk per patient, which equals a 0.9% annual risk per cavernoma. Robinson et al studied 10,435 MR images and found 76 lesions in 66 patients.[41] These patients were followed prospectively for a total of 143 years, and one hemorrhage occurred in this time period, representing ~1% annual risk for hemorrhage per lesion. It is not noted in the article if this hemorrhage was defined as a clinical event or not. Robinson et al could not detect any apparent relation between the size of the cavernoma and the likelihood of hemorrhage when analyzing the cavernomas at the time of the initial MRI examination. It is noteworthy that they did not analyze the risk for hemorrhage by assessing the hemorrhages at the time of the diagnosis as Del Curling et al did,[36] presumably because they realized the potential flaw in such an analysis.

Zabramski et al had a very different approach to the problem.[41] They studied 6 families with familial cavernomas and screened 59 family members, diagnosing 31 patients with cavernomas. The 21 patients who agreed to participate in the study were followed clinically and radiologically every 6 to 12 months in a prospective manner. These 21 patients with a total of 128 cavernomas were followed for a mean of 2.2 years, representing 46 patient years and 282 lesion years. Here three patients experienced exacerbation of their seizure disorders, which was caused by new hemorrhages, representing an annual risk of 1.1%. It is noteworthy that none of the patients experienced any new or aggravated neurologic deficits during the follow-up period; thus, if a neurologic deficit had been the definition of hemorrhage, the risk for hemorrhage would have been 0%.

All the reports in the preceding summary are assessing in a prospective or retrospective manner the annual risk for a cavernoma to cause a clinically significant hemorrhage. The natural course is also analyzed in some articles reporting treatment results following radiosurgery. In these articles, only patients selected for radiosurgery treatments are included, which is a significant selection bias. Will this affect the study results? Let us analyze this further.

We can first divide the results from the articles studying the natural course only and not the results of any treatment in a prospective and a retrospective part. The retrospective incidence of hemorrhages was studied in three articles, and the retrospective analyses summarize 10,063 patient risk years in whom 112 hemorrhagic events were diagnosed, yielding a 1.1% annual incidence of hemorrhages.[37–39] In the prospective studies, 26 hemorrhages in 2045 risk years were found, which translates to a 1.3% annual incidence.[38,39,41–43] If we summarize the pro- and retrospective series, a 1.1% annual incidence will result.

The incidence of pretreatment hemorrhages in the radiosurgically treated patient population is significantly higher. Here, a total of 15,276 risk years was analyzed,[17,21,23,44–48] and 530 hemorrhages found, yielding a 3.5% hemorrhage rate. Because few treat patients with unruptured cavernomas, we cannot exclude that this increased incidence reflects a selection bias rather than a patient population with high-risk cavernomas. We have excluded two publications from this summary,[48,49] as the patients in these studies were included in later publications.[21,48]

In summary, we must conclude that the natural course of cavernomas is poorly known. Based on the published data, the retrospective incidence of hemorrhages is ~1%, and the prospective risk is ~2% if an unselected patient population is studied and 3% risk in a patient population selected for radiosurgery. It is therefore fair to assume that the natural course of a cavernoma is a 2% annual risk for a clinically significant hemorrhage.

Increased Hemorrhage Risk after a Prior Hemorrhage from an Untreated Cavernoma

One of the key findings in the study of Kondziolka et al was that the risk for a hemorrhage increases after an earlier one,[38] as with aneurysms. This finding has been confirmed by others. Unlike aneurysms, this increased risk associated with cavernomas is assumed to be permanent. This could not be analyzed in the Kondziolka study, as the mean follow-up time was less than 3 years. To the best of our knowledge, the very important question of the duration of the increased risk has not been analyzed in any scientific publication. The assumption of an increased risk for an indefinite period of time must, however, be questioned from a purely logical standpoint. The majority, if not all, of diagnosed cavernomas show evidence of hemorrhage, either acute, subacute, or as blood degradation products. If we strictly apply the assumption that the risk is permanently increased if the cavernomas have hemorrhaged earlier, then almost all cavernomas would have an increased risk, which is not supported from the published retrospective data mentioned above. The only way to make these different observations coherent is to assume that the increased risk is temporary and that it resets to the prehemorrhagic level after an unknown number of years.

Comparison of Pre- and Postradiosurgery Hemorrhage Rate

From the preceding discussion, it can be concluded that the natural course of cavernomas is poorly understood. It is therefore tempting to use the pretreatment incidence of hemorrhages as an indicator of the pretreatment risk, instead of the ~2% annual risk as we concluded above and compare it to the posttreatment risk for hemorrhage when the efficacy of radiosurgery is assessed. The pretreatment risk for hemorrhage can be calculated in two ways. The first is to divide the number of hemorrhages by the total number of observation years (method A). This assumes (1) that the patient is born with a cavernoma and (2) that the risk for hemorrhage is constant. It is easy to realize that this cannot be the case, because, if so, it would be common to see cavernoma hemorrhages in children, which is not the case. One way to avoid this problem is to define the date of the first hemorrhage as day one and to calculate the risk for hemorrhage thereafter by adding the number of hemorrhages, excluding the first, and dividing this number with the number of observed years following the first hemorrhage (method B).

We analyzed the differences using method A and found a 3.1 times higher annual incidence of hemorrhage in the articles reporting treatment results as compared with the studies of the natural course of cavernomas only. How can this difference be explained? It is very likely that this reflects a selection bias, presumably because the likelihood is higher to treat a lesion if it has hemorrhaged, and even higher if ruptured several times. In other words, nonbleeders are mostly excluded in the treated patient population, which flaws the analysis. Another example of how important the relations between bleeders and nonbleeders are is to use another way of calculating the incidence of hemorrhage using method A. The annual incidence for hemorrhage (AIH) in a patient population is equals

$$\text{AIH} = b/a,$$

where a is the mean age on the day of treatment and b is the mean number of hemorrhages prior to the day of treatment.

When the equation is studied, it is obvious that the result of method A in a treated patient population more reflects case selection more than the natural course of a cavernoma.

As mentioned earlier, it is tempting to use method B to avoid the assumption of patients being born with the cavernomas and a constant annual risk for rupture. However, because nonhemorrhaged cavernomas will be excluded from the analysis, this method analyzes the incidence of ruptures following a prior hemorrhage only. To be conclusive, one must presume that the timing of treatment is unrelated to prior hemorrhage. In addition, we must assume not only that the patients are randomly selected for treatment, but also that the timing of the treatment is randomly decided. Needless to say, this is not the case. It is obvious that a neurosurgeon is more inclined to treat a lesion that has bled recently, especially if it has ruptured several times before, as compared with an asymptomatic patient with a lesion that has hemorrhaged a long time ago and never again. So, how important is this bias? When we compare the results in the articles analyzing the treatment, an average of 3.5% annual incidence is found if method A is used and 24.8% if method B is used, an increase of a factor of 7. This risk increase cannot be explained by an assumption that these cavernomas are high risk, as it is the same patient population that was analyzed with method A. So, is it possible that the natural course of these cavernomas has become 7 times more dangerous, or is it the bias mentioned above or a combination of the two that explains this difference?

To analyze this further, we have used a random number generator to simulate the incidence of hemorrhages among 2000 virtual cavernomas followed for 10 years (**Table 7.1**). We used the assumption of 1 or 2% annual risk, plus the assumption that the risk was unchanged after a hemorrhage, being increased to 5% for 2 years or being increased to 5% indefinitely. As seen in **Table 7.1,** both methods A and B give accurate results when all virtual patients were studied as both the day of diagnosis and the last day of observation are random parameters. What can be seen with method B is that the risk will asymptotically increase toward the annual post hemorrhage risk with increasing number of observation years when using the assumption that a hemorrhage will constantly increase the risk for future hemorrhages.

Things will start to change if we exclude nonhemorrhagic cavernomas from the study. Using method A, the risk will increase with decreasing number of observation years per patient. As seen in **Table 7.1,** a 10-year observation time results in 10 to 12% annual risk, which is 5–10 times more than the actual risk in this virtual cavernoma patient population. If instead 4000 patients had been followed for 5 years, a calculated annual risk of 26 to 27% would have resulted, which

Table 7.1A Calculation of the risk of hemorrhages in 2000 virtual cavernoma patients followed for 10 years using method A (Table 1A) or B (Table 1B). "H" denotes the number of hemorrhages in the analyzed patient population. The minimum number of hemorrhages to be included in the analysis is given in the columns "patients". The calculations were based on an 1 or 2% annual risk for hemorrhage before the first rupture. The annual hemorrhage risk after the first bleeding was set being unchanged, 5% for the first 2 years or 5% indefintely. As seen, the calculated risk is up to 30 times larger than the real risk, due to flaws in the methods used.

Defined risk for H	patients	H	riskyrs	%	patients	H	riskyrs	%	patients	H	riskyrs	%
1% before, 1% after	all	212	20000	1	≥ 1 H	212	2030	10	≥ 2 H	18	90	20
1% before, 5% 2 yr after	all	225	20000	1	≥ 1 H	225	2030	11	≥ 2 H	44	220	20
1% before, 5% after	all	251	20000	1	≥ 1 H	251	2030	12	≥ 2 H	92	440	21
2% before, 2% after	all	414	20000	2	≥ 1 H	414	3780	11	≥ 2 H	70	340	21
2% before, 5% 2 yr after	all	435	20000	2	≥ 1 H	435	3780	12	≥ 2 H	107	500	21
%2 before, 5% after	all	471	20000	2	≥ 1 H	471	3780	12	≥ 2 H	173	800	22

Table 7.1B

Defined risk for H	patients	H	riskyrs	%	patients	H	riskyrs	%
1% before, 1% after	≥ 1 H	19	919	2	≥ 2 H	19	63	30
1% before, 5% 2 yr after	≥ 1 H	22	919	2	≥ 2 H	22	118	19
1% before, 5% after	≥ 1 H	48	919	5	≥ 2 H	48	266	18
2% before, 2% after	≥ 1 H	36	1707	2	≥ 2 H	36	207	17
2% before, 5% 2 yr after	≥ 1 H	57	1707	3	≥ 2 H	57	287	20
%2 before, 5% after	≥ 1 H	93	1707	5	≥ 2 H	93	506	18

should be compared with the true annual risk of 1 and 2%, respectively. The same skewed result will be seen using method B if only patients having suffered from two hemorrhages or more are included in the analyses.

The results in **Table 7.1** presume that the day of the treatment is a random parameter. It is, however, trivial to conclude that we are much more inclined to recommend treatment for a patient with a cavernoma that has bled numerous times in the past and now has ruptured again as compared with a patient in whom the cavernoma bled 15 years ago and has not bothered the patient since. What happens when we introduce this bias in the model? Let us assume that we will end up treating 50% of the patients with two hemorrhages and all with three hemorrhages or more. Let us further assume that all treatments are performed within a year after the most recent hemorrhage. This assumption is supported by the article by Liu et al, where it is stated that "All 125 patients were treated within 6 months of the initial onset of symptoms."[20] Let us also assume the 1 or 2% annual risk followed by a 5% hemorrhage risk for different lengths of time as mentioned above. By doing so and using model B, the resulting annual incidence of hemorrhages will be calculated as 19 to 34%. Therefore, we can conclude that the resulting annual risk using model B in a selected patient population in which the patients have bled frequently does not coincide with the natural course of the disease.

Changes of the Natural Course after Radiosurgery

To define the merits of any treatment, we must be able to measure or quantify the treatment results. Questions such as, What is the optimal dose? and What can we conclude if a cavernoma needs to be re-treated? are impossible to answer if we cannot define the treatment result per treated lesion. For cavernomas, when the posttreatment hemorrhage rate is the only indicator if the treatment has affected the natural course or not, we cannot define the treatment result per lesion. In the following discussion we will show that it is difficult enough to conclude how much the natural course is affected in a patient population, maybe even impossible to scientifically conclude if the natural course is affected at all. Let us systematically analyze the results: comparison of bleeding rates before and after treatment.

As earlier discussed, this comparison assumes that the patients have harbored the cavernomas since birth, and that the annual risk for hemorrhage is constant and independent of age, prior hemorrhage, and other factors.

So, how high was the posttreatment hemorrhage rate? By adding the information from 16 articles,[4,6–24,43–47,50,51] excluding 3 where the same patient material is within a later publication,[49,50,53] a total of 151 posttreatment hemorrhages in 3210 risk years was found, equals an annual risk of 4.7%. This does not drastically differ from the pretreatment risk of 3.5% found in the same studies using method A or from the 1 to 2% natural course of the disease found in the other articles mentioned above. If anything, the risk is actually higher after as compared with before when using method A.

As we have explained, method B cannot be used in a highly selected patient population, as the pretreatment incidence more reflects patient selection than the natural course of the disease. So, how can we possibly claim that radiosurgery does alter the natural course of the disease? One way is to assume that the risk for a new symptomatic hemorrhage is indefinitely increased after an earlier hemorrhage, and also to assume that there is a 2-year latency between the treatment and the decreased risk for hemorrhage. Our only concern with these assumptions is that we did not see a drastic decrease in the incidence of hemorrhages 2 years or more after the treatment in our own small patient population.[51]

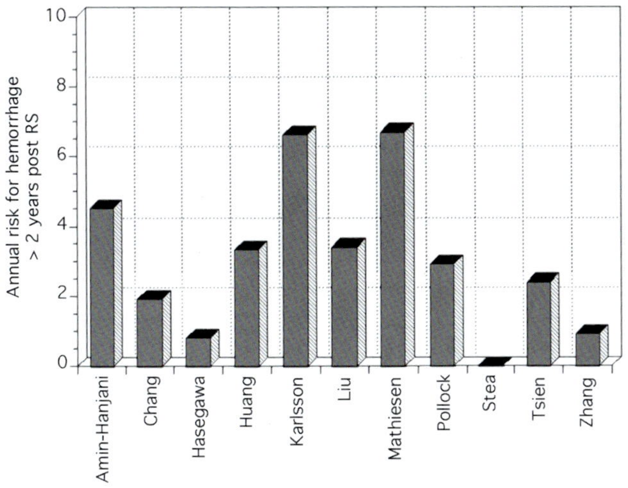

Fig. 7.1 The risk for hemorrhages more than 2 years after the treatment. The risk in most institutions is between 2 and 4%, the exceptions being the Karolinska Institute, Pittsburgh, PA, Syracuse, NY, and Shanghai, China.

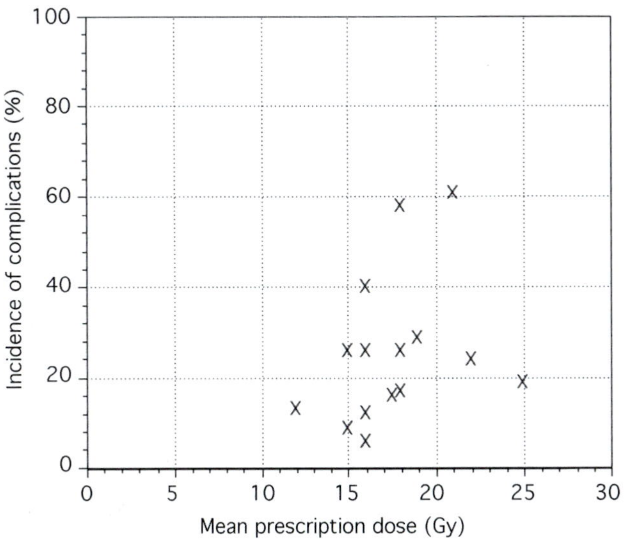

Fig. 7.2 Relationship between mean prescription doses and complication rates at different institutions. As seen, there was a poor correlation between the prescription doses and the complication rates, which is somewhat surprising, as the target volumes were generally small.

Still, let us assume that the risk for hemorrhage in this selected patient material is in the interval between the 2.0 and 3.7% reported earlier, with a mean value of 2.8%, and compare it with the risk for hemorrhage 2 years or more after the treatment. This risk is reported in 11 studies[4,17,18,22–25,45,47,48,51] and illustrated in **Fig. 7.1.** It can be seen that there is a significant difference in the risk of hemorrhages observed in different institutions. It is reasonable to add the number of hemorrhages and risk years, as the number of hemorrhages per study is low. By doing so, a total of 40 hemorrhages in 1478 risk years was found, yielding a 2.7% annual risk for hemorrhage.

In conclusion, the pre- and posttreatment incidence of hemorrhage is of the same magnitude. If we use the 2.8% annual risk as an estimation of the pretreatment risk, it seems that the posttreatment risk is minimally decreased 2 years or more after radiosurgery.

Complications after Radiosurgery for Cavernomas

The patients in the study of Amin-Hajani et al were treated with proton beam radiosurgery, and the prescription doses were based on the 1% risk estimation model developed by Kjellberg.[17] However, the retrospective analysis revealed a 26% incidence of complications. In our own study, the expected number of complications based on our risk estimation model[54] was one patient, yet six complications were observed. Takenaka et al[55] describe a severe undue radiation effect with extensive brain edema, and Amin-Hajani et al[16] note three lethal complications following cavernoma radiosurgery.

The examples above illustrate that the risk for complications is significantly higher when treating a cavernoma as compared with treating an AVM of the same volume using the same dose. They also illustrate that the complications can be more severe than what are seen following AVM radiosurgery. We can therefore expect that a high incidence of complications is reported following radiosurgical treatments of cavernomas. This is also the case. On average, a 26% incidence of complications was reported in the 15 articles analyzed.[17–25,44–48,51,52] Interestingly, there was a significant difference in complication rates between different centers, from 7 to 62%, which is almost a factor of 10 difference. How can this be explained? The first assumption would be that the treatment doses varied significantly from center to center, and that the higher complication rates were seen in centers using higher treatment doses. This was not the case. As seen in **Fig. 7.2,** there is a poor relation between the complication rates and the mean prescription doses used in different centers.

One can argue that the prescription doses are not necessarily related to the irradiation load to the cerebral tissue, and that centers using lower doses treated larger cavernomas. This may be the case, but the relatively small median cavernoma volumes, from 1 to 4 cc in the different studies, does not support this assumption. Still, it is true that we do no know the radiation doses in detail. It may therefore be better to use the treatment response rather than the treatment doses to analyze this further. We know that there is a strong relation between radiation doses and incidence of complications, and we can assume that a dose–response relation exists for cavernomas as well. Thus, with increasing doses we can expect a decreasing posttreatment hemorrhage rate and an increasing complication rate. We can analyze if this is true by plotting the annual incidence of posttreatment hemorrhage against the incidence of complications for different prescription doses. This is shown in **Fig. 7.3.** Here, the incidence of complications was plotted against the annual incidence of posttreatment hemorrhages. As seen, the linear curve fit

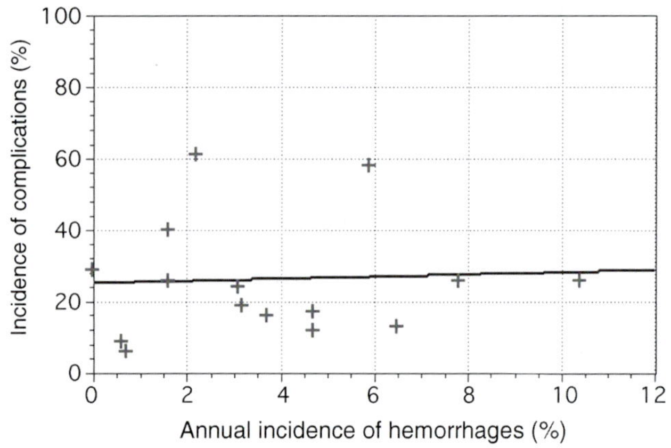

Fig. 7.3 Relationship between posttreatment hemorrhage and complication rates. It could be expected that the complication rate should increase with decreasing hemorrhages rates, assuming a dose–response relation for both the cavernoma and the surrounding brain tissue. This was not seen. In fact, the linear fit suggests an increasing complication rate with an increasing posttreatment incidence of complications.

suggests a negative relation between posttreatment hemorrhages and complications; that is, the lower the posttreatment hemorrhage rate, the lower the complication rate. This does not make sense, and we must therefore assume that the reason for different complication rates in different centers is either incomplete follow-up data or different definitions of complications, hemorrhages, or both in different centers.

Risk–Benefit Relationship and Dose Optimization

Figure 7.3 deserves more attention. As mentioned earlier, we cannot define the treatment response per lesion. Thus, the only way to perform a dose–response analysis is to compare the posttreatment hemorrhage and complication rates. **Figure 7.3** suggests that there is no such relation. This does not exclude a relation between dose and posttreatment hemorrhage rate, but it does indicate to us that the impact of increased doses affects the complication rates more than the hemorrhage rates, and thus that lower rather than higher radiation doses are recommended should cavernomas be treated with radiosurgery. If we summarize the above, the risk–benefit relation is not as favorable for cavernomas as for any other indication. If we compare a $< 1\%$ decrease of the annual risk for hemorrhage to a 20 to 30% complication rate, it will take significantly more than 20 years before the beneficial effect from the treatment exceeds the complication rate. We must conclude, then, that more data are needed before radiosurgery can be recommended for cavernomas. Taking the uncertainty of the natural course of the disease into consideration, a prospective randomized study comparing radiosurgery to no treatment is needed before any scientifically valid conclusions can be drawn. It is our opinion that cavernoma radiosurgery should be used, if at all, as salvage treatment only until such a prospective study has shown a significant benefit from radiosurgical treatment of cavernomas.

◆ The Karolinska Experience with Radiosurgery for Cavernomas

We have published the Karolinska experience in two articles, one from 1998, where the treatment results from 22 cavernoma treatments were published,[51] and one from 2003, where information was shared from 5 cavernoma treatments.[4] In the latter, Mathiesen et al studied central cavernomas managed at the Karolinska Institute. Five of the cavernomas were treated with radiosurgery. Two hemorrhaged after 2 and 6 years, but no information is given about complications.

The fact that, up to and including 1996, only a total of 23 cavernomas were treated at the Karolinska, as compared to 1351 AVMs during the same time period, Drs. Steiner and Lindquist, who were responsible for the radiosurgical treatment of vascular malformations, were far from convinced that radiosurgery was a valuable tool in the management of cavernomas. Their suspicion was also confirmed in our study. Here, 22 patients were followed from 1 to 13 years, with a mean and median follow-up of 6.7 and 8.0 years, respectively. Nine (41%) of the patients experienced a permanent clinical deterioration after the treatment, three from complications, four from hemorrhages, and two from both of them. Six patients developed radiation-induced complications; in five of them the complications were permanent, but two of the five patients suffered from a hemorrhage as well, which contributed to the clinical symptoms. Nine patients hemorrhaged after the treatment. Our conclusion was that "the high incidence of radiation-induced complications does not seem to justify the limited protection the treatment may afford in only exceptional cases. A prospective randomized study is needed before the role of radiosurgery in the management of these lesions can be defined. Until such study has proved differently, a caveat must be raised for the treatment of [cavernous malformation] with [Gamma Knife surgery]." It is clear that this opinion is also valid in 2009. The use of radiosurgery in the management of cavernomas is still controversial. When comparing outcomes from different studies, no relation was found between incidence of complications and post treatment hemorrhages, as illustrated in **Fig. 7.3.** The decrease in the risk for hemorrhage following radiosurgery for cavernomas seems limited. It is, however, clear that the risk for complications is high. In conclusion, radiosurgery should be used, if at all, with care when managing cavernomas, and lower rather than higher doses should be used.

References

1. Karlsson B, Lax I, Yamamoto M, et al. Calculation of isoeffective doses and α/β value by comparing results following radiosurgery and radiotherapy for brain AVMs. J Neurosurg 2006;105:183–189
2. Gonzalez LF, Lekovic G, Eschbacher J, Coons S, Porter R, Spetzler R. Are cavernous sinus hemangiomas and cavernous malformations different entities? Neurosurg Focus 2006;21:e6
3. Johnson P, Wascher T, Golfinos J, Spetzler R. Definition and pathological feature. In: Awad I, Barrow D, eds. Cavernous Malformations. Park Ridge, IL:, American Association of Neurological Surgeons; 1993:1–11
4. Mathiesen T, Edner G, Kihlström L. Deep and brainstem cavernomas: a consecutive 8-year series. J Neurosurg 2003;99(1):31–37

5. Linskey ME, Shekar L. Cavernous sinus hemangiomas: a series, a review and a hypothesis. Neurosurgery 1992;30:101–108
6. Shibata S, Mori K. Effect of radiation therapy on extracerebral cavernous hemangioma in the middle fossa: report of three cases. J Neurosurg 1987;67:919–922
7. Maruishi M, Shima T, Okada Y, Nashida M, Yamane K, and Okita S. cavernous sinus cavernoma treated with radiation therapy–case report. Neurol Med Chir (Tokyo) 1994;34:773–777
8. Iwai Y, Yamanaka K, Nakajima H, Yasui T. Stereotactic radiosurgery for cavernous sinus cavernous hemangioma—case report. Neurol Med Chir (Tokyo) 1999;39:288–290
9. Seo Y, Fukuoka S, Sasaki T, Takanashi M, Hojo A, Nakamura H. Cavernous sinus hemangioma treated with Gamma Knife radiosurgery: usefulness of SPECT for diagnosis—case report. Neurol Med Chir (Tokyo) 2000;40: 575–580
10. Thompson TP, Lunsford L, Flickinger J. Radiosurgery for hemangiomas of the cavernous sinus and orbit: technical case report. Neurosurgery 2000;47:778–783
11. Kida Y, Kobayashi T, Mori Y. Radiosurgery of cavernous hemangiomas in the cavernous sinus. Surg Neurol 2001;56:117–122
12. Nakamura N, Shin M, Tago M, et al. Gamma Knife radiosurgery for cavernous hemangiomas in the cavernous sinus: report of three cases. J Neurosurg 2002;97:477–480
13. Peker S, Kiliç T, Sengöz M, Pamir M. Radiosurgical treatment of cavernous sinus cavernous haemangiomas. Acta Neurochir (Wien) 2004; 146:337–341
14. Bartolomei F, Régis J, Kida Y, et al. Gamma Knife radiosurgery for epilepsy associated with cavernous hemangiomas: a retrospective study of 49 cases. Stereotact Funct Neurosurg 1999;72:22–28
15. Régis J, Bartolomei F, Kida Y, et al. Radiosurgery for epilepsy associated with cavernous malformation: retrospective study in 49 patients. Neurosurgery 2000;47:1091–1097
16. Hsu PW, Chang C, Tseng C, et al. Treatment of epileptogenic cavernomas: surgery versus radiosurgery. Cerebrovasc Dis 2007;24: 116–120
17. Amin-Hanjani S, Ogilvy C, Candia G, Lyons S, Chapman P. Stereotactic radiosurgery for cavernous malformations: Kjellberg's experience with proton beam therapy in 98 cases at the Harvard Cyclotron. Neurosurgery 1998;42:1229–1236
18. Chang SD, Levy R, Adler JJ, Martin D, Krakovitz P, Steinberg G. Stereotactic radiosurgery of angiographically occult vascular malformations: 14-year experience. Neurosurgery 1998;43:213–220
19. Huang Y, Tseng C, Chang C, Wei K, Liao C, and Hsu P. LINAC radiosurgery for intracranial cavernous malformation: 10-year experience. Clin Neurol Neurosurg 2006;108:750–756
20. Kida Y, Kobayashi T, and Tanaka T. Treatment of symptomatic AVOMs with radiosurgery. Acta Neurochir (Wien) 1995;63:68–72
21. Liscák R, Vladyka V, Simonová G, Vymazal J, Novotny JJ. Gamma Knife surgery of brain cavernous hemangiomas. J Neurosurg 2005;102: 207–213
22. Liu KD, Chung W, Wu H, et al. Gamma Knife surgery for cavernous hemangiomas: an analysis of 125 patients. J Neurosurg 2005; 102: 81–86
23. Stea RA, Schicker L, King G, Winfield J. Stereotactic linear radiosurgery for cavernous angiomas. Stereotact Funct Neurosurg 1994; 63:255–265
24. Tsien C, Souhami L, Sadikot A, et al. Stereotactic radiosurgery in the management of angiographically occult vascular malformations. Int J Radiat Oncol Biol Phys 2001;50(1):133–138
25. Zhang N, Pan L, Wang B, Wang E, Dai J, Cai P. Gamma Knife radiosurgery for cavernous hemangiomas. J Neurosurg 2000;93:74–77
26. Chang SD, Steinberg G, Levy R, et al. Microsurgical resection of incompletely obliterated intracranial arteriovenous malformations following stereotactic radiosurgery. Neurol Med Chir (Tokyo) 1998;38: 200–207
27. Chang SD, Shuster D, Steinberg G, Levy R, Frankel K. Stereotactic radiosurgery of arteriovenous malformations: pathologic changes in resected tissue. Clin Neuropathol 1997;16:111–116
28. Elisevich K, Redekop G, Munoz D, Fisher B, Wiese K, Drake C. Neuropathology of intracranial arteriovenous malformations following conventional radiation therapy. Stereotact Funct Neurosurg 1994;63: 250–254
29. Schneider BF, Eberhard D, Steiner L. Histopathology of arteriovenous malformations after Gamma Knife radiosurgery. J Neurosurg 1997;87: 352–357
30. Steinberg GK, Chang S, Levy R, Marks M, Frankel K, Marcellus M. Surgical resection of large incompletely treated intracranial arteriovenous malformations following stereotactic radiosurgery. J Neurosurg 1996; 84:920–928
31. Yamamoto M, Jimbo M, Kobayashi M, et al. Long-term results of radiosurgery for arteriovenous malformation: neurodiagnostic imaging and histological studies of angiographically confirmed nidus obliteration. Surg Neurol 1992;37:219–230
32. Yamamoto M, Jimbo M, Ide M, et al. Gamma Knife radiosurgery for cerebral arteriovenous malformations: an autopsy report focusing on irradiation-induced changes observed in nidus-unrelated arteries. Surg Neurol 1995;44:421–427
33. Szeifert GT, Timperley W, Forster D, Kemeny A. Histopathological changes in cerebral arteriovenous malformations following Gamma Knife radiosurgery. Prog Neurol Surg 2007;20:212–219
34. Gewirtz RJ, Steinberg G, Crowley R, Levy R. Pathological changes in surgically resected angiographically occult vascular malformations after radiation. Neurosurgery 1998;42(4):738–742
35. Nyáry I, Major O, Hanzély Z, Szeifert G. Histopathological findings in a surgically resected thalamic cavernous hemangioma 1 year after 40-Gy irradiation. J Neurosurg 2005;102:56–58
36. Seo Y, Fukuoka S, Takanashi M, et al. Gamma Knife surgery for angiographically occult vascular malformations. Stereotact Funct Neurosurg 1995;64:98–109
37. Del Curling O Jr, Kelly DJ, Elster A, Craven T. An analysis of the natural history of cavernous angiomas. J Neurosurg 1991;75:702–708
38. Kim DS, Park Y, Choi J, Chung S, Lee K. An analysis of the natural history of cavernous malformations. Surg Neurol 1997;48:9–17
39. Kondziolka D, Lunsford LD, Kestle J. The natural history of cerebral cavernous malformations. J Neurosurg 1995;83:820–824
40. Karlsson B, Lindquist C, Johansson A, Steiner L. Annual risk for the first hemorrhage from untreated arteriovenous malformations. Minim Invasive Neurosurg 1997;40:40–46
41. Robinson JR, Awad I, Little J. Natural history of the cavernous angioma. J Neurosurg 1991;75:709–714
42. Zabramski JM, Wascher T, Spetzler R, et al. The natural history of familial cavernous malformations: results of an ongoing study. J Neurosurg 1994;80:422–432
43. Moriarity JL, Wetzel M, Clatterbuck R, et al. The natural history of cavernous malformations: a prospective study of 68 patients. Neurosurgery 1999;44:1166–1174
44. Kida Y, Kobayashi T, Tanaka T. Treatment of symptomatic AOVMs with radiosurgery. Acta Neurochir Suppl (Wien) 1995;63:68–72
45. Huang YC, Tseng C, Chang C, Wei K, Liao C, Hsu P. Linac radiosurgery for intracranial cavernous malformation: 10-year experience. Clin Neurol Neurosurg 2006;108:750–756
46. Kim DG, Choe W, Paek S, Chung H, Kim I, Han D. Radiosurgery of intracranial cavernous malformations. Acta Neurochir (Wien) 2002;144:869–878
47. Pollock BE, Garces Y, Stafford S, Foote R, Schomberg P, Link M. Stereotactic radiosurgery for cavernous malformations. J Neurosurg 2000; 93:987–991
48. Hasegawa T, McInerney J, Kondziolka D, Lee J, Flickinger J, Lunsford L. Long-term results after stereotactic radiosurgery for patients with cavernous malformations. Neurosurgery 2002;50:1190–1198
49. Liscak R, Vladyka V, Simonova G, Vymazal J, Novotny JJ. Gamma Knife radiosurgery of the brain stem cavernomas. Minim Invasive Neurosurg 2000;43:201–207
50. Kondziolka D, Lunsford LD, Flickinger JC, Kestle J. Reduction of hemorrhage risk after stereotactic radiosurgery for cavernous malformations. J Neurosurg 1995;83:825–831
51. Karlsson B, Kihlström L, Lindquist C, Ericson K, Steiner L. Radiosurgery for cavernous malformations. J Neurosurg 1998;88:293–297
52. Mitchell P, Hodgson T, Seaman S, Kemeny A, Forster D. Stereotactic radiosurgery and the risk of haemorrhage from cavernous malformations. Br J Neurosurg 2000;14:96–100
53. Steinberg GK, Levy R, Fabrikant J, Frankel K. Phillips MH. Stereotactic helium ion Bragg peak radiosurgery for angiographically occult intracranial vascular malformations. Stereotact Funct Neurosurg 1991;57:64–71
54. Lax I, Karlsson B. Prediction of complications in Gamma Knife radiosurgery of arteriovenous malformation. Acta Oncol 1996;35:49–55
55. Takenaka N, Imanishi T, Sasaki H, et al. Delayed radiation necrosis with extensive brain edema after Gamma Knife radiosurgery for multiple cerebral cavernous malformations—case report. Neurol Med Chir (Tokyo) 2003;43:391–395

8

Stereotactic Radiosurgery for Meningiomas

Douglas Kondziolka, David Mathieu, Ricky Madhok, John C. Flickinger, and L. Dade Lunsford

Meningiomas are common intracranial tumors that pose a variety of therapeutic challenges because of brain location, size, histologic subtype, and patient characteristics. Over time, craniotomy and tumor resection along with its dural base became the preferred approach for the majority of symptomatic patients.[1] The morbidity of resection was reduced with microneurosurgical technique, better anesthesia, neuronavigation, and improved medical care. However, because these usually benign tumors may be associated closely with critical neural or vascular structures, complete resection may not be feasible.[2–5] Meningiomas adjacent to venous sinuses may be resectable only at the risk of major neurologic deficits caused by venous injury. Elderly or infirm patients often sought alternative approaches. In this chapter we review our experience in the care of over 1000 patients with intracranial meningiomas. We have found that stereotactic radiosurgery safely provided high rates of tumor growth control or regression in patients with small to medium-sized benign tumors.

◆ Patient Characteristics

Over a 20-year period, we performed radiosurgery on 1191 intracranial meningiomas. We recently reviewed the results from the first 972 patients with 1045 tumors managed over the initial 18 years. The brain locations of these tumors are shown in **Table 8.1.** The decision to perform radiosurgery was made in patients with residual or recurrent smaller volume tumors after prior resection, those with symptomatic primary tumors in locations associated with higher risk for resection, those with concomitant medical illnesses or advanced age, in younger patients who chose radiosurgery over other available options, and in younger patients with minimal symptoms or who were asymptomatic but chose against observation. Contraindications or exclusion criteria included large tumor volume (mean diameter > 3.5 cm), tumors with symptomatic optic nerve or chiasmal compression, optic nerve sheath tumors with preserved vision, elderly patients with asymptomatic tumors, and tumors with atypical imaging features and no prior histologic diagnosis. The detailed results from 982 tumors (94%) were available for analysis. Five hundred and four patients (51%) had no prior treatment. Prior surgical resections were usually partial removals (84%). A solitary tumor was present in 818 patients and multiple tumors in 161. Twenty-eight patients had neurofibromatosis type 2. Tumor pathology was known in 511 residual or recurrent tumors. Prior radiotherapy had been delivered to 54 patients (48 after a resection, and 6 had radiotherapy alone);

Table 8.1 Locations of 1045 Intracranial Meningiomas

Location	Number of Tumors
Posterior fossa	
Petroclival	122
Petrous ridge	66
Foramen magnum	22
Other	42
Middle fossa	
Cavernous sinus	306
Sphenoid wing	32
Other	13
Anterior fossa	
Olfactory groove	29
Planum sphenoidale	29
Anterior clinoid	17
Parasellar	13
Convexity	126
Other	
Parasagittal	113
Tentorial notch	40
Torcular	6
Falcine	47
Intraorbital	13
Intraventricular	9

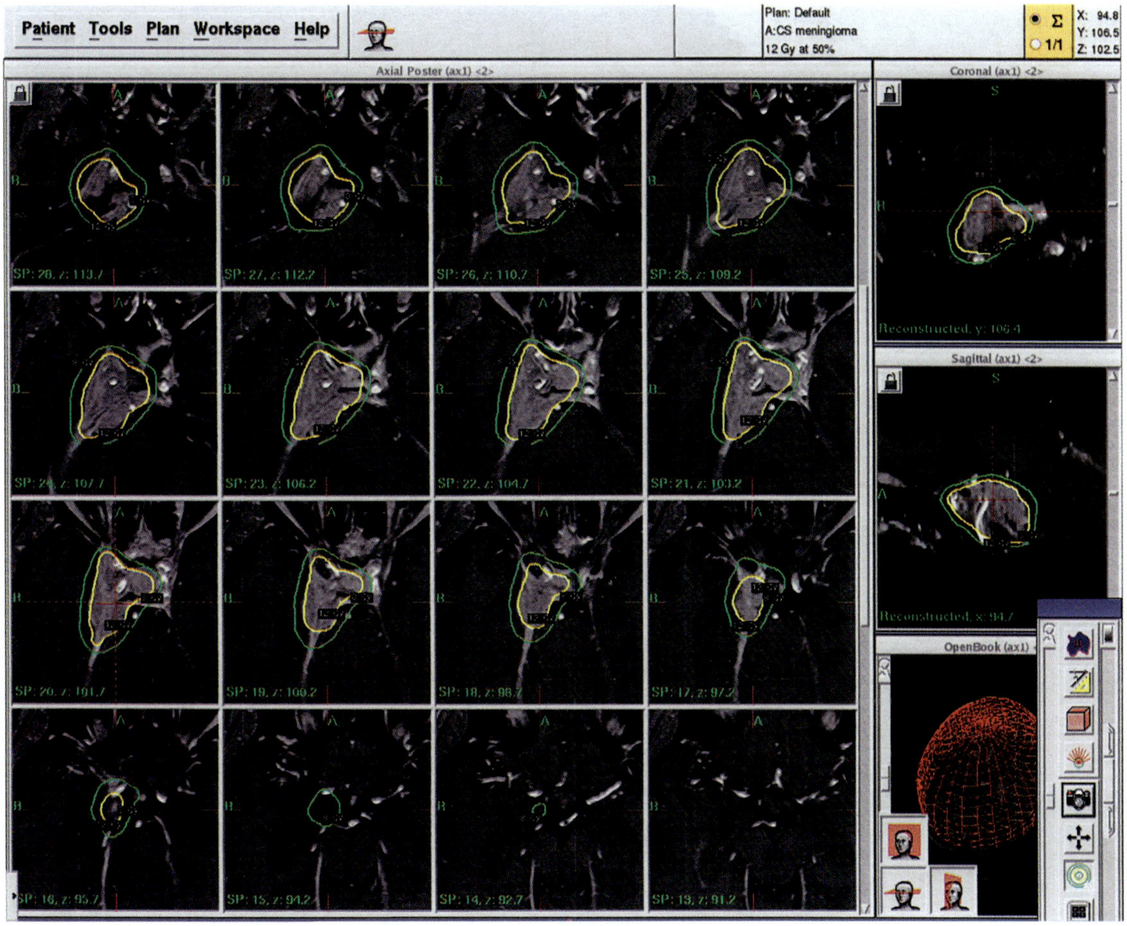

Fig. 8.1 Gamma Knife radiosurgery plan for a 43-year-old woman with a right cavernous sinus meningioma who presented with diplopia. The tumor was planned with 24 isocenters using the Perfexion model Gamma Knife (4, 8, and 16 mm collimators) to deliver a margin dose of 12 Gy and a maximum dose of 24 Gy.

2 patients had prior radiosurgery elsewhere. Eight patients had received chemotherapy. Twenty-five tumors (2.5%) developed after prior fractionated irradiation.

Radiosurgery was performed under local anesthesia with mild sedation as necessary, using a Leksell Gamma Knife (Elekta Instruments AB, Stockholm, Sweden). We have used the Gamma Knife models U, B, C, 4C, and Perfexion for our patients with meningiomas. Radiosurgery was targeted with stereotactic computed tomography (CT) guidance (before 1992) and with magnetic resonance imaging (MRI) since. A mean of 7.5 isocenters were used to provide conformal radiosurgery. The dose received by adjacent critical structures was determined and selective beam blocking used if necessary to restrict the dose fall-off (**Fig. 8.1**). We delivered a mean dose to the tumor margin of 14 Gy and a mean maximum dose of 28 Gy. The mean tumor volume in this series was 7.4 mL. The mean volume receiving ≥ 12 Gy was 8.4 mL. Radiation doses were prescribed to the 50% isodose volume for 886 tumors (85%). For tumors near the optic nerve or chiasm, the average maximal optic dose was 6.4 Gy. After radiosurgery, patients were discharged home within 24 hours, and in recent years on the same day. The median follow-up in this study was 4 years; 842 patients were still living (86%). Follow-up past 5, 7, 10, and 12 years was obtained in 327, 190, 90, and 41 patients, respectively.

◆ Tumor Response to Radiosurgery

Imaging studies after radiosurgery showed that 407 tumors had regressed, 454 were unchanged, and 96 had enlarged, for a raw tumor control rate of 90%. Imaging and clinical follow-up were requested for all patients, but they were not complete for all.

Adjuvant Radiosurgery

Based on prior histopathology, we had 424 World Health Organization (WHO) grade 1 meningiomas in this series, and 384 were available for study. We found that 172 tumors had regressed, 186 were unchanged, and 26 had enlarged for a tumor control rate of 93%, at a median of 4 years. Ninety-one percent of patients were either improved (n = 21) or unchanged ($n = 341$) clinically. Imaging follow-up past 8 and 10 years was obtained in 79 and 53 tumors, respectively, both with a control rate of 91%. Past 10 years, 45 patients were stable, 6 were improved, and 2 were worse. For grade 1 meningiomas, the 5-, 10-, and 15-year actuarial tumor control rates were 97.0 + 1.2%, 87.2 + 4.4%, and 87.2 + 4.4%, respectively. Disease-specific survival was 98.9 + 0.5%, 96.2 + 1.9%, and 96.2 + 1.9%, respectively.

Of 56 WHO grade 2 tumors, 54 were available for review. Sixteen had regressed, 11 were unchanged, and 27 had enlarged for a tumor control rate of 50%, at a median of 2 years. During follow-up, 72% of these patients were stable clinically. Of 31 WHO grade 3 tumors, 29 were reviewed. We found that 4 regressed, 1 was stable, and 24 later enlarged, for a tumor control rate of 17% at a median of 15 months.

Primary Radiosurgery

There were 536 tumors that received radiosurgery as primary management without a prior biopsy (**Fig. 8.2**). All patients had typical imaging features. We were able to evaluate later serial images for 488 tumors. We found that 215 tumors had regressed, 256 were unchanged, and 19 had enlarged for a tumor control rate of 97%, at a median of 4 years. Ninety-three percent of patients with these tumors either improved neurologically ($n = 87$) or remained unchanged ($n = 380$). Imaging follow-up past 8 and 10 years was obtained in 49 and 22 tumors, respectively, with control rates of 94 and 95%. Past 10 years, 16 patients were stable, 3 were improved, and 3 were worse.

Subsequent surgical resection was performed in 51 patients (5.2%) due to local tumor growth or increased symptoms, at an average time of 35 months. Additional fractionated radiotherapy was used in 2.9%, and further radiosurgery was performed in 41 patients (4%), usually for new tumors, at an average of 4 years. No patient developed a radiation-induced tumor.

◆ The Morbidity of Radiosurgery

After radiosurgery, all patients returned to their preoperative activities immediately. Postradiosurgery nausea or other immediate symptoms were rare, although one patient developed

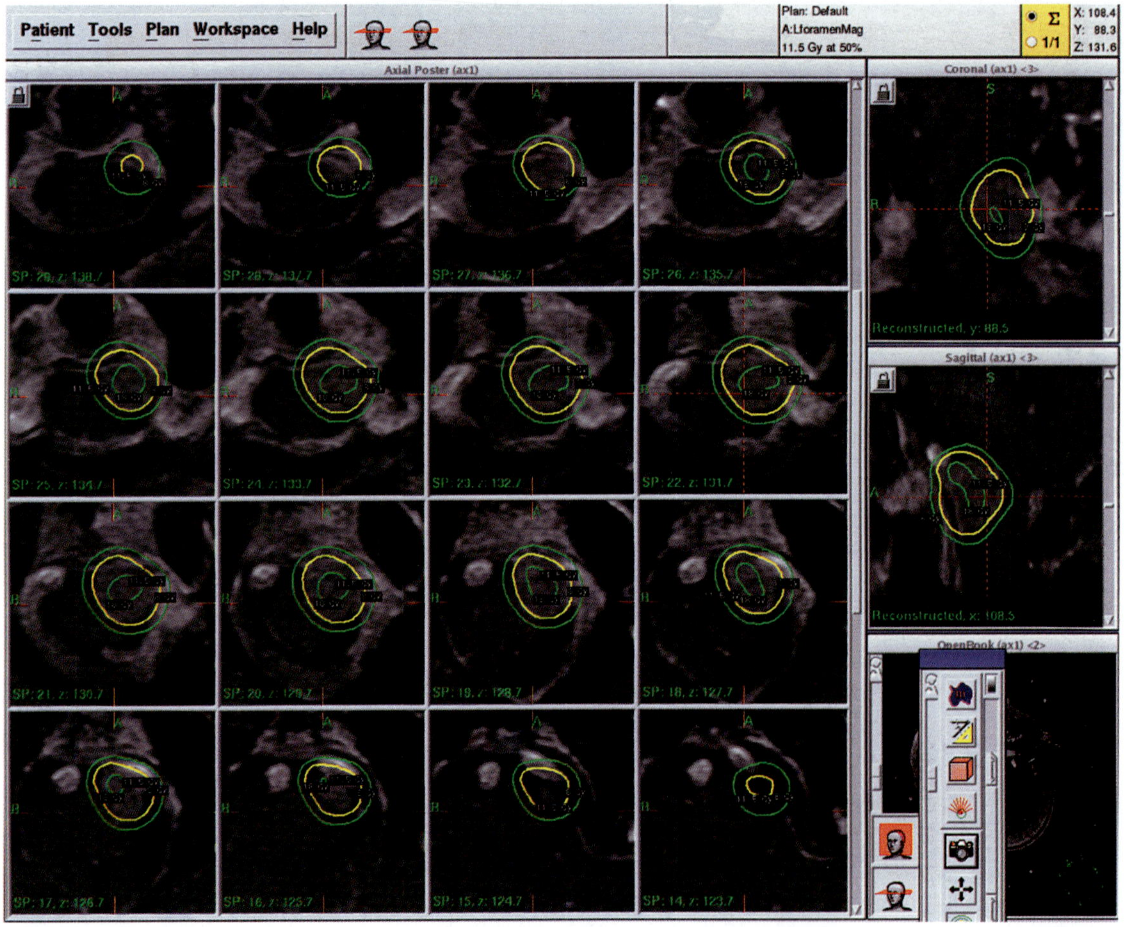

Fig. 8.2 Gamma Knife radiosurgery plan for a 77-year-old woman with an enlarging meningioma at the cervicomedullary junction. The tumor was planned with seven isocenters using the Perfexion model Gamma Knife (4 and 8 mm collimators with sector beam blocking to restrict the dose toward the spinal cord). A margin dose of 11.5 Gy and a maximum dose of 23.0 Gy were delivered.

pneumonia 1 week after radiosurgery and died. A complication attributed to radiosurgery was observed in 76 patients (7.7%), at an average time of 11 months. The morbidity rates for cavernous sinus location and parasagittal locations were 6.3 and 9.7%, respectively. For cavernous sinus tumors, these included cranial nerve deficits in 12 patients. Four of these had diplopia, and two had trigeminal neuropathy (one having neuralgic pain). Six patients had decreased visual acuity, and four of them had prior treatment that included multiple resections ($n = 3$), multiple radiosurgeries ($n = 2$), radiation therapy ($n = 3$), and chemotherapy ($n = 1$).

The 10- and 15-year actuarial complication rates were both 9.1%. Specifically, hydrocephalus was found in 0.4%, a cranial nerve deficit in 3.4%, headaches in 2.2%, seizures in 2.4%, a motor deficit in 1.4%, and a sensory deficit in 0.3%. Complete improvement was noted in 35% of patients who sustained morbidity. Imaging showed interval development of tumoral signal abnormalities determined by long relaxation time MR images in 6.2% of patients, with 4% of the total series having symptomatic imaging changes at an average of 8 months. A ventriculoperitoneal shunt was placed in five patients (0.5%), at an average of 20 months.

Multivariate Analyses

The results of multivariate analyses of survival, disease-free survival, and local control showed that poorer overall survival significantly correlated with increasing WHO grade 0 to 3 (0 for no tissue diagnosis; [$p = 3.9385 \times 10^{-11}$]) and increasing volume ($p = .0407$). Poorer intracranial tumor control correlated with increasing WHO grade 0 to 3, increasing tumor volume, and multiple meningiomas.

Univariate and multivariate analyses of postradiosurgery complications and new imaging changes on MRI were studied. Both volume and 12 Gy volume significantly correlated with the development of postradiosurgery complications and new T2 changes in univariate testing ($p < .0001$), whereas in multivariate analysis, volume correlated with complications.

◆ Indications for Radiosurgery

Over the past 2 decades, the indications for meningioma radiosurgery have expanded to patients with newly diagnosed as opposed to recurrent or residual tumors after initial resection.[6–23] How good are neurosurgeons in making the diagnosis of a benign meningioma based on imaging alone? In long-term follow-up, we found that the initial imaging-based diagnosis of a benign meningioma was not correct in 2.3% (usually proven to be a higher grade meningioma).[24] As primary management, radiosurgery is not appropriate for patients with large meningiomas, for patients with significant symptomatic mass effect, and for patients with optic nerve sheath tumors and preserved vision. Although some surgeons advocate tumor debulking in symptomatic patients (who are then simply followed to see if the residual tumor enlarges), the literature substantiates high recurrence and progression rates after such management. Condra et al found a 70% rate of tumor progression after subtotal resection without fractionated radiation therapy.[25] Other groups have noted the value of postresection irradiation.[26,27] One series found a mean 4 mm annual rate of tumor growth after partial resection of a basal meningioma.[28] We advocate that the entire neoplasm be treated using the most appropriate modalities (when safe and feasible), including complete resection, resection plus radiosurgery for residual tumors, or radiosurgery alone for small-volume tumors in critical locations. We believe that this strategy will provide better long-term outcomes than managing only a portion of the tumor.

Donald Simpson's often cited report described meningioma recurrence rates based on the degree and description of the resection.[29] He reported a 9% recurrence rate after "complete resection" of the tumor and its neoplastic dural base; a 19% recurrence rate when the tumor was "resected" and the dural base only coagulated; a 29% recurrence rate when the tumor itself was removed, but the dura could not be excised or cauterized; and an ~40% recurrence rate when only a subtotal resection was performed. In the modern era, even higher recurrence rates have been noted.[30] Pollock et al studied 136 patients after resection and 62 after radiosurgery with a mean follow-up of 64 months.[31] Their recurrence rates after resection were remarkably similar to the findings of Simpson over 40 years prior. Tumor recurrence was more frequent in the resection group (12% vs 2%; $p = .04$). There was no difference in recurrence rates for patients after a Simpson grade 1 resection, but radiosurgery provided more durable control after grade 2 ($p < .05$) or grade 3–4 resections ($p < .001$).[32] Thus, one could conclude that the results of radiosurgery for a smaller tumor are equal to or better than after a resection, depending on the degree of resection expected. For a "resectable" smaller volume meningioma (i.e., convexity, falcine, or anterior fossa location), other patient factors besides brain location must be considered. We believe that our patient series indicates that radiosurgery can be an effective and safe option for such patients.

Patients undergoing outpatient radiosurgery have not been exposed to the risks related to an open surgical exposure, brain retraction, anesthesia, or a prolonged hospital stay. However, is this of value? In a prior review of 5- to 10-year outcomes in our initial patients, we surveyed patients for their own opinions regarding outcomes.[14] Sixty-five patients answered our questions regarding employment. Twenty-seven patients (42%) were employed at the time of radiosurgery, and 20 remained so (74%). Of 35 patients not employed at radiosurgery, 5 (14%) resumed employment. Patients described their overall level of activity as remaining unchanged in 65%, being increased in 8%, or decreased in 27%. Radiosurgery was described as a "successful" procedure by 67 of 70 patients (96%).[14]

◆ Summary

Stereotactic radiosurgery is a powerful biologic approach for a patient with an intracranial meningioma. It is well tolerated and can be performed on an outpatient basis.[32] Excellent long-term outcomes can be expected in the majority of patients.

References

1. Newman SA. Meningiomas: a quest for the optimum therapy. J Neurosurg 1994;80:191–194
2. Borovich B, Doron Y. Recurrence of intracranial meningiomas: the role played by regional multicentricity. J Neurosurg 1986;64:58–63
3. Kallio M, Sankira R, Hakulinen T, Jaaskelainen J. Factors affecting operative and excess long-term mortality in 935 patients with intracranial meningioma. Neurosurgery 1992;31:2–12
4. Mahmood A, Qureshi NH, Malik GM. Intracranial meningiomas: analysis of recurrence after surgical treatment. Acta Neurochir (Wien) 1994;126:53–58
5. Naumann M, Meixensberger J. Factors influencing meningioma recurrence rate. Acta Neurochir (Wien) 1990;107:108–111
6. Chang SD, Adler J. Treatment of cranial base meningiomas with linear accelerator radiosurgery. Neurosurgery 1997;41:1019–1027
7. DiBiase SJ, Kwok Y, Yovino S, et al. Factors predicting local tumor control after Gamma Knife stereotactic radiosurgery for benign intracranial meningiomas. Int J Radiat Oncol Biol Phys 2004;60:1515–1519
8. Duma CM, Lunsford LD, Kondziolka D, Harsh G, Flickinger JC. Stereotactic radiosurgery of cavernous sinus meningiomas as an addition or alternative to microsurgery. Neurosurgery 1993;32:699–705
9. Friedman WA, Murad G, Bradshaw P, et al. Linear accelerator surgery for meningiomas. J Neurosurg 2005;103:206–209
10. Hakim R, Alexander E, Loeffler JS, et al. Results of linear accelerator-based radiosurgery for intracranial meningiomas. Neurosurgery 1998; 42:446–454
11. Kobayashi T, Kida Y, Mori Y. Long-term results of stereotactic Gamma Knife radiosurgery of meningiomas. Surg Neurol 2001;55:325–331
12. Kondziolka D, Flickinger JC, Perez B. Judicious resection and/or radiosurgery for parasagittal meningiomas: outcomes from the Gamma Knife meningioma study group. Neurosurgery 1998;43:405–414
13. Kondziolka D, Lunsford LD, Coffey RJ, Flickinger J. Stereotactic radiosurgery of meningiomas. J Neurosurg 1991;74:552–559
14. Kondziolka D, Levy E, Niranjan A, Flickinger J, Lunsford LD. Long-term outcomes after meningioma radiosurgery: physicians and patients perspective. J Neurosurg 1999;91:44–50
15. Kreil W, Luggin J, Fuchs I, Weigl V, Eustacchio S, Papaefthymious G. Long-term experience of Gamma Knife radiosurgery for benign skull base meningiomas. J Neurol Neurosurg Psychiatry 2005;76:1425–1430
16. Lee JYK, Niranjan A, McInerney J, Kondziolka D, Flickinger JC, Lunsford LD. Stereotactic radiosurgery provides long-term tumor control of cavernous sinus meningiomas. J Neurosurg 2002;97:65–72
17. Lunsford LD. Contemporary management of meningiomas: radiation therapy as an adjuvant and radiosurgery as an alternative to surgical removal? J Neurosurg 1994;80:187–190
18. Nicolato A, Foroni R, Alessandrini F, Bricolo A, Gerosa M. Radiosurgical treatment of cavernous sinus meningiomas: experience with 122 treated patients. Neurosurgery 2002;51:1153–1161
19. Pendl G, Schrottner O, Eustacchio S, Feichtinger K, Ganz J. Stereotactic radiosurgery of skull base meningiomas. Minim Invasive Neurosurg 1997;40:87–90
20. Pollock BE, Stafford SL. Results of stereotactic radiosurgery for patients with imaging defined cavernous sinus meningiomas. Int J Radiat Oncol Biol Phys 2005;62:1427–1431
21. Roche PH, Regis J, Dufour H, et al. Gamma Knife radiosurgery in the management of cavernous sinus meningiomas. J Neurosurg 2000;93(Suppl 3):68–73
22. Subach BR, Lunsford LD, Kondziolka D, Bissonette D, Flickinger J. Stereotactic radiosurgery for petroclival meningiomas. Neurosurgery 1998;42:437–445
23. Zachenhofer I, Wolfsberger S, Aichholzer M, et al. Gamma Knife radiosurgery for cranial base meningiomas: experience of tumor control, clinical course, and morbidity in a follow-up more than 8 years. Neurosurgery 2006;58:28–36
24. Flickinger JC, Kondziolka D, Maitz A, Lunsford LD. Gamma Knife radiosurgery of imaging-defined intracranial meningioma. Int J Radiat Oncol Biol Phys 2003;56:801–806
25. Condra KS, Buatti J, Mendenhall W, Friedman WA, Marcus R, Rhoton AL. Benign meningiomas: primary treatment selection affects survival. Int J Radiat Oncol Biol Phys 1997;39:427–436
26. Goldsmith BJ, Wara WM, Wilson CB, Larson DA. Postoperative irradiation for subtotally resected meningiomas: a retrospective analysis of 140 patients treated from 1967 to 1990. J Neurosurg 1994;80:195–201
27. Maire JP, Caudry M, Guerin J, et al. Fractionated radiation therapy in the treatment of intracranial meningiomas: local control, functional efficacy, and tolerance in 91 patients. Int J Radiat Oncol Biol Phys 1995;33:315–321
28. Jung HW, Yoo H, Paek SH, Choi KS. Long-term outcome and growth rate of subtotally resected petroclival meningiomas: experience with 38 cases. Neurosurgery 2000;46:567–575
29. Simpson D. The recurrence of intracranial meningiomas after surgical treatment. J Neurol Neurosurg Psychiatry 1957;20:22–39
30. Sankila R, Kallio M, Jaaskelained J, Hakulinen T. Long-term survival of 1986 patients with intracranial meningiomas diagnosed from 1953 to 1984 in Finland. Cancer 1992;70:1568–1576
31. Pollock BE, Stafford SL, Utter A, Giannini C, Schreiner SA. Stereotactic radiosurgery provides equivalent tumor control to Simpson grade 1 resection for patients with small to medium size meningiomas. Int J Radiat Oncol Biol Phys 2003;55:1000–1005
32. Kondziolka D, Nathoo N, Flickinger JC, Niranjan A, Maitz AH, Lunsford LD. Long-term results after radiosurgery for benign intracranial tumors. Neurosurgery 2003;53:815–822

9

Stereotactic Radiosurgery for Pituitary Adenomas

Jay Jagannathan, David J. Schlesinger, Rod J. Oskouian Jr., Nader Pouratian, John A. Jane Jr., Edward R. Laws, Mary Lee Vance, and Jason P. Sheehan

Pituitary adenomas represent 10 to 20% of all primary brain tumors.[1,2] Lesions are broadly classified into two groups, depending on the presence or absence of secreted pituitary hormones. Tumors that secrete an excessive amount of a hormone are associated with various clinical syndromes. The most common secretory adenoma is the prolactinoma, which results in amenorrhea–galactorrhea syndrome and infertility in women and impotence and infertility in men. Growth hormone–secreting pituitary adenomas cause acromegaly in adults and gigantism in children, and tumors secreting adrenocorticotropic hormone (ACTH) cause Cushing's syndrome.

Nonsecretory tumors, which do not secrete biologically active pituitary hormones, account for ~30% of all pituitary adenomas. Adenomas in this group enlarge progressively in the pituitary fossa and often extend beyond the sella turcica.[3] Tumor enlargement may cause local effects, including compression of the optic apparatus and visual field dysfunction. Patients with larger tumors might also have headache from elevated intracranial pressure and hypopituitarism resulting from compression of the normal pituitary gland.

◆ Patient Evaluation

All patients suspected of harboring a pituitary tumor should undergo a complete neurologic, ophthalmologic, endocrinologic, and radiologic workup. This includes formal visual field and acuity testing and a dilated funduscopic examination.[2,4] Each facet of the hypothalamic-pituitary-end organ axis should be assessed. Mild elevations in serum prolactin commonly result from a stalk effect, and levels > 200 ng/mL suggest a prolactin-secreting adenoma. Thyroid function is evaluated by measuring free thyroxine and thyroid-stimulating hormone (TSH). Adrenal function is assessed by a morning serum cortisol and ACTH level. In cases of suspected Cushing's syndrome, a 24-hour urinary free cortisol (UFC) test and a dexamethasone suppression test are performed. Serum growth hormone and insulin like growth factor-1 (IGF-1) levels are measured to evaluate for acromegaly.[5] Oral glucose tolerance with GH measurement is the definitive test in cases of suspected growth hormone–secreting tumors.[6] In children, a radiograph should be obtained to assess bone age in relation to chronological age.

Radiologic evaluation is achieved with thin-slice pre- and postcontrast magnetic resonance (MR) images of the sellar region. Computed tomography (CT) images may be useful to assess the degree of sinus aeration, particularly in younger patients who often have an underpneumatized sphenoid sinus.[7,8]

If a patient has a neurologic deficit attributable to an adenoma, surgery is the initial treatment of choice for all tumors except a prolactinoma. Transsphenoidal surgery (endoscopic or microscopic) allows for the most rapid relief of mass effect and reduction in excessive hormone levels in patients with Cushing disease and acromegaly.[1,4,9–11] This approach is associated with a low rate of complications in the hands of an experienced neurosurgeon.[12]

◆ History and Evolution of Stereotactic Radiosurgery for Pituitary Adenomas

Radiation therapy was originally the adjuvant treatment of choice for recurrent or residual pituitary adenomas, with reports dating to the early 20th century. However, conventional radiotherapy had several limitations. The time to hormonal normalization was slow, and the rate of postprocedural hypopituitarism was high. Side effects of conventional radiation treatment included cognitive difficulty, neuropsychological deficits, visual dysfunction from optic neuropathy, stroke, and damage to other cranial nerves.

The advantage of stereotactic radiosurgery is that it delivers a high and tightly focused dose of radiation to a tumor in a single session. This single-session approach has a clear radiobiological advantage in late-responding tumors such as pituitary adenomas. With the aid of neuroimaging guidance, a steep radiation fall-off, and shielding achieved through blocking patterns, the surrounding tissues are largely spared from the harmful effects of radiation.[13] This is particularly important in pituitary adenomas, as tumors may be located within millimeters of the cavernous sinus and optic apparatus.

Shortly after radiosurgery's development, Lars Leksell treated patients with pituitary tumors using the Gamma Knife (Elekta Instruments AB, Stockholm, Sweden); original localization was achieved through use of plain radiographs of the sella.[14] Since that time, stereotactic radiosurgery with the Gamma Knife or modified linear accelerators (linacs) has been used in thousands of pituitary adenoma patients to control adenoma growth and normalize hormone overproduction.[15–17] At the same time, great attention and effort in the field of stereotactic radiosurgery have been placed on the preservation of surrounding neuronal, vascular, and hormonal structures.

Radiosurgical Treatment Options for Pituitary Tumors

Several radiosurgical treatment options exist for the pituitary, each with potential advantages and limitations. Proton beam radiosurgery was one of the earliest modalities used for the treatment of pituitary tumors.[18,19] This technique takes advantage of the superior dose distribution of protons versus photons, due to the peak in the energy distribution of protons ("Bragg peak") before they come to rest at the treatment depth.[13] This gives the theoretical advantage of producing very little lateral disruption. Proton beam therapy can be used in the treatment of deep-seated lesions in the sella or near the cavernous sinus. Early studies on proton beam radiosurgery were complicated by high rates of hypopituitarism, a factor likely related to the nascent treatment planning of the time.[18] Reports on modern proton beam therapy have a lower rate of hypopituitarism. The major limitation of the technique is that proton beam (cyclotron) facilities are available only at a very limited number of centers worldwide.[20]

In linac-based radiosurgery, multiple radiation arcs are used to crossfire photon beams at a target defined in stereotactic space.[21–23] Most of the current systems use nondynamic techniques in which the patient couch is set at an angle, and the arc is moved around its radius to deliver radiation that enters the skull through many different points. Numerous techniques have been developed to enhance conformity of dose planning and delivery using linac-based systems. These include beam shaping and intensity modulation.[24–26] Newer developments include the introduction of jaws and noncircular and mini- and microleaf collimators.[27] The conformal beam can be delivered with the micromultileaf collimator or conformal blocks.

Gamma Knife radiosurgery usually involves multiple isocenters of different beam diameter to achieve a dose plan that conforms to the irregular three-dimensional volumes of most mass lesions. The total number of isocenters may vary depending on the size, shape, and number of lesions. The most recent version of the Gamma Knife, the Perfexion, combines advances in dose planning, beam collimation, and robotic engineering, and it eliminates the need to set coordinates manually for each isocenter.

No published comparisons of Gamma Knife multiple isocenter techniques, linac or proton beam, have shown a clear advantage of one technique over another with regard to sparing normal tissue, achieving endocrine remission, or reducing complications.[28,29] As with other neurosurgical procedures, the outcome may depend less on the radiosurgical device and more on the experience of the radiosurgical team. To paraphrase neurosurgeon Charles Wilson, it is not just the horse but also the jockey that makes the difference in winning a race.

Radiosurgical Planning and Technique

Cessation of Suppressive Medications

In 2000 Landolt et al reported a significantly lower hormone normalization rate in patients with acromegaly who were receiving antisecretory medications at the time of radiosurgery.[30] The precise mechanism by which antisecretory medications lower hormonal normalization rates is unknown, but it is thought to be related to changes in cell cycling caused by these drugs, potentially decreasing tumor cell radiosensitivity.[30,31] Since 2000, several other groups (e.g., Mayo, Marseille, and the University of Virginia) have documented a counterproductive effect of antisecretory medications on the rate of hormonal normalization following radiosurgery for patients with acromegaly and prolactinomas.[30,32,33] Although the optimal time period to hold antisecretory medications is unclear, published studies have indicated that long-acting somatostatin analogues should probably be discontinued 8 weeks before treatment and resumed 6 to 8 weeks after radiosurgery if the benefit of radiosurgery is to be optimized.[30–34] Based on these reports, many centers have advocated the cessation of antisecretory medications. However, as is true for much of neurosurgical practice, class I evidence is still unavailable to support this treatment approach. Ultimately, the radiosurgical team must weigh the potential risk and benefits of altering antisecretory medication administration. In the absence of antisecretory medication control, a tumor may rarely enlarge, thereby risking adjacent structures (e.g., the optic apparatus), necessitating a lower prescription dose, and making effective treatment more difficult.

Frame Placement

On the day of the treatment, the stereotactic head frame is applied in the standard fashion.[35,36] We find that patients

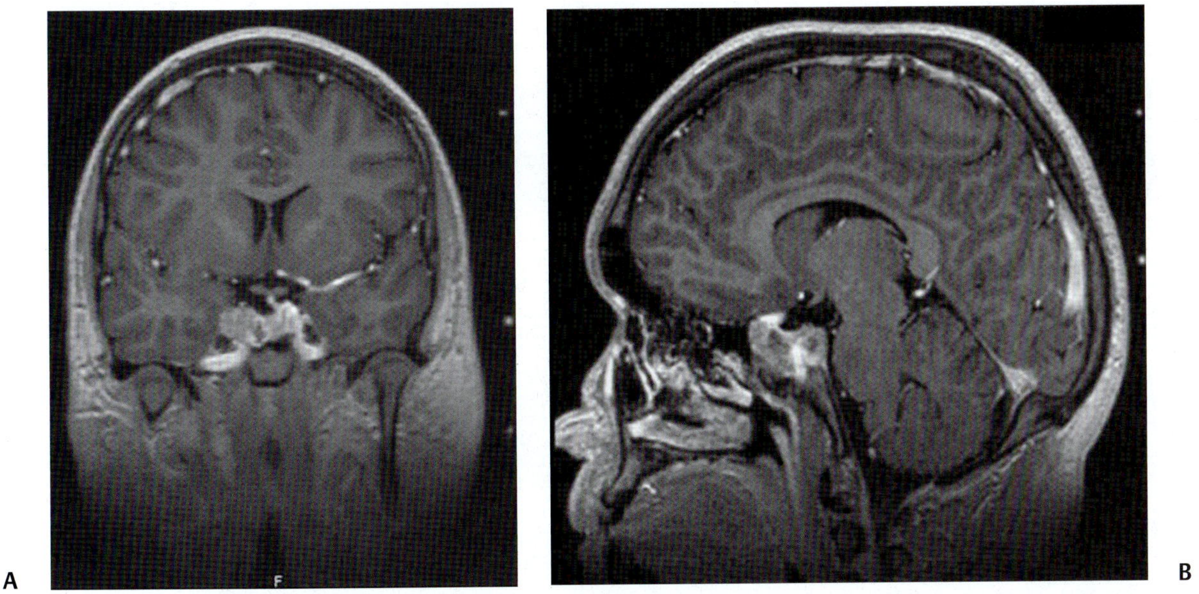

Fig. 9.1 (A) Coronal and (B) sagittal postcontrast magnetic resonance images in an 18-year-old right-handed male with Cushing's disease. The patient presented with rapid visual loss, which improved after transsphenoidal resection. However, he had residual tumor encasing the cavernous sinus and carotid artery, as well as biochemical evidence of persistent Cushing's disease.

are more comfortable when the frame is placed in the operating room using intravenous sedation with an anesthesiologist or nurse anesthetist in attendance. Prior to frame placement, the scalp is prepared with alcohol, and the areas of the pin placements are infiltrated with a long-acting local anesthetic. It is generally useful to use the angle of the optic apparatus as the axis of the frame. This angle approximates a line joining the lateral canthus and the top of the pinna, and it makes identification of the optic nerves, chiasm, and tracts easier by having an image that demonstrates the entire optic apparatus in a single MRI slice.[37]

Radiographic Imaging

Regardless of the radiosurgical modality used, stereotactic radiosurgery requires clear and accurate imaging of that target. Advances in radiographic imaging over the past 20 years have increased the efficacy and safety of radiosurgical treatment of pituitary lesions. Modern imaging consists of an MRI sequence consisting of thin-slice (e.g., 1 mm), postcontrast volume acquisition to define the tumor within the sellar region. In patients with previous surgery, fat suppression techniques can prove useful for differentiating tumor from surgical fat grafts (**Fig. 9.1**). In the pre-MRI era, CT was used routinely, but it is now used only when a patient cannot tolerate an MRI. Positron emission tomography (PET) imaging may also be of value for detecting hypersecretory adenomas; such images can be overlaid on stereotactic tomographic images (e.g., MRI or CT).[38]

Treatment Planning

After the acquisition of images with the stereotactic frame, multiple isocenter dose planning is performed to enclose the borders of the tumor within the prescription isodose line.[39,40] The 50% isodose is the most common prescription isodose line for Gamma Knife radiosurgery because this line is generally where the slope of the radiation fall-off is the steepest (**Fig. 9.2**).[41] However, one should analyze the dose gradient and determine the optimal fall-off isodose, which generally varies between 40 and 60%.[42]

Plugging Strategies

Beam-blocking plug patterns are often used to shift the prescription isodose curves away from the optic apparatus because of the radiosensitivity of this structure. These "plugging patterns" may be generated manually or by using planning software and are then implemented by replacing collimators in the helmet with solid "plugs." The planning software currently in use at most Gamma Knife centers (Leksell GammaPlan versions 5.33–4C; Elekta Instruments, Inc., Norcross, GA) supports two general strategies for plugging: a "merged" plugging strategy and a "custom" plugging strategy. The merged plugging strategy uses the software to create plug patterns for each helmet, which are placed at the union of software-computed patterns for each isocenter. These lowest common denominator patterns for each helmet size are then applied to every isocenter of that size. The advantage of this feature is that much of the work required to define plugging patterns and assign them to isocenters is automated by the software, requiring no plugging pattern changes during treatment other than when changing collimator helmets. The custom plugging strategy involves generating combinations of plugging patterns that are manually applied to one or more isocenters in a dose plan. Isocenters that require similar shielding effects are given similar or identical plugging patterns.[43] With the Gamma

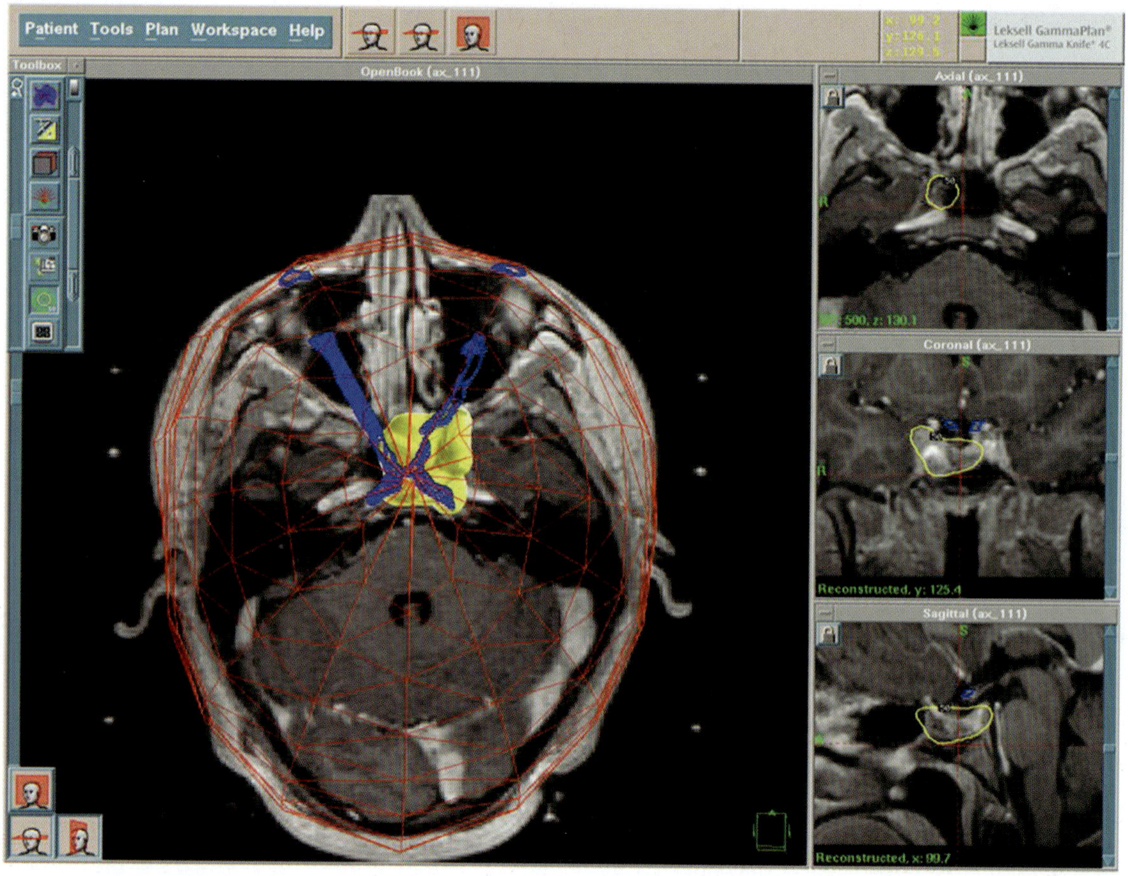

Fig. 9.2 Due to the involvement of the cavernous sinus, the patient underwent Gamma Knife radiosurgery. The three-dimensional dose–volume histograms are demonstrated in this figure, as well as the 50% isodose lines. A margin dose of 22 Gy to the 50% isodose line was prescribed, with a maximum dose of 44 Gy. Fourteen isocenters were used.

Knife Perfexion, plugging can be accomplished by closing off any one or a combination of eight sectors that comprise the 192-source collimator. Sectors are closed in an automated fashion.

The need to use plug patterns can be reduced by adjusting the gamma angle so that the anteroposterior axis of the peripheral isodose curves is parallel to the optic apparatus in the sagittal plane. If the frame is placed parallel to the course of the optic apparatus, then a gamma angle of 72 or 90 degrees may be used. This maneuver takes advantage of the extremely steep fall-off of radiation dorsal to the isocenter. Selection of the prescription dose is based partially on the integrated logistic formula as well as specific strategies for protecting the optic apparatus, controlling tumor growth, and establishing and maintaining normal endocrinologic function.[44,45]

Neuroanatomical Considerations: Radiation Effects on the Optic Apparatus, Cavernous Sinus, and Pituitary Gland

Visual deterioration following radiosurgery is rare and can generally be avoided if the dose to the optic apparatus is restricted to < 8 Gy, although reports of 10 to 12 Gy have been described by some groups.[46] Traditionally, a distance of 3 mm or more between the adenoma and the optic apparatus is desirable. The absolute distance between the optic apparatus is not the limiting factor, but rather defines how steeply the radiation gradient must be constructed so that a tolerable dose is delivered to the optic apparatus while still delivering an effective dose to the adenoma. If an acceptable gradient cannot be constructed, then alternative treatment should be considered. The Gamma Knife Perfexion may allow a distance of as little as 1 to 2 mm.[17,47–50] Ultimately, the tolerable absolute dose permitted likely varies from patient to patient, and it is affected by factors such as previous damage to the optic apparatus by pituitary adenoma compression, ischemic changes, type and timing of previous interventions (e.g., fractionated radiation therapy and surgery), the patient's age, and the presence or absence of other comorbidities.[33,51]

The majority of cranial nerves in the cavernous sinus appear to be more resistant to radiation effects than the optic nerve, but reports of cranial neuropathy, particularly after repeat radiosurgery, are well documented.[51] Although the tolerable limit to the cavernous sinus nerves is unknown, authors have described effective radiosurgical doses of between 19 and 23 Gy to this region without major side

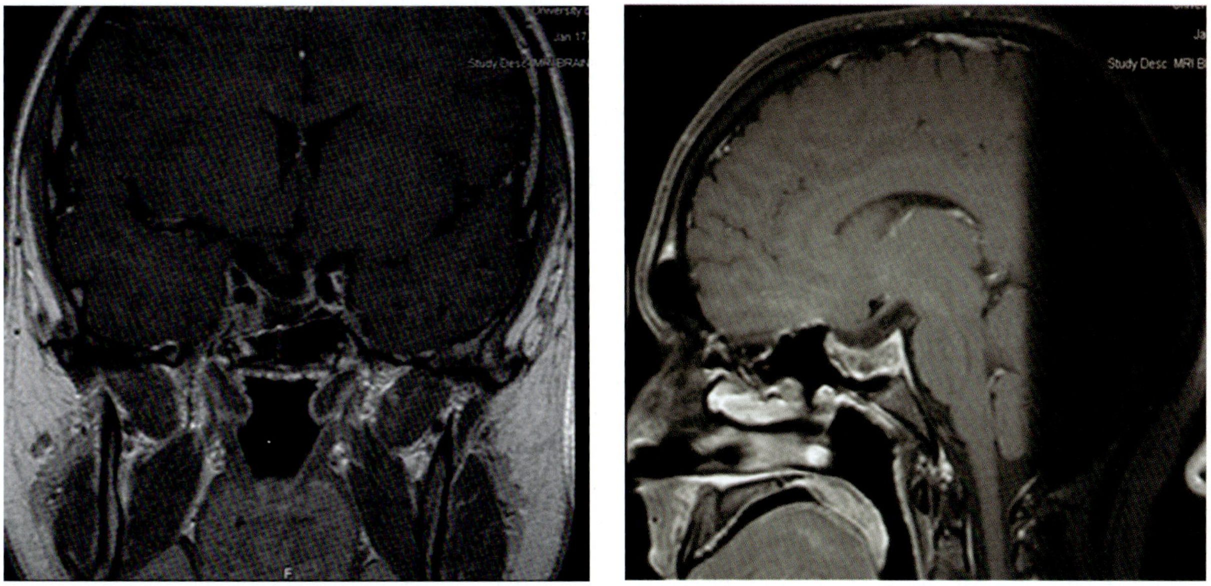

A B

Fig. 9.3 Twenty-four-month postoperative **(A)** coronal and **(B)** sagittal postradiosurgical magnetic resonance images reveal a decrease in tumor volume around the cavernous sinus and carotid artery. The patient had further improvement of his visual function and remains in biochemical remission of Cushing disease.

effects.[17,52–56] Injury to the cavernous segment of the carotid artery is rare after radiosurgery, with a few isolated case reports.[57] In cases where the tumor appears to extend into the cavernous sinus, blocking patterns can be used to deliver radiation while shielding vital structures.

There does not appear to be a direct correlation between the effect on adenoma volume and the endocrine remission rate following radiosurgery.[17,58,59] Fortunately, because most pituitary adenomas are small enough to be well suited for stereotactic radiosurgery, dose–volume considerations are not usually a limiting factor. Because the systemic effects of functioning adenomas can be so devastating, it seems intuitive to deliver a reasonably high dose (≥ 20 Gy to the margin) to allow rapid hormonal normalization and control of tumor growth. For improved rates of hormonal normalization in functioning adenomas, margin dose of 25 or 30 Gy may even be chosen. However, it is not known to what degree a higher margin dose (e.g., 20 vs 30 Gy) will result in delayed hypopituitarism. In cases of functioning adenomas with radiologically identifiable targets in the cavernous sinus, radiosurgical plans can be devised with higher range treatment doses while shielding much of the normal stalk, gland, and optic apparatus. Nonfunctioning pituitary adenomas appear to require a lower radiosurgery treatment dose than functioning adenomas.[48,60–62] The lowest effective dose for a nonfunctioning tumor is not known, but many centers deliver 13 to 15 Gy to the margin.

◆ Effectiveness of Radiosurgery

The goals of stereotactic radiosurgery in the treatment of pituitary tumors are (1) to inactivate tumor cells, thereby controlling tumor growth, and (2) to normalize hormone overproduction in the case of secretory tumors (**Fig. 9.3**). Ideally, these goals are met without damaging the residual normal pituitary gland and surrounding vascular and neuronal structures. Moreover, radiosurgery should be performed in such a way so as to avoid delayed radiation injury and secondary tumor formation.

Radiosurgery for Pituitary Nonfunctioning or Nonsecretory Adenomas

The primary goal of radiosurgery in the treatment of nonfunctioning tumors is to stabilize or reduce adenoma volume, especially for tumors that invade surgically inaccessible areas (i.e., the parasellar region). In nearly all published series, stereotactic radiosurgery afforded excellent control of tumor growth, with a mean tumor control rate of 93% (range 68–100%).[1,15,16,48,63–68] In patients with 4 or more years of follow-up, the mean control rate is 95% (range 83–100%).[62,63,69–74] Some series have even demonstrated improvement in visual function following radiosurgery after shrinkage of the tumor.[47,74–76] Nevertheless, prevention of tumor growth without volume reduction is still considered a successful treatment.

In our experience with 90 patients treated by radiosurgery for nonfunctioning tumors, tumor volume decreased in 59 patients (65.6%), remained unchanged in 24 (26.7%), and increased in 7 (7.8%), at a mean follow-up of 44.9 months.[77] Eight patients were treated with radiosurgery as a primary therapy for medical reasons, or patient preference, and in these patients, a decrease in tumor volume occurred in three (42%); five patients had stabilization of tumor volume (58%) at 34 months' follow-up. In the remaining 82 patients who were treated for recurrent or residual tumor after surgery, a reduction in tumor volume occurred in 56 (68%), no change was detected in 19 (23%), and an increase occurred in 7 (8%). The median time to tumor shrinkage on MRI was 9 months (range 6–48 months) following radiosurgery. This is consistent with a series from 2006 that demonstrated pituitary adenomas were, respectively, 90%, 80%, and 70% of their initial volume at 1, 2, and 3 years following Gamma Knife radiosurgery.[78]

Tumors involving the parasellar space require special consideration, as they would be otherwise untreatable. Of the 61 tumors treated at the University of Virginia that involved the parasellar space, 39 decreased in volume (63%), and 17 remained unchanged (27%).

Radiosurgery for Secretory Adenomas

Reported rates of endocrine remission following radiosurgery for functional pituitary adenomas vary greatly. The wide variance is likely a function of methodology, endocrine criteria used to define remission, study population, and length of follow-up. Most series typically report a higher prescription (margin) dose to patients with functioning adenomas, with a range between 20 and 25 Gy in most reports.[33,51,67,79] Because hormone normalization has been followed by relapse, we prefer the term *remission* to *cure*.

Cushing Disease

Cushing disease is one of the most devastating pituitary disorders and is associated with significant morbidity and premature death. Even after transsphenoidal surgery, up to 30% of patients may have persistent disease.[2,10,60] Most centers define an endocrine remission as a UFC level in the normal range associated with the resolution of clinical stigmata or a series of normal postoperative serum cortisol levels obtained throughout the day.[5,59]

Reported endocrine remission rates following transsphenoidal surgery vary from 10 to 100%, with higher remission rates when radiosurgery follows surgical debulking.[15,16,50,51,71,80–83] In series with at least 10 patients and a median follow-up of 2 years, endocrine remission rates range from 17 to 83%.[71,82–84] Rähn and associates reported their experience at the Karolinska Institute involving 59 patients with Cushing disease who were treated using the Gamma Knife and followed for 2 to 15 years. The efficacy rate of the initial treatment was 50%, with re-treatment eventually providing normalization of cortisol production in 76% of patients.[87]

In our experience treating 107 patients with Cushing disease, the remission rate was 53%, with the rate of remission statistically correlated with tumor volume but not tumor invasion into the cavernous sinus or suprasellar region.[51] The mean prescription (margin) dose in patients with Cushing disease was 23 Gy and is typically lower in patients who had prior radiation. As reported by others, the rate of hormone normalization after radiosurgery for Cushing disease appears to be difficult to predict, with remission occurring as early as 2 months and as late as 8 years.[69,76] Our general experience is that most patients who ultimately have hormonal normalization do so within the first 2 years following radiosurgery, and patients with persistent disease should consider alternative treatments such as adrenalectomy or repeat surgery (although this may be associated with a higher rate of cranial nerve damage).[51]

Nelson's Syndrome

A subset of patients with Cushing disease does not achieve hormone normalization following microsurgery and radiosurgery and require adrenalectomy as a "salvage" treatment for their disease. Although adrenalectomy is the definitive treatment for cortisol overproduction, a small subset of patients may develop Nelson's syndrome, characterized by rapid adenoma growth, hyperpigmentation, and tumor invasion into the parasellar structures.[88]

There are relatively few studies detailing the results of radiosurgery for Nelson's syndrome.[1,64,71,89–93] These studies report a mean tumor dose from between 12.0 and 28.7 Gy and an endocrine remission rate ranging from 0 to 36%, although only a minority of these studies defined what was meant by endocrine remission. Even cases where endocrine remission was not achieved, tumor growth control rates were favorable, ranging from 82 to 100%.

Pollock and Young reported on 11 patients who underwent Gamma Knife surgery for Nelson's syndrome.[92] They reported control of tumor growth in 9 of 11 patients, with ACTH normalization in 4 patients (36%). Our experience involves 23 patients with at least 6 months' follow-up and a rate of tumor control of 90%. Decrease in ACTH levels occurred in 67% of patients with elevation, but normalization occurred in only four patients.[91]

Acromegaly

Just as the endocrine criteria for remission in Cushing's disease remain the subject of debate, the criteria for remission in acromegaly have also been inconsistent. The most widely accepted guidelines for a remission in acromegaly consist of a growth hormone level < 1 ng/mL in response to an oral glucose challenge and a normal serum IGF-1 when matched for age and gender.[6,86]

Remission rates following radiosurgery for acromegaly vary widely from 0 to 100%, with the majority patients achieving tumor growth control.[30,32,34,50,94–98] Jezkova et al reported a remission rate of 50% at 42 months' follow-up in 96 patients with acromegaly who received radiosurgery.[99] Nearly one third of these patients, however, had radiosurgery as a primary treatment, without surgical extirpation of the adenoma. Pollock et al[32] demonstrated a remission rate of 50% in 46 patients who were treated with radiosurgery for acromegaly, with a higher remission rate in patients who were off suppressive medications at the time of radiosurgery. Our (unpublished) experience with 135 patients with mean follow-up of 57 months demonstrates a remission rate of 59% in patients off suppressive medications compared with 37% in patients receiving a suppressive medication (most commonly octreotide). In both groups, the mean prescription dose was 22 Gy. As a result of this finding, we currently recommend a cessation of somatostatin analogue medication 8 weeks before and for 8 weeks after Gamma Knife radiosurgery.

Prolactinoma

In patients with prolactinomas, the criteria to define endocrine remission are generally consistent, with most studies defining a remission as a patient who has a normal serum prolactin level while off antisecretory medications. In published studies of radiosurgery for prolactinomas, the mean radiosurgical dose to the tumor margin has varied from 13.3 to 33.0 Gy, and remission rates varied from 0 to 84%.[1,31,33,67,79,100,101] Variations in success rate are likely related to the radiosurgical dose delivered to the tumor. Witt et al noted no remission with a margin dose of 19 Gy.[49,50] Pan et al reported a 52% endocrine "cure" rate and a prescription dose of 30 Gy in a retrospective study of 128 patients in whom Gamma Knife surgery was used as a first-line treatment for prolactinomas.[102] Though this report boasts a large sample size, its applicability is limited by the fact that Gamma Knife surgery was used as a first-line treatment, which is atypical in most centers, because prolactinomas are usually responsive to medical treatment and, at least in the United States, radiosurgery is not used as a first-line treatment for prolactinomas.[103]

We typically use radiosurgery as a salvage treatment for prolactinomas after failure of medical and/or surgical treatment. Of the 23 patients treated at our institution, normalization of prolactin levels occurred in 26%, at an average time of 24.5 months, with a prescription (margin) dose of 19 Gy.[33] Consistent with the work of Landolt and Lomax, we also found that the remission rate was lower in patients receiving an antisecretory medication at the time of radiosurgery.[31]

◆ Complications

Side effects following radiosurgery for pituitary adenomas are typically rare. However, the latency of such effects may be long (i.e., > 10 years) and warrants continued neurologic, endocrine, and radiological follow-up. The most common problem after radiosurgery is new hypopituitarism. Well-respected groups have reported a low incidence (0–36%) of pituitary dysfunction following radiosurgery.[17,51,104,105] This incidence is likely higher when patients are followed long term, with the Karolinska Institute reporting a 72% incidence of hypopituitarism when patients were followed for more than 10 years.[69] We have observed an overall risk of 20 to 30% for development of hypopituitarism following radiosurgery.

Ultimately, the total dose prescribed and the prescription (margin) dose are likely the major factors determining the risk and onset of radiation-induced hypopituitarism. The growth hormone axis is the most sensitive to the late effects of radiation, with the radiation-induced defect occurring largely at the hypothalamic level.[106,107] The gonadotropin and corticotropin axes are the next most sensitive to radiation damage, and the TSH axis is least sensitive. Diabetes insipidus is extremely uncommon after radiosurgery, with only sporadic case reports.[108]

Cranial neuropathies following Gamma Knife surgery are exceedingly rare following the first procedure, although the incidence may increase on re-treatment.[51] Visual injury in general can be avoided if the dose to the optic apparatus is restricted to < 8 Gy (see discussion above).

Injury to the cavernous segment of the carotid artery or brain parenchymal is uncommon following radiosurgery. The exact incidence of radiosurgery-induced neoplasms is unknown at present. To date, there are no reports of radiation-induced neoplasms following radiosurgery to treat a pituitary adenoma.

◆ Prognosis and Follow-Up

Prognosis for a pituitary adenoma is dependent on the preradiosurgical status, comorbid conditions, adenoma size and extension, and functional nature of the tumor. Patients being treated for pituitary adenomas must be followed long term with serial clinical, ophthalmologic, endocrine, and radiological evaluations after radiosurgery. In particular, height, weight, and pubertal status must be carefully monitored in relevant age groups. Serial visual field examinations and screening should be performed. Questioning directed at assessing hormone function (screening for hypothyroidism, adrenal insufficiency, diabetes insipidus, etc.) should be directed to the patient and family. Serial testing of adrenal, thyroid function, and growth hormone status (with IGF-1 levels and provocative testing when applicable) should be undertaken. Patients with functioning tumors should be investigated as appropriate (e.g., 24-hour UFC testing in patients with Cushing disease). Patients receiving hormone replacement should have their replacement therapy adjusted as necessary. Finally, serial MRI should be performed to assess for tumor recurrence. Generally, initial postradiosurgical neuroimaging is performed 6 months following treatment and yearly thereafter (or more frequently as indicated). Endocrine and ophthalmologic follow-up should typically occur at these same time points.

◆ Developments in Radiosurgery for Pituitary Adenomas

The CyberKnife (Accuray Inc., Sunnyvale, CA), developed in 1997, overcomes the need for rigid target fixation, as it is mounted on a maneuverable robotic manipulator and tracks the target with the aid of real-time guidance.[85,109] Early experience with these techniques has been promising for nonfunctioning adenomas, with a growth control rate of 95% and a lower prescription dose (14–16 Gy) than described for established radiosurgical modalities such as the Gamma Knife.[110] For secretory adenomas, early remission rates appear to be comparable to Gamma Knife surgery, with a low (9.5%) rate of endocrinopathy at 12 months posttreatment.[110–112] Restoration of visual function in patients with perioptic tumors has also been described.[111] Ultimately, longer follow-up and information on the rate of complications and recurrences will determine the efficacy of this newer treatment method.

Intensity modulated radiotherapy combines two advanced concepts to deliver three-dimensional conformal radiation therapy: (1) inverse treatment planning with optimization by computer and (2) computer-controlled intensity modulation of the radiation beam during treatment.[113] In addition, other linac-based radiosurgical devices such as the Trilogy (Varian Medical Systems, Inc., Palo Alto, CA), Synergy (Elekta), Novalis (BrainLAB AG, Feldkirchen, Germany), and Tomo therapy (TomoTherapy Inc., Madison, WI) may be useful to treat pituitary adenomas. However, long-term results with such devices are not currently available.

◆ Summary

Stereotactic radiosurgery is a safe and effective modality in the treatment of patients with a recurrent or residual pituitary adenoma. In most patients, radiosurgery controls adenoma growth and reduces or normalizes hormone overproduction. Several challenges persist, including the optimal timing of administration of antisecretory medications, the identification of other factors that can improve the response of adenomas to radiosurgery, and the optimal target of the adenoma.

References

1. Laws ER Jr., Vance ML. Radiosurgery for pituitary tumors and craniopharyngiomas. Neurosurg Clin N Am 1999;10:327–336
2. Laws ER, Sheehan JP. Pituitary Surgery: A Modern Approach. Basel and New York: Karger; 2006
3. Kovács K, Horvath E, Universities Associated for Research and Education in Pathology. Tumors of the Pituitary Gland. Washington, DC: Armed Forces Institute of Pathology; 1986.
4. Laws ER Jr. Recurrent pituitary adenomas. In: A L, M V, P R, eds. Pituitary Adenomas. Edinburgh: Churchill-Livingtone; 1996: 385–394
5. Nieman LK. Medical therapy of Cushing's disease. Pituitary 2002; 5:77–82
6. Vance ML. Endocrinological evaluation of acromegaly. J Neurosurg 1998;89:499–500
7. Jagannathan J, Dumont AS, Jane JA Jr., Laws ER Jr. Pediatric sellar tumors: diagnostic procedures and management. Neurosurg Focus 2005;18:E6
8. Kanter AS, Diallo AO, Jane JA Jr., et al. Single-center experience with pediatric Cushing's disease. J Neurosurg 2005;103:413–420
9. Laws ER Jr., Ebersold M. The results of transsphenoidal surgery in specific clinical entities. In: Laws ER Jr., Randall R, EB K, eds. Management of Pituitary Adenomas and Related Lesions with Emphasis on Transsphenoidal Microsurgery. New York: Appleton-Century-Croft; 1982:277–305
10. Laws ER Jr., Fode NC, Redmond MJ. Transsphenoidal surgery following unsuccessful prior therapy: an assessment of benefits and risks in 158 patients. J Neurosurg 1985;63:823–829
11. Laws ER, Vance ML, Thapar K. Pituitary surgery for the management of acromegaly. Horm Res 2000;53(Suppl 3):71–75
12. Ciric I, Ragin A, Baumgartner C, Pierce D. Complications of transsphenoidal surgery: results of a national survey, review of the literature, and personal experience. Neurosurgery 1997;40:225–236
13. Lyman JT, Phillips MH, Frankel KA, Levy RP, Fabrikant JI. Radiation physics for particle beam radiosurgery. Neurosurg Clin N Am 1992; 3:1–8
14. Leksell L. The stereotaxic method and radiosurgery of the brain. Acta Chir Scand 1951;102:316–319
15. Izawa M, Hayashi M, Nakaya K, et al. Gamma Knife radiosurgery for pituitary adenomas. J Neurosurg 2000;93(Suppl 3):19–22
16. Jackson IM, Noren G. Gamma Knife radiosurgery for pituitary tumours. Best Pract Res Clin Endocrinol Metab 1999;13:461–469
17. Sheehan JP, Jagannathan J, Pouratian N, Steiner L. Stereotactic radiosurgery for pituitary adenomas: a review of the literature and our experience. Front Horm Res 2006;34:185–205
18. Braunstein GD, Loriaux DL. Proton-beam therapy. N Engl J Med 1971; 284:332–333
19. Dawson DM, Dingman JF. Hazards of proton-beam pituitary irradiation. N Engl J Med 1970;282:1434
20. Ronson BB, Schulte RW, Han KP, Loredo LN, Slater JM, Slater JD. Fractionated proton beam irradiation of pituitary adenomas. Int J Radiat Oncol Biol Phys 2006;64:425–434
21. Podgorsak EB, Pike GB, Pla M, Olivier A, Souhami L. Radiosurgery with photon beams: physical aspects and adequacy of linear accelerators. Radiother Oncol 1990;17:349–358
22. Popescu GF, Rodgers JE, von Hanwehr R. Optimization of dose distribution for linac-based radiosurgery using elliptical collimators. Acta Neurochir Suppl (Wien) 1995;63:35–39
23. Schell MC, Smith V, Larson DA, Wu A, Flickinger JC. Evaluation of radiosurgery techniques with cumulative dose volume histograms in linac-based stereotactic external beam irradiation. Int J Radiat Oncol Biol Phys 1991;20:1325–1330
24. Andrews DW, Suarez O, Goldman HW, et al. Stereotactic radiosurgery and fractionated stereotactic radiotherapy for the treatment of acoustic schwannomas: comparative observations of 125 patients treated at one institution. Int J Radiat Oncol Biol Phys 2001;50:1265–1278
25. Dong L, Shiu A, Tung S, Hogstrom K. A pencil-beam photon dose algorithm for stereotactic radiosurgery using a miniature multileaf collimator. Med Phys 1998;25:841–850
26. Glasgow GP, Corrigan KW. Installation of 60Co 100 cm source-to-axis distance teletherapy units in vaults designed for 80-cm units. Health Phys 1995;68:411–415
27. Wang S, Wang R, Zhang X, Lin C, Wong Z, Li X. Dose distributions of linac-based radiosurgery for pineal region mass. Sheng Wu Yi Xue Gong Cheng Xue Za Zhi 1997;14:279–282
28. Cheung JY, Yu KN, Ho RT, Yu CP. Monte Carlo calculations and GafChromic film measurements for plugged collimator helmets of Leksell Gamma Knife unit. Med Phys 1999;26:1252–1256
29. Yu C, Luxton G, Jozsef G, Apuzzo ML, Petrovich Z. Dosimetric comparison of three photon radiosurgery techniques for an elongated ellipsoid target. Int J Radiat Oncol Biol Phys 1999;45:817–826
30. Landolt AM, Haller D, Lomax N, et al. Octreotide may act as a radioprotective agent in acromegaly. J Clin Endocrinol Metab 2000;85:1287–1289
31. Landolt AM, Lomax N. Gamma Knife radiosurgery for prolactinomas. J Neurosurg 2000;93(Suppl 3):14–18
32. Pollock BE, Jacob JT, Brown PD, Nippoldt TB. Radiosurgery of growth hormone-producing pituitary adenomas: factors associated with biochemical remission. J Neurosurg 2007;106:833–838
33. Pouratian N, Sheehan J, Jagannathan J, Laws ER Jr., Steiner L, Vance ML. Gamma Knife radiosurgery for medically and surgically refractory prolactinomas. Neurosurgery 2006;59:255–266
34. Landolt AM, Haller D, Lomax N, et al. Stereotactic radiosurgery for recurrent surgically treated acromegaly: comparison with fractionated radiotherapy. J Neurosurg 1998;88:1002–1008
35. Galloway RL, Maciunas RJ. Stereotactic neurosurgery. Crit Rev Biomed Eng 1990;18:181–205
36. Walton L, Hampshire A, Roper A, et al. Development of a relocatable frame technique for Gamma Knife radiosurgery: technical note. J Neurosurg 2000;93(Suppl 3):198–202
37. Hayashi M, Taira T, Chernov M, et al. Gamma Knife surgery for cancer pain-pituitary gland-stalk ablation: a multicenter prospective protocol since 2002. J Neurosurg 2002;97:433–437
38. Levivier M, Massager N, Wikler D, Devriendt D, Goldman S. Integration of functional imaging in radiosurgery: the example of PET scan. Prog Neurol Surg 2007;20:68–81
39. Alexander E III, Loeffler JS. Radiosurgery using a modified linear accelerator. Neurosurg Clin N Am 1992;3:167–190
40. Flickinger JC, Lunsford LD, Wu A, Maitz AH, Kalend AM. Treatment planning for Gamma Knife radiosurgery with multiple isocenters. Int J Radiat Oncol Biol Phys 1990;18:1495–1501
41. Wu A, Lindner G, Maitz AH, et al. Physics of Gamma Knife approach on convergent beams in stereotactic radiosurgery. Int J Radiat Oncol Biol Phys 1990;18:941–949

42. Paddick I. A simple scoring ratio to index the conformity of radiosurgical treatment plans: technical note. J Neurosurg 2000;93(Suppl 3): 219–222
43. Schlesinger DSJ, Sheehan JP. Shielding strategies for Gamma Knife surgery of pituitary adenomas. J Neurosurg 2006;105(Suppl):241–248
44. Flickinger JC. An integrated logistic formula for prediction of complications from radiosurgery. Int J Radiat Oncol Biol Phys 1989;17:879–885
45. Flickinger JC, Lunsford LD, Kondziolka D. Dose prescription and dose-volume effects in radiosurgery. Neurosurg Clin N Am 1992;3:51–59
46. Leber KA, Bergloff J, Pendl G. Dose-response tolerance of the visual pathways and cranial nerves of the cavernous sinus to stereotactic radiosurgery. J Neurosurg 1998;88:43–50
47. Chen JC, Giannotta SL, Yu C, Petrovich Z, Levy ML, Apuzzo ML. Radiosurgical management of benign cavernous sinus tumors: dose profiles and acute complications. Neurosurgery 2001;48:1022–1030
48. Lim YL, Leem W, Kim TS, Rhee BA, Kim GK. Four years' experiences in the treatment of pituitary adenomas with Gamma Knife radiosurgery. Stereotact Funct Neurosurg 1998;70(Suppl 1):95–109
49. Witt TC. Stereotactic radiosurgery for pituitary tumors. Neurosurg Focus 2003;14:e10
50. Witt TC, Kondziolka D, Flickinger JC, Lunsford LD. Gamma Knife radiosurgery for pituitary tumors. In: Lunsford LD, Kondziolka D, Flickinger J, eds. Gamma Knife Brain Surgery Progress in Neurological Surgery. Basel: Karger; 1998:114–127
51. Jagannathan J, Sheehan JP, Pouratian N, Laws ER, Steiner L, Vance ML. Gamma Knife surgery for Cushing's disease. J Neurosurg 2007;106: 980–987
52. Kuo JS, Chen JC, Yu C, et al. Gamma Knife radiosurgery for benign cavernous sinus tumors: quantitative analysis of treatment outcomes. Neurosurgery 2004;54:1385–1393
53. Liu AL, Wang C, Sun S, Wang M, Liu P. Gamma Knife radiosurgery for tumors involving the cavernous sinus. Stereotact Funct Neurosurg 2005;83:45–51
54. Nakamura N, Shin M, Tago M, et al. Gamma Knife radiosurgery for cavernous hemangiomas in the cavernous sinus: report of three cases. J Neurosurg 2002;97:477–480
55. Peker S, Kilic T, Sengoz M, Pamir MN. Radiosurgical treatment of cavernous sinus cavernous haemangiomas. Acta Neurochir (Wien) 2004;146:337–341, discussion 34
56. Sheehan JP, Kondziolka D, Flickinger J, Lunsford LD. Radiosurgery for residual or recurrent nonfunctioning pituitary adenoma. J Neurosurg 2002;97:408–414
57. Lim YJ, Leem W, Park JT, Kim TS, Rhee BA, Kim GK. Cerebral infarction with ICA occlusion after Gamma Knife radiosurgery for pituitary adenoma: a case report. Stereotact Funct Neurosurg 1999;72(Suppl 1):132–139
58. Sheehan JM, Lopes MB, Sheehan JP, Ellegala D, Webb KM, Laws ER Jr. Results of transsphenoidal surgery for Cushing's disease in patients with no histologically confirmed tumor. Neurosurgery 2000;47: 33–39
59. Sheehan JM, Vance ML, Sheehan JP, Ellegala DB, Laws ER Jr. Radiosurgery for Cushing's disease after failed transsphenoidal surgery. J Neurosurg 2000;93:738–742
60. Mampalam TJ, Tyrrell JB, Wilson CB. Transsphenoidal microsurgery for Cushing disease: a report of 216 cases. Ann Intern Med 1988;109:487–493
61. Martinez R, Bravo G, Burzaco J, Rey G. Pituitary tumors and Gamma Knife surgery: clinical experience with more than two years of follow-up. Stereotact Funct Neurosurg 1998;70(Suppl 1):110–118
62. Shin M, Kurita H, Sasaki T, et al. Stereotactic radiosurgery for pituitary adenoma invading the cavernous sinus. J Neurosurg 2000; 93(Suppl 3):2–5
63. Feigl GC, Bonelli CM, Berghold A, Mokry M. Effects of Gamma Knife radiosurgery of pituitary adenomas on pituitary function. J Neurosurg 2002;97:415–421
64. Ganz JC, Backlund EO, Thorsen FA. The effects of Gamma Knife surgery of pituitary adenomas on tumor growth and endocrinopathies. Stereotact Funct Neurosurg 1993;61(Suppl 1):30–37
65. Hayashi M, Izawa M, Hiyama H, et al. Gamma Knife radiosurgery for pituitary adenomas. Stereotact Funct Neurosurg 1999;72(Suppl 1): 111–118
66. Inoue HK, Kohga H, Hirato M, et al. Pituitary adenomas treated by microsurgery with or without Gamma Knife surgery: experience in 122 cases. Stereotact Funct Neurosurg 1999;72(Suppl 1):125–131
67. Kim SH, Huh R, Chang JW, Park YG, Chung SS. Gamma Knife radiosurgery for functioning pituitary adenomas. Stereotact Funct Neurosurg 1999;72(Suppl 1):101–110
68. Losa M, Valle M, Mortini P, et al. Gamma Knife surgery for treatment of residual nonfunctioning pituitary adenomas after surgical debulking. J Neurosurg 2004;100:438–444
69. Hoybye C, Grenback E, Rahn T, Degerblad M, Thoren M, Hulting AL. Adrenocorticotropic hormone-producing pituitary tumors: 12- to 22-year follow-up after treatment with stereotactic radiosurgery. Neurosurgery 2001;49:284–291
70. Ikeda H, Jokura H, Yoshimoto T. Transsphenoidal surgery and adjuvant Gamma Knife treatment for growth hormone-secreting pituitary adenoma. J Neurosurg 2001;95:285–291
71. Kobayashi T, Kida Y, Mori Y. Gamma Knife radiosurgery in the treatment of Cushing disease: long-term results. J Neurosurg 2002;97: 422–428
72. Mokry M, Ramschak-Schwarzer S, Simbrunner J, Ganz JC, Pendl G. A six-year experience with the postoperative radiosurgical management of pituitary adenomas. Stereotact Funct Neurosurg 1999; 72(Suppl 1):88–100
73. Wowra B, Stummer W. Efficacy of Gamma Knife radiosurgery for nonfunctioning pituitary adenomas: a quantitative follow-up with magnetic resonance imaging-based volumetric analysis. J Neurosurg 2002;97:429–432
74. Yoon SC, Suh TS, Jang HS, et al. Clinical results of 24 pituitary macroadenomas with linac-based stereotactic radiosurgery. Int J Radiat Oncol Biol Phys 1998;41:849–853
75. Abe T, Yamamoto M, Taniyama M, Tanioka D, Izumiyama H, Matsumoto K. Early palliation of oculomotor nerve palsy following Gamma Knife radiosurgery for pituitary adenoma. Eur Neurol 2002;47:61–63
76. Hayashi M, Taira T, Ochiai T, et al. Gamma Knife surgery of the pituitary: new treatment for thalamic pain syndrome. J Neurosurg 2005; 102(Suppl):38–41
77. Mingione V, Yen CP, Vance ML, et al. Gamma Knife surgery in the treatment of nonsecretory pituitary macroadenoma. J Neurosurg 2006;104:876–883
78. Pamir MN, Peker S. Microvascular decompression for trigeminal neuralgia: a long-term follow-up study. Minim Invasive Neurosurg 2006;49:342–346
79. Kim MS, Lee SI, Sim JH. Gamma Knife radiosurgery for functioning pituitary microadenoma. Stereotact Funct Neurosurg 1999;72(Suppl 1): 119–124
80. Arnaldi G, Angeli A, Atkinson AB, et al. Diagnosis and complications of Cushing's syndrome: a consensus statement. J Clin Endocrinol Metab 2003;88:5593–5602
81. Chu JW, Matthias DF, Belanoff J, Schatzberg A, Hoffman AR, Feldman D. Successful long-term treatment of refractory Cushing's disease with high-dose mifepristone (RU 486). J Clin Endocrinol Metab 2001;86:3568–3573
82. Morange-Ramos I, Regis J, Dufour H, et al. Gamma Knife surgery for secreting pituitary adenomas. Acta Neurochir (Wien) 1998;140: 437–443
83. Petrovich Z, Yu C, Giannotta SL, Zee CS, Apuzzo ML. Gamma Knife radiosurgery for pituitary adenoma: early results. Neurosurgery 2003;53:51–61
84. Mahmoud-Ahmed AS, Suh JH. Radiation therapy for Cushing's disease: a review. Pituitary 2002;5:175–180
85. Chang SD, Murphy M, Geis P, et al. Clinical experience with image-guided robotic radiosurgery (the CyberKnife) in the treatment of brain and spinal cord tumors. Neurol Med Chir (Tokyo) 1998;38: 780–783
86. Giustina A, Barkan A, Casanueva FF, et al. Criteria for cure of acromegaly: a consensus statement. J Clin Endocrinol Metab 2000; 85:526–529
87. Rähn T, Thoren M, Hall K, Backlund EO. Stereotactic radiosurgery in Cushing's syndrome: acute radiation effects. Surg Neurol 1980;14: 85–92
88. Nagesser SK, van Seters AP, Kievit J, Hermans J, Krans HM, van de Velde CJ. Long-term results of total adrenalectomy for Cushing's disease. World J Surg 2000;24:108–113
89. Ganz JC. Gamma Knife radiosurgery and its possible relationship to malignancy: a review. J Neurosurg 2002;97:644–652
90. Levy RP, Fabrikant JI, Frankel KA, et al. Heavy-charged-particle radiosurgery of the pituitary gland: clinical results of 840 patients. Stereotact Funct Neurosurg 1991;57:22–35

91. Mauermann WJ, Sheehan JP, Chernavvsky DR, Laws ER, Steiner L, Vance ML. Gamma Knife surgery for adrenocorticotropic hormone-producing pituitary adenomas after bilateral adrenalectomy. J Neurosurg 2007; 106:988–993
92. Pollock BE, Young WF Jr. Stereotactic radiosurgery for patients with ACTH-producing pituitary adenomas after prior adrenalectomy. Int J Radiat Oncol Biol Phys 2002;54:839–841
93. Wolffenbuttel BH, Kitz K, Beuls EM. Beneficial Gamma Knife radiosurgery in a patient with Nelson's syndrome. Clin Neurol Neurosurg 1998;100:60–63
94. Buchfelder M, Fahlbusch R, Schott W, Honegger J. Long-term follow-up results in hormonally active pituitary adenomas after primary successful transsphenoidal surgery. Acta Neurochir Suppl (Wien) 1991;53:72–76
95. Cozzi R, Barausse M, Asnaghi D, Dallabonzana D, Lodrini S, Attanasio R. Failure of radiotherapy in acromegaly. Eur J Endocrinol 2001;145: 717–72
96. Freda PU. How effective are current therapies for acromegaly? Growth Horm IGF Res 2003;13(Suppl A):S144–S151
97. Fukuoka S, Ito T, Takanashi M, Hojo A, Nakamura H. Gamma Knife radiosurgery for growth hormone-secreting pituitary adenomas invading the cavernous sinus. Stereotact Funct Neurosurg 2001;76:213–217
98. Horvath E, Kovacs K, Scheithauer BW, et al. Pituitary adenomas producing growth hormone, prolactin, and one or more glycoprotein hormones: a histologic, immunohistochemical, and ultrastructural study of four surgically removed tumors. Ultrastruct Pathol 1983;5:171–183
99. Jezkova J, Marek J, Hana V, et al. Gamma Knife radiosurgery for acromegaly—long-term experience. Clin Endocrinol (Oxf) 2006;64: 588–595
100. Post KD, Habas JE. Comparison of long-term results between prolactin-secreting adenomas and ACTH-secreting adenomas. Can J Neurol Sci 1990;17:74–77
101. Yildiz F, Zorlu F, Erbas T, Atahan L. Radiotherapy in the management of giant pituitary adenomas. Radiother Oncol 1999;52:233–237
102. Pan L, Zhang N, Wang EM, Wang BJ, Dai JZ, Cai PW. Gamma Knife radiosurgery as a primary treatment for prolactinomas. J Neurosurg 2000;93(Suppl 3):10–13
103. Molitch ME. Pathologic hyperprolactinemia. Endocrinol Metab Clin North Am 1992;21:877–901
104. Jane JA Jr., Vance ML, Woodburn CJ, Laws ER Jr. Stereotactic radiosurgery for hypersecreting pituitary tumors: part of a multimodality approach. Neurosurg Focus 2003;14:e12
105. Pollock BE, Kondziolka D, Lunsford LD, Flickinger JC. Stereotactic radiosurgery for pituitary adenomas: imaging, visual and endocrine results. Acta Neurochir Suppl (Wien) 1994;62:33–38
106. Blacklay A, Grossman A, Ross RJ, et al. Cranial irradiation for cerebral and nasopharyngeal tumours in children: evidence for the production of a hypothalamic defect in growth hormone release. J Endocrinol 1986;108:25–29
107. Shalet SM. Radiation and pituitary dysfunction. N Engl J Med 1993; 328:131–133
108. Piedra MP, Brown PD, Carpenter PC, Link MJ. Resolution of diabetes insipidus following Gamma Knife surgery for a solitary metastasis to the pituitary stalk: case report. J Neurosurg 2004;101: 1053–1056
109. Adler JR Jr., Chang SD, Murphy MJ, Doty J, Geis P, Hancock SL. The CyberKnife: a frameless robotic system for radiosurgery. Stereotact Funct Neurosurg 1997;69:124–128
110. Kajiwara K, Saito K, Yoshikawa K, et al. Image-guided stereotactic radiosurgery with the CyberKnife for pituitary adenomas. Minim Invasive Neurosurg 2005;48:91–96
111. Adler JR Jr., Gibbs IC, Puataweepong P, Chang SD. Visual field preservation after multisession CyberKnife radiosurgery for perioptic lesions. Neurosurgery 2006;59:244–254
112. Pham CJ, Chang SD, Gibbs IC, Jones P, Heilbrun MP, Adler JR Jr. Preliminary visual field preservation after staged CyberKnife radiosurgery for perioptic lesions. Neurosurgery 2004;54:799–810
113. Purdy JA. Intensity-modulated radiation therapy. Int J Radiat Oncol Biol Phys 1996;35:845–846

10

Stereotactic Radiosurgery for Skull Base Chordomas and Chondrosarcomas

Jean-Louis Habrand, Stéphanie Bolle, Régis Ferrand, and Georges Noel

Skull base chondrosarcomas and chordomas are very rare neoplasms that share similarities that justify a joint study on these entities: both can be located in the skull base or along the spinal axis; both share an indolent course in the majority of cases; both are highly invasive locally; and in the long run, a fatal outcome is inevitable if they are not adequately managed. From a therapeutic standpoint, both are formidable challenges for neurosurgeons and radiation oncologists, due to their invasiveness, proximity to vital structures, and sensitivity to therapeutic irradiation. Nonetheless, considerable progress has been achieved over the past decade or so in the outcome of both tumor types, due to the development of safer extensive skull base resections, combined with innovative radiosurgery and radiotherapy approaches, especially proton therapy. This chapter focuses on this latter technique.

◆ Epidemiology and Pathogenesis

Chondrosarcomas

Chondrosarcomas are very rare neoplasms that account for 0.5 case per million[1] and ~1 per 1000 malignancies in the head and neck region. They generally occur in the 2nd and 3rd decade of life with no predilection for gender. Anatomically, the skull base ranks generally behind more common presentations in the nasal/paranasal cavities, the mandible, or the orbits. Within the skull base, they tend to arise more frequently off the midline in the petrous bone, parasellar area, or cerebellopontine angle. Macroscopically, they frequently present as large lesions destroying existing bone. Microscopically, they have been divided into "conventional," mesenchymal, clear cell, and "dedifferentiated" variants (World Health Organization classification).[2] The common low-grade variant exhibits a lobulated appearance with frequent central necrosis and calcifications, associated with well-differentiated hyaline cartilage, and a myxoid ground substance. In higher grade variants, cartilage architecture is generally lost and associated with increased cellularity, mitoses, and larger nuclear sizes. Grading exerts a considerable prognostic impact. Indeed, 50 to 60% of chondrosarcomas are classified as low-grade (grade 1) lesions based on the nuclear appearance and cellularity, with the remaining lesions classified as grade 2 or 3. The very rare "mesenchymal" and "undifferentiated" variants include, respectively, highly undifferentiated small round cells and high-grade noncartilaginous sarcomas. Immunohistochemically, most of them display positive staining for mesenchymal antigens (vimentin) and sometimes for neuroepithelial antigens (S100 protein) and glial fibrillary acidic protein (GFAP). These features can help differentiate other low-grade malignancies, such as chordomas. More recently, genetic alterations have been described in association with chondrosarcomas: they consist of alterations of genes involved in tumor suppression, proliferation regulation, cell cycle regulation and differentiation, and repair. They are located on chromosomes 5, 9, 11, 13, 17, and 19.

Chondrosarcomas can be either primary or secondary lesions, depending on whether they arise in a previously normal bone or in a benign precursor, such as enchondroma. The risk of malignant transformation is quite low in cases of isolated foci but greater in cases of widespread congenital enchondromatoses: the multiple enchondromatosis (Ollier disease) carries a 25 to 30% risk of developing into secondary mesenchymal malignancies; the Mafucci syndrome, which combines Ollier bony anomalies and soft tissue angiomas, carries a 25 to 50% risk of developing into secondary polymorphic malignancies.

Chordomas

Chordomas are also very rare neoplasms, found in < 1% of autopsy-verified central nervous system (CNS) tumor processes, representing ~1 case per million.[1] The mean age is ~45 to 50 years, with cases described as early as 3 years and as late as 80 years, and a predilection is seen for males. They likely originate from remnants of the notochord, an embryonic structure located along the craniovertebral axis, which serves as primitive backbone support of the body and regresses by the 6th week of development. Their jelly-like appearance led early scientists to postulate links with the intervertebral disk, known as the nucleus pulposus. More recently, the role of the notochord in the embryonic formation of the dorsal and ventral roots of the spinal cord was emphasized.[3] Chordomas can arise anywhere along the primitive notochord, with ~45 to 50% of cases described in the sacrum, 35 to 40% in the skull base, and 15% along the spine. Anatomically, intracranial sites affect the midline, especially the spheno-occipital junction, but "aberrant" locations (i.e., sphenoid, maxillary, and frontal sinuses) have been reported. Macroscopically, chordomas are lobulated in appearance with gelatinous processes. Histologically, cells are arranged in sheets or cords or float singly within an abundant myxoid stroma (that can be confused with myxoid chondrosarcoma). Typically, they contain abundant pale, vacuolated cytoplasm ("physaliphorous") and moderate nuclear atypias. In the chondroid variant, which has the reputation of a more indolent course, some areas may mimic hyaline or myxoid cartilage, a feature likely to cause confusion with true chondrosarcomas. The dedifferentiated (including high-grade sarcoma areas) and "highly cellular" variants are extremely rare and distinctly aggressive.

By immunohistochemistry, most of them display polymorphic positive stainings for epithelial (cytokeratin, epithelial membrane antigen), neuroepithelial (S100 protein), and mesenchymal (vimentin) antigens. Genetic alterations consist of gains in chromosomes 5, 7, 12, and 20 and losses of 1 and 3. These have been linked to alterations of tumor suppressor genes, mismatched repairs, and oncogenes.

◆ Patient Presentation

Symptoms are generally insidious and nonspecific. Half of the patients present with ocular symptoms linked to oculomotor palsy (i.e., diplopia) or compression of the visual pathway (bitemporal hemianopia). Headaches, which occur typically in the retro-orbital and occipital regions, are also common at presentation. Snoring can be reported when a nasopharyngeal or pharyngeal mass is present. These symptoms are frequently neglected by the clinicians and the patients themselves. Generally, they require specific imaging after several years while they have been deteriorating. Radiologically, computed tomography (CT) scans and magnetic resonance imaging (MRI) are the most useful modalities for assessing tumor extension. Chondrosarcomas appear on CT scans as large off-midline lesions destroying bone, with calcifications and rather well-defined margins. On MRI, the appearance is generally hypointense on T1-weighted images and strongly hyperintense on T2-weighted images. They usually enhance contrast medium poorly due to their hypovascularity. For chordomas, CT imaging is superior for detecting bony destruction, whereas MRI is useful for assessing the diagnosis and for defining tumor extension; typically, the tumor displays a lobulated, "honeycomb" appearance on contrast-enhanced images and is located in the clival area, which displaces or even distorts the brainstem posteriorly and the optic pathway superiorly[1,4] (**Fig. 10.1**). On T1-weighted images, the tumor demonstrates an intermediate to low signal with foci of hyperintensity that can represent residual osseous fragments, calcifications, or proteinacous or hemorrhagic fluid. On T2-weighted images, it demonstrates very high signal intensity arranged with low signal septa. Chordomas usually enhance the contrast medium slightly. The evolution of both diseases is generally slow although invariably lethal if not appropriately managed. Following therapy, imaging is crucial to assess tumor control. The radiologic aspects remain frequently stable for months or years and should not be interpreted as local failure. The malignant nature of chordomas is supported by the reports of distant hematogenous foci (nodal, pulmonary, hepatic, cutaneous, etc.), not to mention second synchronous or metachronous primaries located within the clival bone or in the CNS. Failures have been described along the surgical route, as well as within the abdominal wall where fat was removed during surgery.[5,6]

◆ Management

Skull base chordomas and chondrosarcomas require advanced radiosurgery or radiotherapeutical technologies capable of delivering high-dose, high-precision radiation. Although radiosurgery can be used, this chapter will focus on proton therapy for treating skull base sarcomas.

A considerable tumor burden generally persists after surgery. Both diseases are notorious for being highly radioresistant, and they both frequently abut sensitive anatomical structures (e.g., optic nerve, chiasm, brainstem, and spinal cord) whose injury could be lethal or highly damaging. Dose fractionation may provide biological advantages in terms of tumor sensitivity and normal organ repair mechanisms. These are the numerous reasons why proton therapy has become a major therapeutical tool since the mid-1970s.

Proton Therapy

Physical and Biological Properties

In contrast with photon beams, which are exponentially absorbed in matter, charged particles, such as electrons and protons, exhibit a finite range. Because the mass of protons is 2000-fold that of electrons, they carry considerably higher kinetic energy (at equal velocity); therefore, a vastly greater release of energy is obtained as they are slowing down. Furthermore, these "projectiles" are barely deflected

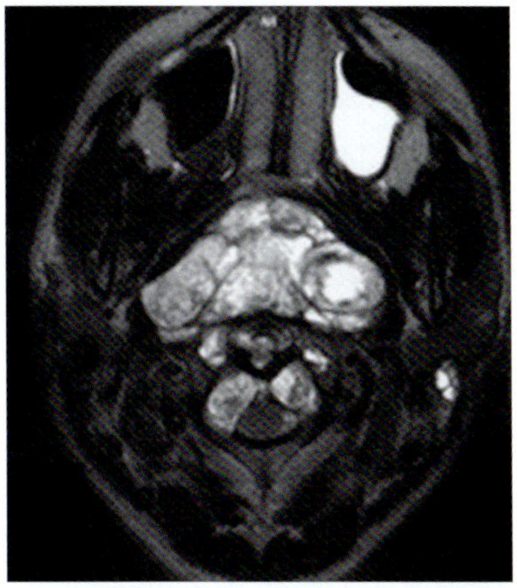

Fig. 10.1 Preoperative imaging in a 17-year-old adolescent with a clival chordoma. Considerable extension is seen to the nasopharynx and the entire skull base.

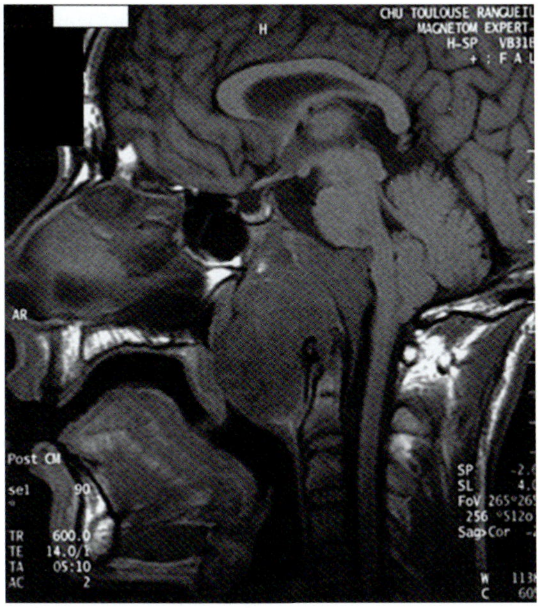

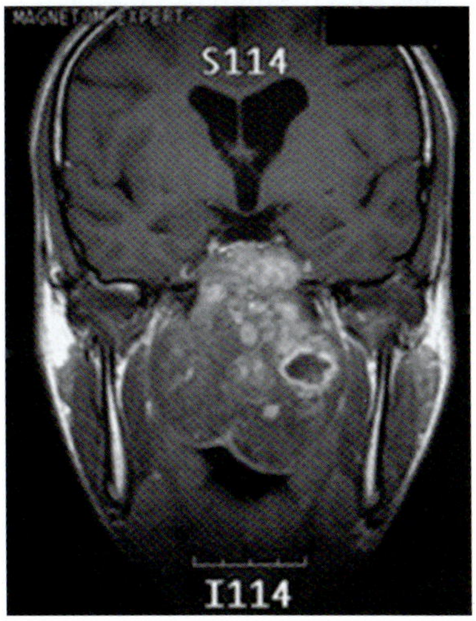

during the process, which translates into a sharp lateral "penumbra" on dose profiles.[7]

Monoenergetic proton beams generated in large accelerators such as synchrotrons produce particles exhibiting a highly uniform range (roughly 1%) and deep penetration (~15–30 cm in water-equivalent material). These properties translate into the so-called Bragg curve: (1) relatively limited interactions in their initial path and limited dose-absorption and (2) a steep rise toward the end of their range, followed by a sharp fall-off of radiation dose. A slight increase in the relative biological effectiveness (RBE) along the beam's path that requires appropriate correction of the physical dose (by 10%) has been reported.[8]

The "pristine" Bragg peak does not exceed a few millimeters at midheight and needs to be "spread out" to encompass thick lesions. The drawback, however, is an increase in the entrance dose. In practice, this disadvantage can be overcome by using multiple angularly separated beams, which is facilitated by using an isocentric gantry, and by technologies under development, such as spot scanning. The latter approach, which is available in the Paul Scherrer Institute, Villigen, Switzerland, improves the modulation of each field by delivering actively modulated small "beamlets."[9]

It should be pointed out that the stopping power of different tissues for protons differs substantially as a function of their density; for example, major corrections are required when the beam passes from bones to soft tissues (i.e., water equivalent) and even more to air cavities. These differences can be "compensated" for by interposing Lucite "compensators" within the beam path in the passive scattering approach or by using the more recent spot-scanning technology without an additional compensator.

Technical Aspects

Early proton facilities were established on university campuses (e.g., centre de Protonthérapie d'Orsay, Orsay, France) or in nuclear research centers (e.g., the Paul Scherrer Institute). These facilities featured simple technology—fixed beam, passive scattering, handmade compensators, for example.[10] Recently, hospital-based facilities have been developed, especially in the United States and Japan. This became possible because modern accelerators are somewhat more compact than their earlier counterparts. Although synchrotrons seem to be the most appropriate accelerators for producing protons of high (i.e., 200–250 MeV) and variable energies, recently interest has been directed to modified cyclotrons, which can achieve excellent performances at relatively low cost ("isochronous" cyclotrons). Newer technology features sophisticated beam delivery systems, including isocentric gantries that help set up complex beam arrangements but are still considerably space consuming. Approximately 25 centers worldwide have implemented a clinical program.

Patient Setup and Alignment

We will briefly discuss the procedure implemented at the Orsay center. The patient can be lying supine or seated (**Fig. 10.2**). A thick custom-made thermoplastic mask is used for immobilization purposes. A bite block can be used concomitantly in compliant patients to avoid head tilt movements. Final accuracy largely depends on stereotactic alignment, based on the implantation of four or five radiopaque nonferromagnetic fiducial markers in the outer skull under local anesthesia. Orthogonal x-ray films are compared with digitally reconstructed radiographs before each daily session to check alignment and repeated for each field. The fiducial markers allow appropriate translation and angular corrections using an original computer program (ROTAPLUS) developed at the Institut Curie d'Orsay Proton Therapy Center. Appropriate corrections are made using a high-precision robotic chair or a couch. Setup accuracy has been verified to < 1 mm in the X, Y, and Z directions and 1 degree for the rotation parameter. Proton therapy treatment time averages 25 minutes, with 20 minutes for the patient setup and 5 minutes for irradiation itself. Possible displacement during the irradiation session is minimized by the visualization of magnified landmarks drawn on the mask or on a TV monitor or of special external marks on an infrared camera. Most treatments are conducted in a conventionally fractionated way (i.e., 30 to 40 daily fractions of 2 CGE cobalt gray equivalent [CGE] = physical dose in Gy + 10% dose for RBE).

Treatment Planning and Simulation

Treatment planning and simulation are conducted using high-definition fused CT-MRI images recorded in the treatment position. Three-dimensional (3D) treatment plans, including dose–volume histograms, are generated using "homemade" software (ISIS) recently upgraded by the DOSIsoft (Cachan, France). Proton beam arrangement generally combines six or seven noncoplanar beams that can be matched using both their lateral and distal penumbras (beam "patching") (**Fig. 10.3**). In adults, approximately half of the treatment is delivered using photons and the other half with protons (**Fig. 10.4**). This does not seem to compromise tumor coverage compared with protons alone.[11] Children are exclusively treated with protons to maximize the shielding of normal structures even in the "low" and "medium" dose regions.

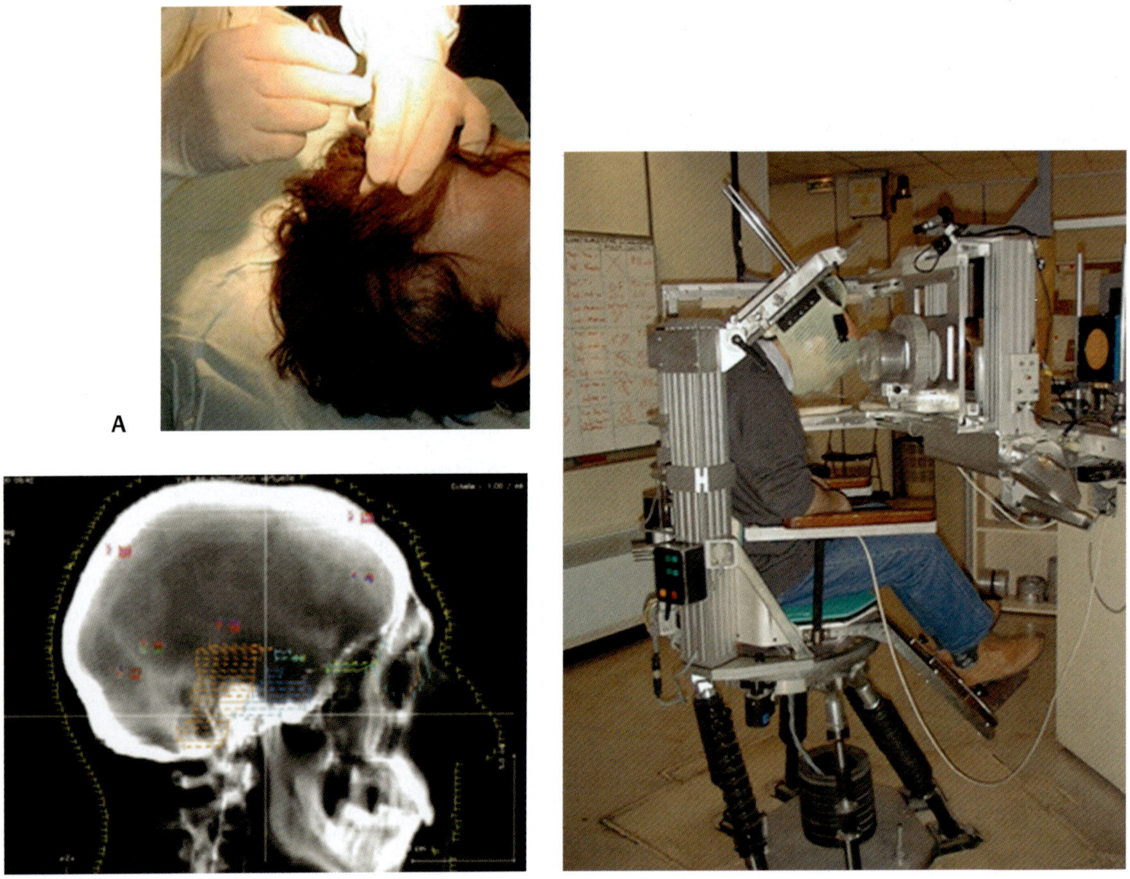

A B C

Fig. 10.2 Patient's preparation and setup before fractionated proton beam therapy. **(A)** Implantation of intracranial fiducial markers, **(B)** digitally reconstructed radiographs used for alignment, and **(C)** patient with thermoplastic mask in robotic chair.

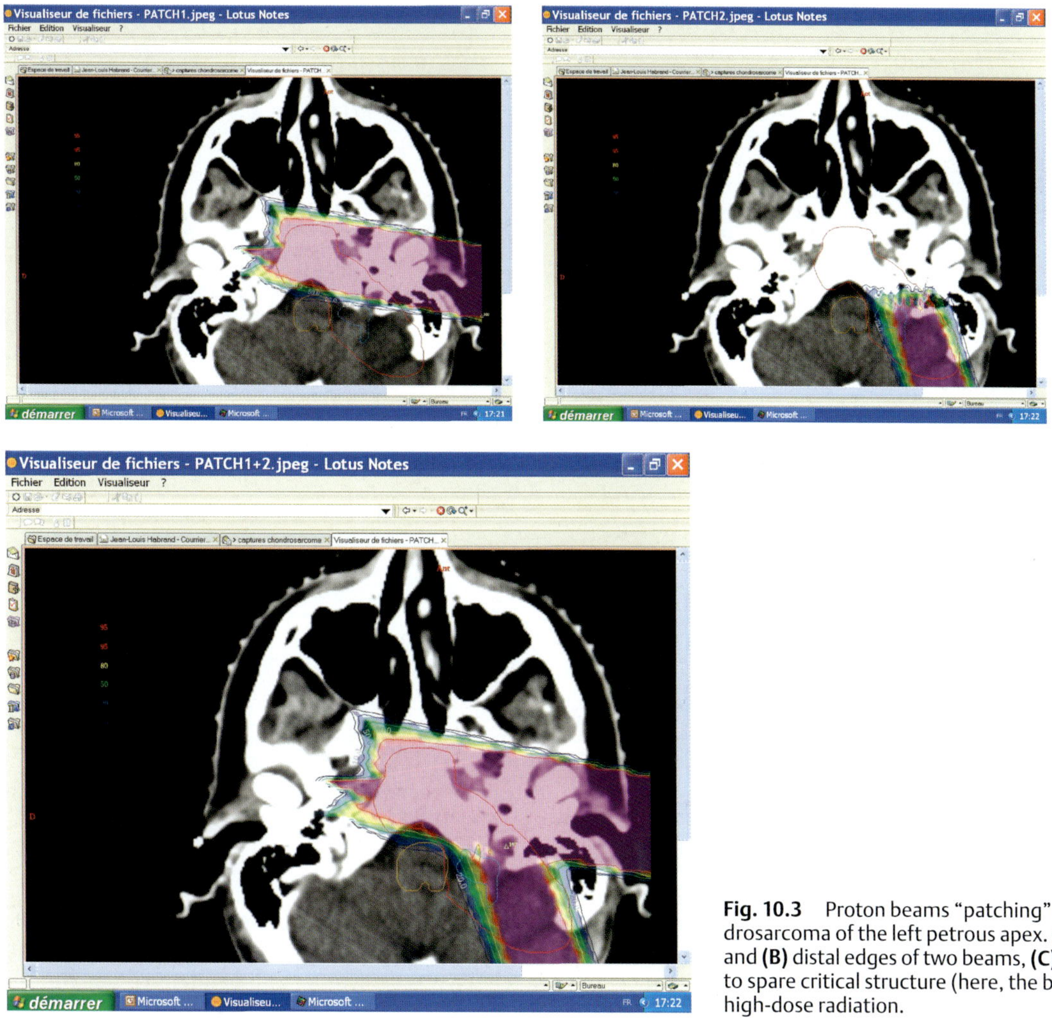

Fig. 10.3 Proton beams "patching" in a low-grade chondrosarcoma of the left petrous apex. **(A)** Abutment of lateral and **(B)** distal edges of two beams, **(C)** with dose summation, to spare critical structure (here, the brainstem) from high-dose radiation.

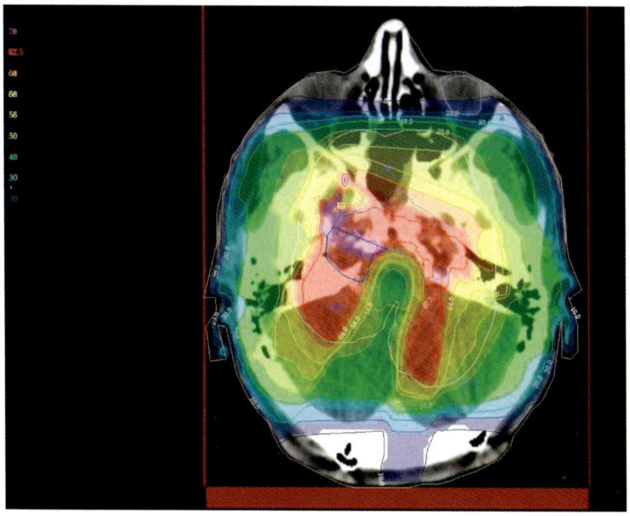

Fig. 10.4 Same patient as in **Fig. 10.1.** Dose distribution with fractionated photon-proton beams therapy (prescribed: 70 CGE to the tumor in 35 fractions over 7.5 weeks). Typical "horseshoe" dose distribution of the high-dose region is seen around the brainstem.

Clinical Results

The Bragg peak with its sharp lateral and distal dose fall-off was theoretically proven to be of major interest in such challenging situations; this led to early clinical experiments in the Department of Radiation Oncology, Massachusetts General Hospital (Boston) in the late 1970s.[12] Local control soared to 59–100%. The main series[13–18] are summarized in **Table 10.1.**[13–18] Most failures are seen within 3 years and are correlated with various prognosticators; the strongest one appears to be the pathological type, with chondrosarcomas faring better than chordomas (chordoma: 59–78%; chondrosarcoma: 78–100%).[12,14,19–22] Despite its better reputation, the chondroid variant has probably a poorer outcome,[23] like the mesenchymal chondrosarcoma.[24] Preliminary data suggest a correlation with the expression of cellular growth factors and with extracellular matrix enzymes in tumor progression.[25,26] Equally prognostic, but less convincingly, were the tumor volume,[16] anatomical situation (cervical and foramen magnum being worse),[27] and gender (exclusively in the case of chordomas, with female patients having a less favorable

Table 10.1 Chordomas and Chondrosarcomas of the Skull Base and Upper Cervical Spine Treated with Proton Therapy

Authors	Tumors	No. of Cases	Dose (Range)/dpf	Results
Hug et al[13]	CH and CS	58	71 CGE (65–79)	Med f-up: 33 m 5-y LC/OS: CH: 59%/79% CS: 75%/100%
Munzenrider and Liebsch[14]	CH and CS	621	67 CGE (66–83)/1.8 CGE	Med f-up: 41 m 10-y LC/OS: CH: 54%/54% CS: 94%/88%
Noel et al[15]	CH and CS	67	67 CGE (60–70)/2 CGE	Med f-up: 29 m 3-y LC/4-y OS: CH: 71%/88% CS: 85%/75%
Igaki et al[16]	CH	13	72 CGE (63–95)	Med f-up: 69.3 m 5-y LC/OS: 46%/66.7%
Weber et al[17]	CH and CS	29	68–74 CGE	Med f-up: 29 m 3-y LC/OS: Med CH: 87.5%/93.8% CS: 100%/93.8%
Habrand et al[18]	CH and CS (ped)	30	68.3 (54.6–71.0)/1.8 CGE	Med f-up: 26.5 m 5-y PFS/OS: CH: 77%/81% CS:100%/100%

Abbreviations: bid, twice a day; CGE, cobalt gray equivalent; CH, chordoma; CS, chondrosarcoma; dpf, dose per fraction; f-up, follow-up period; LC, local control; med, median; m, months; OS, overall survival; ped, pediatric; PFS, progression-free survival; y, years.

outcome).[28] The reason for the latter finding is unknown. Chordomas express hormone receptors (estrogen, progesterone, and androgen) but inconstantly, and differently from one patient to another. Links with sexual chromosomes or genes involved in notochord development are purely speculative. A link with the Ki67 labeling index score, an estimate of tumor doubling time, has been reported.[24] As far as therapeutic factors are concerned, the impact of quality of resection, as well as of escalating doses of radiation > 70 CGE, remains controversial[12–15,21,29]: 26% versus 58% in the Boston series, although the main reason for limiting the dose to the tumor appeared to be the proximity of an organ at risk, a factor related to dose uniformity within the gross tumor volume (GTV, i.e., macroscopic residue).[21,30]

Toxicity

Although relatively few side effects have been reported, a valuable database has been collected, particularly by the Boston group, on dose, volume, and risk estimates for normal organs that are routinely included in the irradiated volume. It should be remembered that all those data concern patients treated with "conventional" fractionation (i.e., doses of ~2 CGE per fraction). Risks associated with single proton fractions do not differ from alternative techniques of radiosurgery and will not be detailed here.

Concerning temporal lobes, the 2- and 5-year complication rates (i.e., clinical and/or radiologic symptoms of radionecrosis) have been established as 8 to 13%, respectively, following doses of 66 and 72 CGE. Surprisingly, the male gender was seen as an independent risk factor.[31]

Glosser et al did not observe any early or late cognitive side effects related to doses up to 66 CGE in adult patients. However, half of the patients had psychomotor speed impairments and symptoms of depression or anxiety.[32]

The risk of brainstem injury was estimated by Debus et al as 12% at 10 years, with a mean 10 months' delay (maximum 3 years). This risk was correlated with the number of previous surgical procedures, a dose > 60 CGE, and associated diabetes mellitus.[33]

Cervical spinal cord toxicity was reported to be close to 15% minor and 5% major injuries for doses ranging from 55 to 58 CGE at the cord center and up to 70 CGE at its surface. The number of previous surgical procedures seemed to be the only prognosticator.[34]

Radiation-related hypothalamus–pituitary endocrine damages were estimated at 10 years:[35] 84% for hyperprolactinemia, 63% for hypothyroidism, 36% for hypogonadism, and 28% for hypoadrenalism. The growth hormone was not routinely evaluated. No patient sustained radiotherapy-induced alteration of the posterior pituitary. The minimum and maximum doses to the pituitary and the maximum dose to the hypothalamus were correlated with multiple deficits (50, 70, and 50 CGE, respectively).

Clearly, neurovisual impairments are a major concern in escalated-dose skull base protocols (along with brainstem toxicity), due to their dramatic impact on the quality of life of patients who generally have an extended life expectancy. This risk has strongly influenced our group's approach to the management of skull base sarcomas. Patients with a tumor abutting the visual pathway are generally offered a limited reoperation to remove at least 1 or 2 mm of this extension. Given the sharp proton lateral penumbra (15%/mm), this means a 5 to 10 CGE drop toward the critical structure. The estimated risk appraised by Habrand et al was ~10% at 55 CGE and ≥ 20% at > 60 CGE.[36] Kim et al demonstrated that beam patching increased this risk if field abutments concerned nerves or chiasm.[37] Several series point out the predisposing role of underlying vasculopathies related to diabetes mellitus and high blood pressure.[36]

Permanent hearing loss is a symptom frequently related to cochlear injury.[14,20,38] Schoenthaler et al showed that in two thirds of patients suffering from hearing loss, the dose had exceeded 62.7 CGE.[38]

The other cranial nerves were found to be relatively "radioresistant," as evidenced by Munzenrider and Liebsch.[14] In Urie et al's detailed analysis of 27 patients, based on anatomical nerve reconstructions, the risk was set to 3%, with a mean 74 months' interval. Using logistic regression, they estimated a risk of 1% at 60 CGE and 5% at 70 CGE for the "common" cranial nerves.[39]

Using a model based on radioprotection data, Miralbell et al estimated that a substantial reduction in the risk of carcinogenesis could be expected from the use of protons due to a reduction in the integral dose to the entire body.[40] This is a major concern in children.

◆ Alternate Approaches

Surgery and Conventional Radiotherapy

Surgery

Because the skull base is an anatomically complex structure, the skull base tumors can hide easily in the crevices that interconnect the intra- and extracranial spaces and intermingle with important neurovascular structures. Often total resection of these tumors is not possible,[41] making some form of postoperative radiotherapy necessary. Even in series in which surgery alone remains predominant, the results appear conflicting, which could reflect selection biases, such as tumor volume or "aggressiveness" of the procedure. Five-year recurrence-free survival (RFS) rates in chondrosarcomas/chordomas was 90%/65% in the Gay series (20% irradiated), at the price of substantial toxicity (cerebrospinal fluid [CSF] leakage, meningitis, and loss of Karnofsky performance status).[42] For chordomas, the 10-year RFS rates were 42% in patients operated on upfront and 26% following reoperation in the Tzortzidis et al series.[43] For chondrosarcomas, the outcome looks better:[44,45] 5-/10-year overall survival (OS) rates of 93%/84% in the Crockard et al series. In our experience, surgery plays a crucial role in combination with high-dose radiotherapy. The rationale is not only to reduce tumor burden, but also to improve dose distribution by separating tumor from critical structures (especially the brainstem and optic pathway) by at least 2 to 3 mm (**Fig. 10.5**). Repeated minimal resections can also play a role in the palliative armamentarium.[46]

External Beam Fractionated Radiotherapy (EBFRT)

The main series[47–51] are presented in **Table 10.2.** In the case of radiation therapy, based on old data, nonconformal two-dimensional radiotherapy at doses not exceeding 55 Gy yielded a 5-year local control rate of 17 to 33%[49,52,53] and an OS rate of 33 to 90%.[54–58]

Since the early 1990s, radiotherapy has evolved toward 3D conformal approaches based on CT scan. More recent literature generally reports on doses escalated to ~60 Gy, given in four or five weekly sessions at a rate of 2 Gy per session. Outcomes do not appear to have been dramatically altered: disease-free survival (DFS) and OS rates attaining 23% and 54% at 5 years, respectively, in a Canadian series of cranial and mobile spine chondrosarcomas;[8] 17% and 38%, respectively, in a Spanish series;[49] and 23% and 35% in a Turkish study.[51] Outcomes following surgical resection and/or conventional radiotherapy are somewhat better in chondrosarcomas with local control attaining 40 to 60% and survival 70 to 85% in tumors located in the head and neck region, with mixed histopathologies.[55–57,59] Series on doses exceeding 60 Gy delivered fractionatedly demonstrated a trend toward improved results, although the experience with photon therapy is still limited.[45,47,60]

Radiosurgery Alone or Combined with External Beam Fractionated Radiotherapy

The main series[61–68] are displayed in **Table 10.3**. Doses in the range of 14 to 19 Gy have been administered in single fractions, alone, or combined with stereotactically guided fractionated radiotherapy, an approach based on noninvasive frames. The fractionated component is delivered between 50 and 65 Gy, with the lowest range corresponding to patients supplemented with a radiosurgery boost. Clinical experience remains very limited in terms of the low number of patients and short follow-up periods. Most series also seem to concentrate on small lesions (i.e., ≤ 20 mm).[66] Historically for radiosurgery, the lesion needs to be 3 to 5 mm away from the optic chiasm or nerves. However, with current radiosurgical devices, such as the Gamma Knife Perfexion (Elekta Instruments AB, Stockholm, Sweden), the rostral extent of the tumor can be even closer to the optic apparatus and still be treated using radiosurgery. At the moment, outcomes appear to be conflicting for chordomas (~30–80% local control) and more encouraging for chondrosarcomas. A substantial amount of late toxicity has been reported, especially when EBFRT is associated with radiosurgery, by the order of 35%.[62]

The CyberKnife (Accuray Inc., Sunnyvale, CA), a technology based on a fully rotational embarked low-energy linear accelerator (with respiratory tracking capabilities as far as

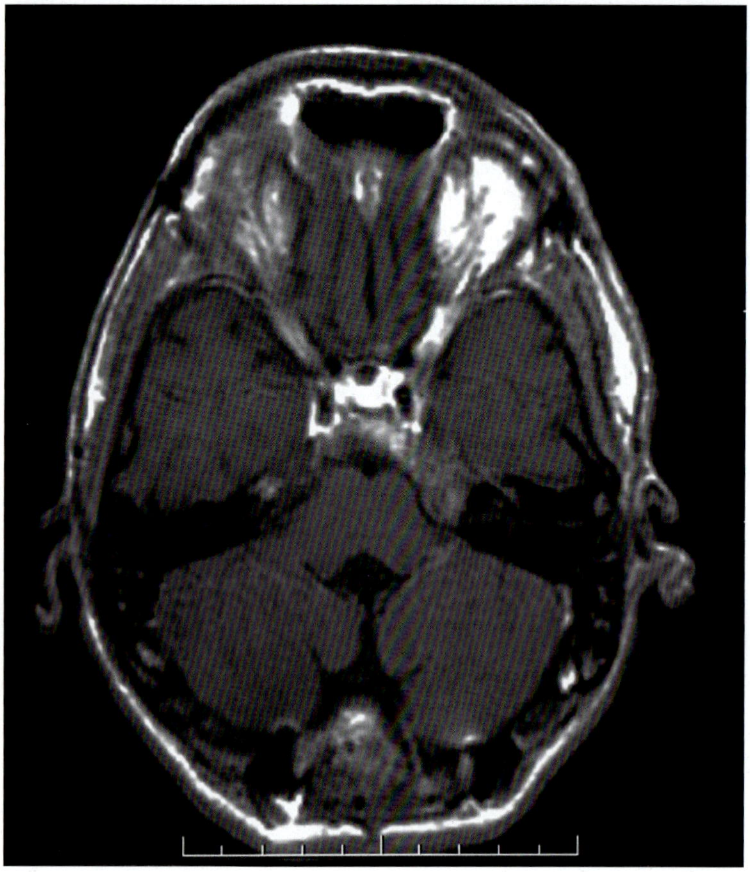

Fig. 10.5 Same patient as in Fig. 10.1. Postoperative aspect. Minimal residual is seen in the left cerebellopontine angle.

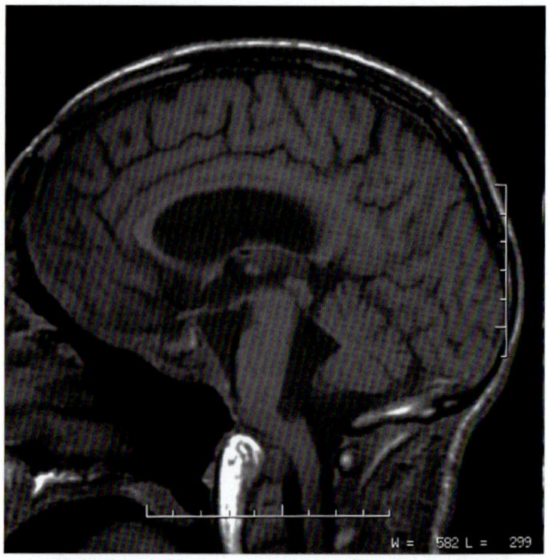

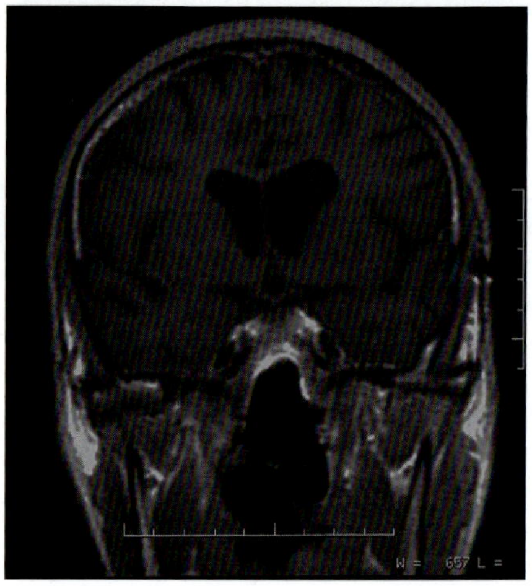

extracranial targets) coupled with a versatile couch, could also play an increasing role in this setting. Target stereotactic positioning and tracking require both invasive and cutaneous fiducial markers. So far the CyberKnife has mainly proven useful for spinal/paraspinal metastases and for primaries that are refractory to previous irradiation. The main limitation lies in the protracted duration of treatment sessions that are still compatible with minimal dose fractionation.

Table 10.2 Chordomas and Chondrosarcomas Treated by Conventional Photon Radiotherapy

Authors	Tumors	No. of Cases	Management	Dose (Range)/dpf	Results
Foweraker et al[47]	CH and CS	12	EBFRT	64.3 Gy (60–65)/1.66 Gy	Med f-up: 38 m 5-y DFS/OS: CH: 80%/62% CS: 100%/100%
Catton et al[48]	CH	48	EBFRT	50 Gy (25–60)/2 Gy (1 Gy bid in 8)	5-y OS: 54% 5-y PFS: 23%
Romero et al[49]	CH	18	EBFRT	50.1 Gy (29.9–64.8) /1.5–2.0 Gy (1.0–1.5 Gy bid in 8)	5-y PFS: 17% 5-y OS: 38%
Magrini et al[50]	CH	15	EBFRT		5-y OS: 58% 10-y PFS: 25%
Zorlu et al[51]	CH	18	EBFRT	60 Gy (50–64)/2 Gy	Med f-up: 43.2 m 5-y PFS: 23% 5-y OS: 35%

Abbreviations: bid, twice a day; CH, chordoma; CS, chondrosarcoma; DFS, disease-free survival; dpf, dose per fraction; EBFRT, external beam fractionated radiotherapy; f-up, follow-up period; m, months; med, median; OS, overall survival; ped, pediatric; PFS, progression-free survival; y, year.

Table 10.3 Chordoma and Chondrosarcoma of the Skull Base and Upper Cervical Spine Treated with Radiosurgery

Author	Tumors	No. of Cases	Technique	Dose/Dractionation	Results
Feigl et al[61]	CH and CS	13	GKS	17 Gy (14–18), SD	Med f-up: 17 m LC: 14%/15%
Krishnan et al[62]	CH and CS	29	GKS ± EBFRT	15 Gy (10–20), SD ± 50.4 Gy (45–54)/C	Med f-up: 4.8 y 5-y LC: CH/CS 32%/100%
Debus et al[63]	CH and CS	45	FSRT – linac	64.9–66.6 Gy/C	Mean f-up: 19–27 m 5-y LC/OS: CH: 50%/82% CS: 100%/100%
Gwak et al[64]	CH and CS	9	CBK (primary + reirradiation)	21.0–43.6 Gy/3–5 f	Med f-up: 24 m LC: 8%/9%
Chang et al[65]	CH	10	linac or CBK	19.4 Gy (18–24)	Mean f-up: 4 y LC: 8%/10%
Hasegawa et al[66]	CH and CS	37	GKS	14 Gy	Mean f-up: 59 m 10-y LC/OS: 67%/53%
Martin et al[67]	CH and CS	28	GKS	16 Gy	5-y LC/OS: CH: 62.9%/62.9% CS: 80%/ NA
Cho et al[68]	CH and CS	30	EBFRT ± GKS	EBFRT: 60.22 Gy (50.4–39.6)/C GKS 17 Gy (15–20)/SD	Mean f-up: 56 m 5-y PFS/OS: CH: 40%/80% CS: 80%/100%

Abbreviations: bid, twice a day; C, conventional fractionation (i.e., 5 daily sessions/wk of 2 Gy each); CBK, cyberknife; CH, chordoma; CS, chondrosarcomas; dpf, dose per fraction; EBFRT, external beam fractionated radiotherapy; FSRT, fractionated stereotactic radiotherapy; f-up, follow-up period; GKS, gamma knife surgery; LC, local control; linac, linear accelerator; med, median; m, months; OS, overall survival; ped, pediatric; PFS, progression-free survival; SD, single dose; y, year; NA, nonassessed.

Gwak et al reported on nine patients with chordomas treated to 21.0 to 43.6 Gy in three to five fractions in which eight of the nine patients were locally controlled.[64] The reverse was two of nine cases of cervical myelopathies. It is certainly too premature to draw any conclusions about the value of this technical innovation.

Light Ion Treatment

These particles (especially carbon ions) combine a dose distribution akin to that of protons, with interesting biological properties. With an RBE of 4, they could prove to be attractive in highly radioresistant lesions, such as chordomas and chondrosarcomas. In addition, a higher dose per fraction of light ions does not seem as toxic as an equivalent dose of photons and therefore could be used in hypofractionated radiation courses. Only two centers worldwide are currently operational (Darmstadt, Germany, and Chiba, Japan), plus a center with the capacity to deliver both protons and ions (Yogo, Japan). These centers use new 3D-scanning particle delivery modes that further improve the dose conformality.[69] Following pioneering work conducted in Berkeley,[70] the GSI (Darmstadt, Germany) group achieved 80 and 70% local control at 3 and 5 years of follow-up, respectively, in a series of 96 cases of chordomas treated with a dose of 60 CGE, in 20 × 3 CGE fractions, over 3 weeks.[71] Toxicity consisted of optic neuropathy (4.1%) and temporal lobe injury (7.2%). The outcome was 96.2 and 89.8% at 3 and 4 years, respectively, in 54 patients with chondrosarcomas. Late toxicity was minor in five patients and severe in one.[72]

Medical Treatments

Chordomas and classical-type chondrosarcomas are notorious for their lack of chemosensitivity. The group at the Medical University, Vienna, Austria reported a case of prolonged survival in an advanced chordoma case by the combination of reirradiation, chemotherapy (doxorubicin), and antiangiogenic agents (isotretinoin, interferon-α, and thalidomide).[73] There are also reports on the use of imatinib (Glivec), a kinase inhibitor,[74] and of razoxane,[75] a radiosensitizing agent.

◆ Management of Chordomas and Chondrosarcomas in Children

Clinical experience of skull base chordomas and chondrosarcomas is extremely limited in children. Using protons alone or predominantly, the Boston and Orsay groups have undoubtedly the largest experience with similar results, by the order of 80% local control/OS in chordomas and 100% in chondrosarcomas.[76] These results could surpass those reported in adults, although very young children have been excluded from our own series due to the lack of capabilities until recently for delivering general anesthesia at the cyclotron site. Very young age poses specific problems associated with major concerns regarding tolerance of normal structures to radiotherapy and possibly unusually aggressive histological subtypes (i.e., dedifferentiated or "highly cellular").

◆ Summary

In summary, skull base chondrosarcomas and chordomas are rare and histologically low-grade malignancies that are frequently highly extensive loco-regionally. These tumours have greatly benefited from recent neurosurgical and radiotherapeutical innovations, and more modestly, in advanced or recurrent presentations, from biological agents and chemotherapy. A management combining maximal resection followed by stereotactically guided high-dose fractionated proton therapy has been extensively explored by oncological groups in the United States, Japan, and Europe, and is generally regarded as the "gold-standard" of therapy. A long-term outcome in excess of 90% in chondrosarcomas and 70% in chordomas can be reasonably expected using such an approach, at the price of a minimal toxicity. The appraisal of very long term outcome, prognostic factors, optimal doses of radiotherapy, emerging technologies (cyberknife, carbon ion, etc.) are still under evaluation.

Acknowledgments We are indebted to all the physicians, physicists, technologists, and dosimetrists involved in the Orsay intracranial proton program and to Lorna Sainte-Ange for editing the manuscript.

References

1. Halperin EC, Perez CA, Brady LW, eds. Principles and Practice of Radiation Oncology. 5th ed. Philadelphia: Lippincott Williams & Wilkins; 2008;1–9
2. Fletcher DM, Unni KK, Mertens F, eds. Pathology and Genetics: Tumors of Soft Tissue and Bone. Lyon: IARC press Pub; 2002; 247–251
3. Halperin EC. Why is female sex an independent predictor of shortened overall survival after proton/photon radiation therapy for skull base chordomas? Int J Radiat Oncol Biol Phys 1997;38: 225–230
4. Bonneville F, Savatovsky J, Chiras J. Imaging of cerebellopontine angle lesions: an update, II: Intra-axial lesions, skull base lesions that may invade the CPA region, and non-enhancing extra-axial lesions. Eur Radiol 2007;17(11):2908–2920
5. Arnautovic KI, Al-Mefty O. Surgical seeding of chordomas. J Neurosurg 2001;95(5):798–803
6. Fischbein NJ, Kaplan MJ, Holliday RA, Dillon WP. Recurrence of clival chordoma along the surgical pathway. AJNR Am J Neuroradiol 2000; 21(3):578–583
7. Bonnett DE. Current developments in proton therapy: a review. Phys Med Biol 1993;38:1371–1392
8. Paganetti H, Niemierko A, Ancukiewicz M, et al. Relative biological effectiveness (RBE) values for proton beam therapy. Int J Radiat Oncol Biol Phys 2002;53:407–421
9. Goitein M, Lomax AJ, Pedroni ES. Treating cancer with protons: physics fighting cancer. Physics Today 2002;55(9):45–50. Available at: http://www.physicstoday.org
10. Chu WT, Ludewigt BA, Renner TR. Instrumentation for treatment of cancer using protons and light-ions beams. Rev Sci Instrum 1993;64: 2055–2122
11. Feuvret L, Noel O, Weber DC, et al. A treatment planning comparison of combined photon-proton beams versus proton beams-only for the treatment of skull base tumors. Int J Radiat Oncol Biol Phys 2007; 69(3):944–954
12. Austin-Seymour M, Munzenrider J, Goitein M, et al. Fractionated proton radiation therapy of chordoma and low-grade chondrosarcoma of the base of the skull. J Neurosurg 1989;70:13–17
13. Hug EB, Loredo LN, Slater JD, et al. Proton radiation therapy for chordomas and chondrosarcomas of the skull base. J Neurosurg 1999;91: 432–439
14. Munzenrider JE, Liebsch NJ. Proton therapy for tumors of the skull base. Strahlenther Onkol 1999;175(Suppl 2):57–63
15. Noel G, Habrand JL, Mammar H, et al. Combination of photon and proton radiation therapy for chordomas and chondrosarcomas of the skull base: the Centre de Protontherapie d'Orsay experience. Int J Radiat Oncol Biol Phys 2001;51:392–398
16. Igaki H, Tokuuye K, Okomura T, et al. Clinical results of proton beam therapy for skull base chordoma. Int J Radiat Oncol Biol Phys 2004; 60(4):1120–1126
17. Weber DC, Rutz HP, Pedroni ES, et al. Results of spot-scanning proton radiation therapy for chordoma and chondrosarcoma of the skull base: the Paul Scherrer Institut experience. Int J Radiat Oncol Biol Phys 2005;63(2):401–409
18. Habrand JL, Schneider R, Alapetite C, et al. Proton therapy in pediatric skull base and cervical canal low-grade bone malignancies. Int J Radiat Oncol Biol Phys 2008;17(3):672–675
19. Austin JP, Urie MM, Cardenosa G, Munzenrider JE. Probable causes of recurrence in patients with chordoma and chondrosarcoma of the base of skull and cervical spine. Int J Radiat Oncol Biol Phys 1993; 25:439–444
20. Hug EB, Slater JD. Proton radiation therapy for chordomas and chondrosarcomas of the skull base. Neurosurg Clin N Am 2000;11:627–638
21. Noel G, Feuvret L, Ferrand R, Boisserie G, Mazeron JJ, Habrand JL. Radiotherapeutic factors in the management of cervical-basal chordomas and chondrosarcomas. Neurosurgery 2004;55:1252–1260
22. Berson AM, Castro JR, Petti P, et al. Charged particle irradiation of chordoma and chondrosarcoma of the base of skull and cervical spine: the Lawrence Berkeley Laboratory experience. Int J Radiat Oncol Biol Phys 1988;15:559–565
23. Almefty K, Pravdenkova S, Colli BO, Al-Mefty O, Godken M. Chordoma and chondrosarcoma: similar, but quite different, skull base tumors. Cancer 2007;110(11):2457–2477
24. Crockard HA, Steel T, Plowman N, et al. A multidisciplinary team approach to skull base chordomas. J Neurosurg 2001;95(2):175–183
25. Naka T, Kuester D, Boltze C, et al. Expression of hepatocyte growth factor and c-MET in skull base chordoma. Cancer 2008;112(1):104–110
26. Naka T, Kuester D, Boltze C, et al. Expression of matrix metalloproteinases-1, -2, and -9; tissue inhibitors of matrix metalloproteinases-1 and -2; cathepsine B; urokinase plasminogen activator; and plasminogen activator inhibitor, type I in skull base chordoma. Hum Pathol 2008;39(2):217–223
27. Colli B, Al-Mefty O. Chordomas of the craniocervical junction: follow-up review and prognostic factors. J Neurosurg 2001;95(6):933–943
28. Muthukumar N, Kondziolka D, Lunsford LD, Flickinger JC. Stereotactic radiosurgery for chordoma and chondrosarcoma: further experiences. Int J Radiat Oncol Biol Phys 1998;41:387–392
29. Suit HD, Goitein M, Munzenrider J, et al. Definitive radiation therapy for chordoma and chondrosarcoma of base of skull and cervical spine. J Neurosurg 1982;56:377–385
30. Terahara A, Niemierko A, Goitein M, et al. Analysis of the relationship between tumor dose inhomogeneity and local control in patients with skull base chordoma. Int J Radiat Oncol Biol Phys 1999;45:351–358
31. Santoni R, Liebsch N, Finkelstein DM, et al. Temporal lobe (TL) damage following surgery and high-dose photon and proton irradiation in 96 patients affected by chordomas and chondrosarcomas of the base of the skull. Int J Radiat Oncol Biol Phys 1998;41:59–68
32. Glosser G, McManus P, Munzenrider J, et al. Neuropsychological function in adults after high dose fractionated radiation therapy of skull base tumors. Int J Radiat Oncol Biol Phys 1997;38:231–239
33. Debus J, Schultz-Ertner D, Schad L, et al. Stereotactic fractionated radiotherapy for chordomas and chondrosarcomas of the skull base. Int J Radiat Oncol Biol Phys 2000;47(3):591–596
34. Marucci L, Niemierko A, Liebsch N, Aboubaker F, Liu MCC, Munzenrider JE. Spinal cord tolerance to high dose fractionated 3D conformal proton-photon irradiation as evaluated by equivalent uniform dose

and dose volume histogram analysis. Int J Radiat Oncol Biol Phys 2004;59(2):551–555

35. Pai HH, Thornton A, Katznelson L, et al. Hypothalamic/pituitary function following high-dose conformal radiotherapy to the base of the skull: demonstration of a dose-effect relationship using dose-volume histogram analysis. Int J Radiat Oncol Biol Phys 2001;49(4): 1079–1092
36. Habrand IL, Austin-Seymour M, Birnbaum S, et al. Neurovisual outcome following proton radiation therapy. Int J Radiat Oncol Biol Phys 1989;16:1601–1606
37. Kim J, Munzenrider JE, Maas A, et al. Optic neuropathy following combined proton and photon radiotherapy for base of skull tumors. Int J Radiat Oncol Biol Phys 1997;39:272
38. Schoenthaler R, Fullerton B, Maas A, et al. Relationship between dose to auditory pathways and audiological outcomes in skull-base tumor patients receiving high-dose proton-photon radiotherapy. Int J Radiat Oncol Biol Phys 1996;36:291, abstr 2026
39. Urie MM, Fullerton B, Tatsuzaki H, et al. A dose response analysis of injury to cranial nerves and/or nuclei following proton beam radiation therapy. Int J Radiat Oncol Biol Phys 1992;23:27–39
40. Miralbell R, Lomax A, Cella L, Schneider U. Potential reduction of the incidence of radiation-induced second cancers by using proton beams in the treatment of pediatric tumors. Int J Radiat Oncol Biol Phys 2002;54:824–829
41. Nguyen-Huynh A, Blevins NH, Jackler RK. The challenges of revision skull base surgery. Otolaryngol Clin North Am 2006;39(4):783–799
42. Gay E, Sekhar LN, Rubinstein E, et al. Chordomas and chondrosarcomas of the cranial base: results and follow-up of 60 patients. Neurosurgery 1995;36:887–896
43. Tzortzidis F, Elahi F, Wright D, Natarajan SK, Sekhar LN. Patient outcome at long-term follow-up after aggressive microsurgical resection of cranial base chordomas. Neurosurgery 2006;59(2):230–237
44. Tzortzidis F, Elahi F, Wright D, Temkin N, Natarajan SK, Sekhar LN. Patient outcome at long-term follow-up after aggressive microsurgical resection of cranial base chondrosarcomas. Neurosurgery 2006;58(6): 1090–1098
45. Crockard HA, Cheeseman A, Steel T, et al. A multidisciplinary approach to skull base chondrosarcomas. J Neurosurg 2001;95(2):184–189
46. Kyoshima K, Oikawa S, Kanaji M, et al. Repeat operations in the management of clival chordomas: palliative surgery. J Clin Neurosci 2003;10(5):571–578
47. Foweraker KL, Burton KE, Maynard SE, et al. High-dose radiotherapy in the management of chordoma and chondrosarcoma of the skull base and cervical spine, I: Clinical outcomes. Clin Oncol 2007;19: 509–516
48. Catton C, O'Sullivan B, Bekk R, et al. Chordoma: long-term follow-up after radical photon irradiation. Radiother Oncol 1996;41(1):67–72
49. Romero J, Cardenes H, La Torre A, et al. Chordoma: results of radiation therapy in eighteen patients. Radiother Oncol 1993;29(1):27–32
50. Magrini SM, Papi MG, Marletta F, et al. Chordoma: natural history, treatment and prognosis. The Florence radiotherapy department experience (1956–1990) and a critical review of the literature. Acta Oncol 1992;31(8):847–851
51. Zorlu F, Gürkaynak M, Yildiz F, Oge K, Atahan L. Conventional external radiotherapy in the management of clivus chordoma with overt residual disease. Neurol Sci 2000;21(4):203–207
52. Fuller DB, Bloom JG. Radiotherapy for chordoma. Int J Radiat Oncol Biol Phys 1988;15:331–339
53. Keisch ME, Garcia DM, Shibuya RB. Retrospective long-term follow-up analysis in 21 patients with chordomas of various sites treated at a single institution. J Neurosurg 1991;75:374–377
54. Forsyth PA, Cascino TL, Shaw EG, et al. Intracranial chordomas: a clinicopathological and prognostic study of 51 cases. J Neurosurg 1993;78: 741–747
55. Mark RJ, Tran LM, Sercarz J, Fu YS, Calcaterra TC, Parker RG. Chondrosarcoma of the head and neck: the UCLA experience, 1955–1988. Am J Clin Oncol 1993;16:232–237
56. Ruark DS, Schlehaider UK, Shah JP. Chondrosarcomas of the head and neck. World J Surg 1992;16:1010–1015
57. Saito K, Unni KK, Wollan PC, Lund BA. Chondrosarcoma of the jaw and facial bones. Cancer 1995;76:1550–1558
58. Samii A, Gerganov VM, Herold C, et al. Chordomas of the skull base: surgical management and outcome. J Neurosurg 2007;107(2): 319–324
59. Oghalai JS, Buxbaum JL, Jackler RK, McDermott MW. Skull base chondrosarcoma originating from the petroclival junction. Otol Neurotol 2005;26(5):1052–1060
60. Tai PTH, Craighead P, Bagdon F. Optimization of radiotherapy for patients with cranial chordoma. Cancer 1995;75(3):749–756
61. Feigl GC, Bundschuh O, Charabachi A, et al. Evaluation of a new concept for the management of skull base chordoma and chondrosarcomas. J Neurosurg 2005;102(Suppl):165–170
62. Krishnan S, Foote RL, Brown PD, Pollock BE, Link MJ, Garces YI. Radiosurgery for cranial base chordomas and chondrosarcoma. Neurosurgery 2005;56(4):777–784
63. Debus J, Hug EB, Liebsch NJ, et al. Brainstem tolerance to conformal radiotherapy of skull base tumors. Int J Radiat Oncol Biol Phys 1997;39:967–975
64. Gwak HS, Yoo HJ, Youn SM, et al. Hypofractionated stereotactic radiation therapy for skull base and upper cervical chordoma and chondrosarcoma: preliminary results. Stereotact Funct Neurosurg 2005;83(5–6):233–243
65. Chang SD, Martin DP, Lee E, Adler JR Jr. Stereotactic radiosurgery and hypofractionated stereotactic radiotherapy for residual or recurrent cranial base and cervical chordomas. Neurosurg Focus 2001;10(3):E5,10.3
66. Hasegawa T, Ishii D, Kida Y, Yoshimoto M, Iizuka H. Gamma Knife surgery for skull base chordomas and chondrosarcomas. J Neurosurg 2007;107(4):752–757
67. Martin JJ, Niranjan A, Kondziolka D, Flinckinger JC, Lozanne KA, Lunsford LD. Radiosurgery for chordomas and chondrosarcomas of the skull base. J Neurosurg 2007;107(4):758–764
68. Cho YH, Kim JH, Khang SK, Lee JK, Kim CJ. Chordomas and chondrosarcomas of the skull base: comparative analysis of clinical results in 30 patients. Neurosurg Rev 2008;31(1):35–43
69. Schulz-Ertner D, Haberer T, Scholz M, et al. Acute radiation-induced toxicity of heavy ion radiotherapy delivered with intensity modulated pencil beam scanning in patients with base of skull tumors. Radiother Oncol 2002;64(2):189–195
70. Castro JR, Linstadt DE, Bahary JP, et al. Experience in charged particle irradiation of tumors of the skull base: 1977–1992. Int J Radiat Oncol Biol Phys 1994;29:647–655
71. Schulz-Ertner D, Karger CP, Feuerhake A, et al. Effectiveness of carbon ion radiotherapy in the treatment of skull-base chordomas. Int J Radiat Oncol Biol Phys 2007;68(2):449–457
72. Schulz-Ertner D, Nikoghosyan A, Hof H, et al. Carbon ion radiotherapy of skull base chondrosarcomas. Int J Radiat Oncol Biol Phys 2007; 67(1):171–177
73. Schönegger K, Gelpi E, Prayer D, et al. Recurrent and metastatic clivus chordoma: systemic palliative therapy retards disease progression. Anticancer Drugs 2005;16(10):1139–1143
74. Casali PG, Stacchiotti S, Sangalli C, Olmi P, Gronchi A. Chordoma. Curr Opin Oncol 2007;19(4):367–370
75. Rhomberg W, Böhler FK, Novak H, Dertinger S, Breitfellnzer G. A small prospective study of chordomas treated with radiotherapy and razoxane. Strahlenther Onkol 2003;179(4):249–253
76. Hoch BL, Nielsen GP, Liebsch NJ, Rosenberg AE. Base of skull chordomas in children and adolescents: a clinicopathologic study of 73 cases. Am J Surg Pathol 2006;30(7):811–818

11

Stereotactic Radiosurgery for Glomus Tumors

Jeffrey T. Jacob, Michael J. Link, Robert L. Foote, and Bruce E. Pollock

Glomus tumors arise from the paraganglia of the chemoreceptor system and occur in both intracranial and extracranial locations. Glomus tumors represent ~0.01% of all tumors diagnosed in humans.[1–3] Greer et al reported an incidence of 8.6 cases per 100,000 new patients.[4] Glomus jugulare tumors and glomus tympanicum lesions are the two most common sites of intracranial occurrence. Women are affected approximately 2 to 5 times more frequently than are men. Local invasion of adjacent structures and the effect of tumor mass cause symptoms associated with this tumor. Neurovascular structures within the hypoglossal canal, jugular foramen, and temporal bone can be affected. Their intimate association with the lower cranial nerves and inner ear complicates their management, because injuries to these structures can cause significant morbidity and functional disability.[5]

The optimum treatment of glomus tumors remains controversial. Although the majority of tumors are histologically benign, these tumors are characterized by unpredictable biological behavior. Typically arising from glomus bodies located in the dome of the jugular bulb, this neoplasm is intimately associated with critical neurovascular structures at the skull base. Successful treatments have included surgical resection, embolization, external beam fractionated radiotherapy (EBFRT), and a combination of these modalities.[4,6] Early treatment of patients with glomus tumors focused on limited resection combined with radiation therapy or radiation therapy alone. The relative inaccessibility of the jugular bulb region, the potential for damage to the surrounding structures, and the vascular nature of these tumors dictated a treatment that was, for the most part, consistent with palliation. Surgery has been most frequently performed in young patients or for patients with complete loss of cranial nerve function. Gross total surgical resection has been accomplished in 0 to 90% of cases in reported series.[7–14] EBFRT has been used in elderly patients and for symptomatic tumors that were considered unresectable, were incompletely resected, or had recurred after resection.[15–18] Control of glomus tumors after EBFRT has ranged from 85 to 100%, with complication rates of 0 to 10%. Complications associated with EBFRT have included necrosis of the temporal bone or brain, mastoiditis, and other local tissue injury.

◆ Radiosurgery for Glomus Tumors

Rationale for Radiosurgery

As an alternative to surgical resection or EBFRT, radiosurgery has been used to manage patients with glomus tumors in the hope of achieving high tumor control rates and symptom response similar to those seen with EBFRT.[19–32] Radiosurgery is commonly performed for patients with benign intracranial tumors, and long-term growth control has been demonstrated for patients with vestibular schwannomas and meningiomas.[33,34] Improved neuroimaging and dose-planning software has contributed greatly to the reduction in cranial nerve deficits after radiosurgery of skull base tumors. Radiosurgery has less general radiation exposure compared with EBRT, and radiosurgery is typically performed in a single session rather than over 5 to 6 weeks.

Early Reports

In 1999 Eustacchio et al reported 10 patients having radiosurgery for glomus tumors.[19] Radiosurgery was the primary treatment for the majority ($n = 7$) of the patients. At a median follow-up of 37.6 months, four patients had tumors that decreased in size, whereas six patients had tumors that remained stable. In a series published by Jordan et al in 2000, eight patients who were deemed unsuitable for surgery were treated with stereotactic radiosurgery.[25] The mean follow-up duration was 27 months, and no patient had an increase in the size of the tumor. One patient experienced intractable vertigo requiring hospitalization after radiosurgery. Saringer et al reported on 13 patients in 2001, with none showing evidence of tumor growth.[30] Two patients experienced radiation-induced cranial neuropathies, both of which were transient. More recent studies have supported the findings of early reports on the efficacy and safety of glomus tumor radiosurgery.[20,21,23,26,31,32] Of note, four patients from the Cleveland Clinic series (23%) showed evidence of tumor expansion after radiosurgery.[32] Three out of these four patients improved clinically. Likely this finding relates to the methodology used to determine tumor size after radiosurgery. In this series, volumetric analyses of tumor volumes were calculated rather than simply comparing linear measurements before and after radiosurgery. The phenomenon of temporary tumor expansion after radiosurgery is well documented after vestibular schwannoma radiosurgery and is not an indicator of a failed procedure.[35]

Mayo Clinic Experience

In 1997 Foote et al published our first report on glomus tumor radiosurgery.[22] This preliminary study evaluated the acute and intermediate toxicities associated with radiosurgery for patients with unresectable or subtotally resected glomus tumors. No radiation-induced complications were noted, and eight of nine tumors remained stable in size at a median follow-up duration of 20 months. More recently, Pollock reported on 42 patients with glomus tumors who underwent Gamma Knife (Elekta Instruments AB, Stockholm, Sweden) surgery at the Mayo Clinic.[29] The mean follow-up for 39 evaluable patients was 44 months (range 6–149). After radiosurgery, 12 tumors (31%) decreased in size, 26 tumors (67%) were unchanged, and 1 tumor enlarged. This patient underwent repeat radiosurgery. The progression-free survival (PFS) rate after radiosurgery was 100% at 3 and 7 years and 75% at 10 years. Six patients (15%) developed new deficits (hearing loss: $n = 3$; facial numbness and hearing loss: $n = 1$; vocal cord paralysis and hearing loss: $n = 1$; temporary imbalance/vertigo: $n = 1$). For 26 patients with testable hearing before radiosurgery, hearing preservation was achieved in 86% and 81% at 1 and 4 years, respectively. No patient developed a new lower cranial nerve deficit after single radiosurgery; the patient having repeat radiosurgery had a new vocal cord paralysis 1 year after his second procedure.

Between March 1990 and October 2007, 57 patients with glomus tumors underwent Gamma Knife surgery at our center. The mean patient age was 58.5 years (range 18–88). Twenty-three patients (40%) had undergone one or more tumor resections prior to surgery. We used an average of 8.1 isocenters of radiation (range 1–19) to cover a mean tumor volume of 14.1 cc (range 1.2–70.3). The mean tumor margin dose was 15.3 Gy (range 12–18); the mean maximum radiation dose was 32.2 Gy (range 24–40). Imaging follow-up was available in 54 patients at a mean of 48 months after the procedure. Fifty-three tumors either decreased ($n = 14$, 26%) or were unchanged ($n = 39$, 72%) in size after radiosurgery (**Fig. 11.1**). One patient showed tumor progression 99 months after radiosurgery and underwent repeat radiosurgery. There has been no evidence of tumor progression after his repeat procedure. Overall, PFS in our series is now 100% at 3 and 7 years and 83% at 10 years (**Fig. 11.2**).

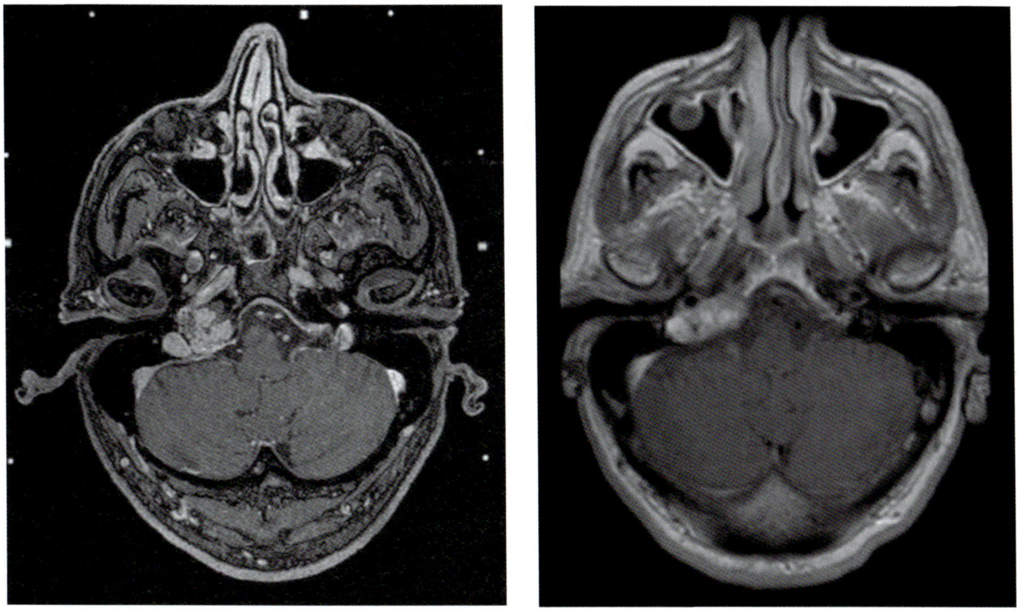

A B

Fig. 11.1 Axial postgadolinium magnetic resonance imaging (MRI) of a 62-year-old man diagnosed with a right-sided glomus jugulare tumor after developing hoarseness and tongue weakness. **(A)** MRI at the time of radiosurgery. The tumor margin dose was 16 Gy. **(B)** MRI 84 months after radiosurgery showing the tumor to be decreased in size.

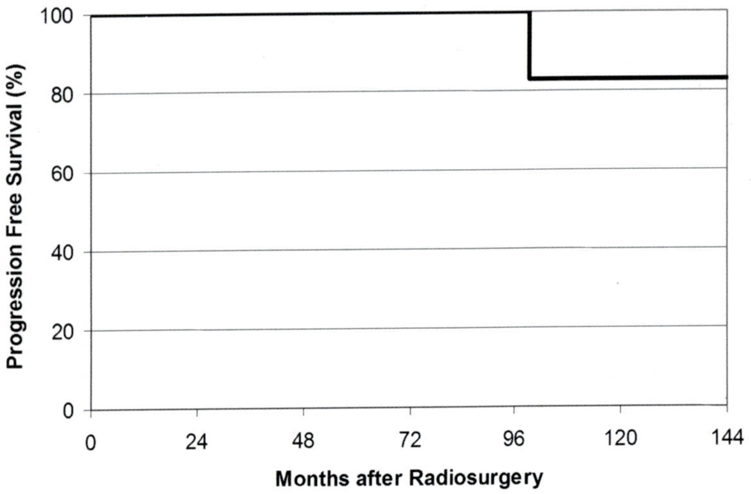

Fig. 11.2 Progression-free survival of 54 patients after glomus tumor radiosurgery. The mean follow-up was 48 months.

Recent Reports

A summary of the studies on glomus tumor radiosurgery published after 1999, including our updated information, shows a tumor growth control rate of 94% (**Table 11.1**). In these studies, 204 patients received a mean dose of 16.4 Gy. The mean follow-up of this collective series was 46 months. As with most of the series involving EBFRT, the follow-up period for these studies is short for a benign tumor. Clearly, more long-term studies are needed to determine PFS rates at 10 and 20 years, especially because more recent patients have been treated with lower radiation doses. It has been shown that tumor cells persist after radiation therapy.[24] Therefore, it is critical to see whether patients who undergo radiosurgery, who almost always have demonstrable tumor on follow-up imaging, show delayed progression at more extended follow-up intervals. Notably, in our series and in the series of Eustacchio et al, which had a mean follow-up of 86 months, patients have been shown to have progressive tumors at 7 years and 8 years, respectively.[20,29] Nevertheless, the information available to date shows that radiosurgery is a viable treatment option for patients with intracranial glomus tumors, particularly if they are older or have recurrent tumors after prior resection.

Complications

Radiosurgery is able to afford local tumor control with low morbidity and essentially zero mortality. All case series reviewed have demonstrated neurologic improvement or stability in the vast majority of patients.[19–32] The most common complication following radiosurgery for glomus tumors is hearing loss, affecting as many as 54% of patients. Although the vestibulocochlear nerve is exposed to radiation during radiosurgery of these tumors, the high rate of hearing loss may also relate to radiation exposure of the cochlea and other temporal bone structures.[36,37] Lower cranial dysfunction is extremely rare. Other complications are nausea, vomiting, and dizziness/vestibular dysfunction. With time, neurologic improvement was noted in some patients with regard to their tinnitus, vertigo, balance, hearing, dysphagia, cranial nerve dysfunction, and headache. In the report by Saringer et al, two patients experienced transient facial or glossopharyngeal neuropathies due to radiation injury, one

Table 11.1 Recent Publications on Glomus Tumor Radiosurgery

Authors	Treatment	Mean F-up (Months)	No. Pts.	%Tumor Size Decreased or Stable	Margin Dose (Median) Gy	Maximum Dose (Median) Gy
Liscak et al[28]	GKS	24	66	95	10–30 (26.5)	20–60 (32)
Jordan et al[25]	GKS	27	8	88	12–20 (16.3)	22.0–46.5 (33)
Saringer et al[30]	GKS	50	13	100	9–14 (12)	22–35 (24)
Eustacchio et al[20]	GKS	86	19	95	12–20 (14)	24–40 (30)
Sheehan et al[31]	GKS	35	8	100	12–18 (15)	24–36 (30)
Gerosa et al[23]	GKS	51	20	100	15–24 (17.5)	NA
Varma et al[32]	GKS	45	17	76	13–18 (15)	23.6–36.0 (29)
Present series, 2008	GKS	49	57	98	12–18 (15.2)	24.0–37.5 (32.2)
Combined data		46	208	94	16.4	30

Abbreviations: GKS, Gamma Knife surgery; NA, TK.

at 1 month and the other at 1 year after radiosurgery.[30] Both conditions completely resolved within 6 months after treatment with corticosteroid treatment. Neither the target volume nor the radiation dose was associated with the incidence of cranial neuropathies. One patient in the study by Jordan et al experienced immediate onset of severe vertigo after radiosurgery that resolved after 11 months.[25] Overall, complication rates in radiosurgical series are low, and neurologic deterioration was observed in no more than 6% of patients. Given the low rate of cranial neuropathies seen in the literature, it would appear that radiosurgical margin doses between 14 and 16 Gy are safe and effective.

Indications for Glomus Tumor Radiosurgery

Clinical factors that must be weighed in the decision-making process for resection or radiosurgery include the patient's age, tumor size, rate of growth in serial neuroimaging, symptoms, neurologic deficits, and overall health. Despite the refinements of microsurgical technique and intraoperative cranial nerve monitoring, a truly radical surgical removal is not the rule for these tumors due to their vascular structure and their extremely critical location. The morbidity associated with resection of glomus tumors remains considerable and includes cerebrospinal fluid leakage, facial weakness, hearing loss, and ataxia. However, the most devastating complication is damage to the lower cranial nerves. An article by Netterville and Civantos on rehabilitation from glossopharyngeal, vagus, and accessory nerve deficits after neurotologic skull base surgery affirmed the significance of such deficits.[38] They said that "the time required to return to a reasonably enjoyable diet often extends to one year postoperatively. A few never attain the goal of enjoyable intake and continue to struggle to maintain adequate nutrition. The latter situation is the rule, not the exception, in the elderly population." Ojemann in an editorial on skull base surgery also commented on the functional consequences of a lower cranial injury relative to other cranial nerve deficits:" If the patient has a high probability of being cured of the tumor or of having a useful life significantly lengthened or more serious disabilities relieved, then the loss of facial nerve function or hearing is acceptable. On the other hand, the loss of ninth and 10th cranial nerve function is one of the most serious neurologic disabilities for a patient. . . . There is a real question as to whether one should electively give this disability to a patient."[5] Finally, most reported surgical series describe postoperative mortality of 4 to 6%.[7,13] This is particularly true for the so-called complex glomus jugulare tumors as described by Al-Mefty and Teixeira characterized by one or more unfavorable criteria: giant size, multifocality, malignant oncotypes, and catecholamine secretion.[7]

Young patients with large tumors causing significant mass effect should undergo resection with or without preoperative embolization.[7,13,14] Although complete resection is always the goal, a subtotal resection is acceptable if total resection would cause an undue risk of morbidity or mortality. Residual or recurrent tumor following resection can then be treated with radiosurgery once the patient has recovered from surgery. Patients with smaller tumors can be safely treated primarily with radiosurgery if there is a clear diagnosis of a glomus tumor based on the patient's history, clinical examination, and neuroimaging studies. Previously, patients with cervical tumor extension were required to undergo resection due to the limitations of the radiosurgical devices. More recently, use of the CyberKnife (Accuray Inc., Sunnyvale, CA) and the Leksell Gamma Knife Perfexion (Elekta Instruments, Inc., Norcross, GA) permits radiosurgery to be performed safely for select cervical lesions.[39–41] Another consideration that favors resection over radiosurgery are patients with significant effects from catecholamine-secreting tumors. Although such cases are rare, representing ~1% of patients with intracranial glomus tumors, resection provides a rapid reduction in circulating catecholamine levels, making medical management of these patients much simpler. Our experience with two patients with catecholamine-secreting tumors mimics what we have noted after radiosurgery of hormone-secreting pituitary adenomas (**Fig. 11.3**).[42,43] Biochemical remission is

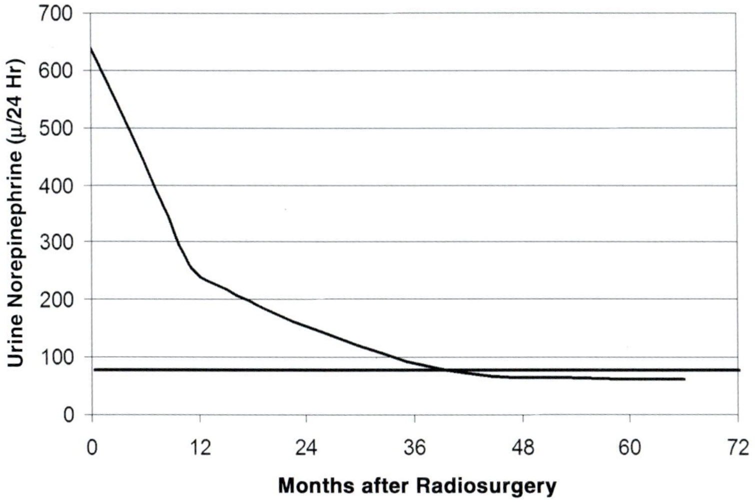

Fig. 11.3 Graph showing the 24-hour urine norepinephrine levels of a 47-year-old woman with a catecholamine-secreting tumor having radiosurgery after prior surgery. Her catecholamine levels became normal 42 months after radiosurgery.

frequently achieved, but the time frame required is usually several years after radiosurgery.

Issues to Consider in Deciding to Do Glomus Tumor Radiosurgery

Stereotactic radiosurgery proved to be a safe and effective option for patients with glomus tumors. Nonetheless, the decision to perform radiosurgery for these patients must take into account several facts. First, although malignant paragangliomas do occur, the overwhelming majority of patients have benign tumors that grow very slowly. In fact, patients have been reported who have survived decades without any treatment.[44,45] Consequently, observation rather than radiosurgery is reasonable for elderly patients whose tumors are small and have not enlarged on serial imaging. Second, due to the often slow growth rate of these tumors and the fact that less than one half of treated tumors have been demonstrated to decrease in size after radiosurgery, some argue that radiosurgery may slow the growth of these tumors, but after some interval, they will again become active and begin to enlarge. This same argument has been forwarded regarding the use of fractionated radiation therapy for glomus tumors.[24,46] It is possible that in patients not showing a reduction in tumor size after radiosurgery, we are simply seeing the natural history of these tumors that may remain quiescent for decades even without treatment. However, 40% of our patients had enlarging tumors documented by serial imaging prior to radiosurgery. Nonetheless, we remain concerned that the only failure we have noted to date did so at 99 months after the procedure and received a tumor margin dose of only 12 Gy. Based on our experience, we typically treat patients with glomus tumors with a margin dose of 14 or 15 Gy, recognizing the cochlea is an organ at risk and precautions are taken to minimize its radiation exposure. Close open-ended follow-up is still needed before we can more accurately define the PFS rate after glomus tumor radiosurgery. Lastly, younger patients with benign tumors need to understand that radiation-induced neoplasms may occur after radiosurgery.[47,48] Even though the chance of this complication remains unclear for a variety of methodological reasons, it is fair to state at this point that the risk of a radiation-induced neoplasm after radiosurgery is at least a log factor less than the 2 to 3% chance following EBFRT of benign tumors.[49,50]

References

1. Lack EE, Cubilla AL, Woodruff JM, Farr HW. Paragangliomas of the head and neck region: a clinical study of 69 patients. Cancer 1977; 39:397–409
2. Mariman EC, van Beersum SE, Cremers CW, van Baars FM, Ropers HH. Analysis of a second family with hereditary non-chromaffin paragangliomas locates the underlying gene at the proximal region of chromosome 11q. Hum Genet 1993;91:357–361
3. Heth J. The basic science of glomus jugulare tumors. Neurosurg Focus 2004;17:E2:6–11
4. Greer JA, Cody TR, Weiland LH. Neoplasms of the temporal bone. J Otolaryngol 1976;5:391–398
5. Ojemann RG. Skull-base surgery: a perspective. J Neurosurg 1992;76: 569–570
6. Gstoettner W, Matula C, Hamzavi J, Kornfehl J, Czerny C. Long-term results of different treatment modalities in 37 patients with glomus jugulare tumors. Eur Arch Otorhinolaryngol 1999;256:351–355
7. Al-Mefty O, Teixeira A. Complex tumors of the glomus jugulare: criteria, treatment, and outcome. J Neurosurg 2002;97:1356–1366
8. Anand VK, Leonetti JP, al-Mefty O. Neurovascular considerations in surgery of glomus tumors with intracranial extensions. Laryngoscope 1993;103:722–728
9. Briner HR, Linder TE, Pauw B, Fisch U. Long-term results of surgery for temporal bone paragangliomas. Laryngoscope 1999;109:577–583
10. Gjuric M, Seidinger L, Wigand ME. Long-term results of surgery for temporal bone paraganglioma. Skull Base Surg 1996;6:147–152
11. Green JD Jr., Brackmann DE, Nguyen CD, Arriaga MA, Telischi FF, De la Cruz A. Surgical management of previously untreated glomus jugulare tumors. Laryngoscope 1994;104:917–921
12. Patel SJ, Sekhar LN, Cass SP, Hirsch BE. Combined approaches for resection of extensive glomus jugulare tumors: a review of 12 cases. J Neurosurg 1994;80:1026–1038
13. Watkins LD, Mendoza N, Cheesman AD, Symon L. Glomus jugulare tumours: a review of 61 cases. Acta Neurochir (Wien) 1994;130: 66–70
14. Woods CI, Strasnick B, Jackson CG. Surgery for glomus tumors: the Otology Group experience. Laryngoscope 1993;103:65–70
15. Cole JM, Beiler D. Long-term results of treatment for glomus jugulare and glomus vagale tumors with radiotherapy. Laryngoscope 1994;104: 1461–1465
16. de Jong AL, Coker NJ, Jenkins HA, Goepfert H, Alford BR. Radiation therapy in the management of paragangliomas of the temporal bone. Am J Otol 1995;16:283–289
17. Larner JM, Hahn SS, Spaulding CA, Constable WC. Glomus jugulare tumors: long-term control by radiation therapy. Cancer 1992;69: 1813–1817
18. Skolyszewski J, Korzeniowski S, Pszon J. Results of radiotherapy in chemodectoma of the temporal bone. Acta Oncol 1991;30:847–849
19. Eustacchio S, Leber K, Trummer M, Unger F, Pendl G. Gamma Knife radiosurgery for glomus jugulare tumours. Acta Neurochir (Wien) 1999;141:811–818
20. Eustacchio S, Trummer M, Unger F, Schrottner O, Sutter B, Pendl G. The role of Gamma Knife radiosurgery in the management of glomus jugular tumours. Acta Neurochir Suppl (Wien) 2002;84:91–97
21. Feigenberg SJ, Mendenhall WM, Hinerman RW, Amdur RJ, Friedman WA, Antonelli PJ. Radiosurgery for paraganglioma of the temporal bone. Head Neck 2002;24:384–389
22. Foote RL, Pollock BE, Gorman DA, et al. Glomus jugulare tumor: tumor control and complications after stereotactic radiosurgery. Head Neck 2002;24:332–338
23. Gerosa M, Visca A, Rizzo P, Foroni R, Nicolato A, Bricolo A. Glomus jugulare tumors: the option of Gamma Knife radiosurgery. Neurosurgery 2006;59:561–569
24. Gottfried ON, Liu JK, Couldwell WT. Comparison of radiosurgery and conventional surgery for the treatment of glomus jugulare tumors. Neurosurg Focus 2004;17:E4:22–30
25. Jordan JA, Roland PS, McManus C, Weiner RL, Giller CA. Stereotactic radiosurgery for glomus jugulare tumors. Laryngoscope 2000;110: 35–38
26. Lim M, Gibbs IC, Adler JR Jr., Martin DP, Chang SD. The efficacy of linear accelerator stereotactic radiosurgery in treating glomus jugulare tumors. Technol Cancer Res Treat 2003;2:261–265
27. Liscak R, Vladyka V, Simonova G, Vymazal J, Janouskova L. Leksell Gamma Knife radiosurgery of the tumor glomus jugulare and tympanicum. Stereotact Funct Neurosurg 1998;70(Suppl 1):152–160
28. Liscak R, Vladyka V, Wowra B, et al. Gamma Knife radiosurgery of the glomus jugulare tumour: early multicentre experience. Acta Neurochir (Wien) 1999;141:1141–1146
29. Pollock BE. Stereotactic radiosurgery in patients with glomus jugulare tumors. Neurosurg Focus 2004;17:E10:63–67
30. Saringer W, Khayal H, Ertl A, Schoeggl A, Kitz K. Efficiency of Gamma Knife radiosurgery in the treatment of glomus jugulare tumors. Minim Invasive Neurosurg 2001;44:141–146
31. Sheehan J, Kondziolka D, Flickinger J, Lunsford LD. Gamma Knife surgery for glomus jugulare tumors: an intermediate report on efficacy and safety. J Neurosurg 2005;102(Suppl):241–246

32. Varma A, Nathoo N, Neyman G, et al. Gamma Knife radiosurgery for glomus jugulare tumors: volumetric analysis in 17 patients. Neurosurgery 2006;59:1030–1036
33. Kondziolka D, Lunsford LD, McLaughlin MR, Flickinger JC. Long-term outcomes after radiosurgery for acoustic neuromas. N Engl J Med 1998;339:1426–1433
34. Stafford SL, Pollock BE, Foote RL, Gorman DA, Schomberg PJ, Leavitt JA. Meningioma radiosurgery: tumor control, outcomes, and complications in 190 consecutive patients. Neurosurgery 2001;49:1029–1038
35. Pollock BE. Management of vestibular schwannomas that enlarge after stereotactic radiosurgery: treatment recommendations based on a 15-year experience. Neurosurgery 2006;58:241–247
36. Linskey ME, Johnstone PA, O'Leary M, Goetsch S. Radiation exposure of normal temporal bone structures during stereotactically guided Gamma Knife surgery for vestibular schwannomas. J Neurosurg 2003;98:800–806
37. Thomas C, Di Maio S, Ma R, et al. Hearing preservation following fractionated stereotactic radiotherapy for vestibular schwannomas: prognostic implications of cochlear dose. J Neurosurg 2007;107:917–926
38. Netterville JL, Civantos FJ. Rehabilitation of cranial nerve deficits after neurotologic skull base surgery. Laryngoscope 1993;103:45–54
39. Chang SD, Adler JR. Robotics and radiosurgery—the CyberKnife. Stereotact Funct Neurosurg 2001;76:204–208
40. Gerszten PC, Ozhasoglu C, Burton SA, Kalnicki S, Welch WC. Feasibility of frameless single-fraction stereotactic radiosurgery for spinal lesions. Neurosurg Focus 2002;13:E4:1–6
41. Lindquist C, Paddick I. The Leksell Gamma Knife Perfexion and comparisons with its predecessors. Neurosurgery 2007; 61(3, Suppl):130–140
42. Pollock BE, Nippoldt TB, Stafford SL, Foote RL, Abboud CF. Stereotactic radiosurgery for patients with hormone producing pituitary adenomas: factors associated with endocrine normalization. J Neurosurg 2002;97:525–530
43. Pollock BE, Jacob JT, Brown PD, Nippoldt TB. Radiosurgery of growth hormone producing pituitary adenomas: factors associated with endocrine cure. J Neurosurg 2007;106:833–838
44. Steinberg N, Holz WG. Glomus jugularis tumors. Arch Otolaryngol 1965;82:387–394
45. Van der Mey AG, Frijns JH, Cornelisse CJ, et al. Does intervention improve the natural course of glomus tumors? A series of 108 patients seen in a 32-year period. Ann Otol Rhinol Laryngol 1992;101: 635–642
46. Brackmann DE, House WF, Terry R, Scanlan RL. Glomus jugulare tumors: effect of irradiation. Trans Am Acad Ophthalmol Otolaryngol 1972;76:1423–1431
47. Loeffler JS, Niemierko A, Chapman PH. Second tumors after radiosurgery: tip of the iceberg or a bump in the road? Neurosurgery 2003;52:1436–1440
48. Rowe J, Grainger A, Walton L, Silocks P, Radatz M, Kemeny A. Risk of malignancy after Gamma Knife stereotactic radiosurgery. Neurosurgery 2007;60:60–66
49. Breen P, Flickinger JC, Kondziolka D, et al. Radiotherapy for nonfunctional pituitary adenoma: analysis of long-term tumor control. J Neurosurg 1998;89:933–938
50. Minniti G, Traish D, Ashley S, et al. Risk of second brain tumor after conservative surgery and radiotherapy for pituitary adenoma: update after an additional 10 years. J Clin Endocrinol Metab 2005;90: 800–804

12

Stereotactic Radiosurgery for Vestibular Schwannomas

Nicolas Massager and Marc Levivier

Vestibular schwannomas, also referred to as acoustic neuromas, are relatively rare tumors, representing < 10% of primary brain tumors. The incidence of vestibular schwannomas is estimated to be 10 per 1,000,000 people per year, representing ~2000 to 2500 new cases diagnosed each year in the United States. With the advent and widespread availability of magnetic resonance imaging (MRI), vestibular schwannomas are diagnosed more frequently and at earlier stages of presentation. The patients are generally 40 to 59 years old, with a slight female preponderance. Histologically, vestibular schwannomas result from benign proliferations of Schwann cells arising from the myelin sheath, mostly of one of the vestibular branches of the eighth cranial nerve (CN VIII). These tumors develop either in the internal auditory canal or in the cerebellopontine angle. Although their histological characteristics are benign and their behavior is noninvasive, vestibular schwannomas create a problem because of their proximity to the brainstem and multiple cranial nerves. Mass effect exerted on these structures results in the common presenting symptoms of hearing loss (95–98% of cases), tinnitus (63–70%), disequilibrium (61–67%), facial numbness (9–29%), facial weakness (5–10%), otalgia (9%), and altered taste sensation (2–6%). Deafness leads to the diagnosis of vestibular schwannoma in 95% of cases, and the most frequently obtained audiologic curve shows a major hearing loss in the 1000 to 4000 Hz frequency, sometimes rising to 8000 Hz. Several hypotheses have been proposed to explain the loss of hearing: (1) direct compression of nerve fibers by the tumor, creating a conduction block, followed by degeneration of nerve fibers; (2) compression or thrombosis of the internal auditory artery, causing deafness of the endocochlear type, sometimes of sudden origin; (3) biochemical modifications of endo- and perilymphatic fluids; and (4) destruction of the cochlea by the tumor (rare and mostly seen in cases of neurofibromatosis).[1]

◆ Evolution of Radiosurgery Technique

In 1971 Dr. Lars Leksell published the indications for and technique of vestibular schwannoma radiosurgery, as first performed in a patient in 1969.[2] In the application of his initial concept of radiosurgery described in 1951,[3] Leksell used the first generation of the Gamma Knife (Elekta Instruments AB, Stockholm, Sweden) unit with 179 cobalt 60 radiation beams to target the tumor using air or contrast encephalography. A comprehensive evaluation of the initial Swedish series of 14 patients was reported by Noren et al in 1983.[4] The modern era of vestibular schwannoma radiosurgery was ushered in at the University of Pittsburgh under Dr. L. D. Lunsford using a 201-source Gamma Knife unit and high-resolution imaging techniques. In 1988, Kamerer and Lunsford published their early experience of nine patients treated with this technique.[5]

In the early 1990s, radiosurgical techniques evolved considerably. These changes included improvements in four different fields:

1. *Stereotactic imaging improved significantly.* Tumor imaging with computed tomography (CT), and later MRI, replaced pneumencephalography and angiography, which allowed precise visualization of the whole tumor by today's standards. The intracanalicular portion of the vestibular schwannoma was seen and could be targeted accurately.
2. *Dosimetric planning progressed considerably with the use of computers.* Because treatment-planning computer programs were faster and fully integrated with imaging, highly conformal multiisocenter treatment plans could be performed. Later years saw the introduction of inverse treatment planning in the treatment-planning computer program, wherein the computer itself was programmed to create a dosimetric planning based on three-dimensional tracing of the tumor volume.

3. *Improvement in the mechanical precision and automatization of beam delivery.* The new generations of radiosurgical devices included robotic systems for patient positioning during radiation treatment.[6] These robotic systems increased the accuracy of beam delivery according to the planned dose distribution.[7] Moreover, automatization of the changes in patient positioning has facilitated the use of highly conformational planning using a large number of small-diameter isocenters.
4. *Reduction of the prescription doses for vestibular schwannoma radiosurgery.* Initially, minimum tumor doses of 16 to 20 Gy were prescribed, according to tumor volume. To reduce the incidence of facial paresis and increase preservation of hearing, prescription doses were lowered slowly. The most commonly used prescription dose today is in the range of 12 to 13 Gy, with a lower morbidity and no compromise in tumor control so far.[8,9]

◆ Management Options for Vestibular Schwannomas

Patients with vestibular schwannomas have several treatment options, including observation, microsurgical resection, stereotactic radiosurgery, and fractionated radiation therapy. The decision can be difficult for some patients and easier for others; each therapeutic procedure has its own indications, limitations, results, and morbidity. Individual treatment decisions should take into account the patient's age, past medical history, tumor size, hearing status, and extent of symptoms. We believe that observation can be a good option only for very old patients or for patients with asymptomatic and small-sized tumors. Hence, a significant tumor growth is found in the majority of patients with vestibular schwannomas who choose observation.[10] Microsurgical resection is mainly indicated for patients with large tumors (Koos grade IV) that have caused neurologic deficits from brainstem compression or when pathologic examination is required because tumor imaging is not characteristic of vestibular schwannoma. The consequence of surgery is often total loss of unilateral hearing and partial or total loss of unilateral facial nerve function. Within this context, stereotactic radiosurgery provides an attractive alternative to surgical resection. Radiosurgery is used for small or medium-sized vestibular schwannomas with the goals of preserved neurologic function and prevention of tumor growth. The long-term outcome of Gamma Knife radiosurgery has proven its role in the primary or adjuvant management (e.g., after subtotal removal or recurrence) of this tumor.[8,9] Fractionated radiotherapy has been suggested as an alternative treatment option for selected patients with larger tumors for whom microsurgery may not be feasible or for some patients in an attempt to preserve cranial nerve function.[11]

◆ The Brussels Gamma Knife Center Experience

The Brussels Gamma Knife Center was inaugurated in January 2000. Between January 2000 and December 2007, 300 patients with a vestibular schwannoma were treated by Gamma Knife radiosurgery in our center located on the campus of the University Hospital Erasme, Brussels, Belgium (**Table 12.1**). The median patient age was

Table 12.1 Results of Vestibular Schwannoma Radiosurgery at the Gamma Knife Center of Brussels, 2000–2007

Preoperative data		
No. of patients	300	
Age		
Median	54 years	
SD	15 years	
Range	11–88 years	
Sex		
Male	153	
Female	147	
Location		
Left	162	
Right	138	
Prior surgery		
Yes	33	11%
No	267	89%
Hearing status		
Serviceable	168	56%
Nonserviceable	132	44%
Treatment data		
Tumor volume		
Mean	1520 mm^3	
SD	1,664 mm^3	
Range	11–8300 mm^3	
No. of shots		
Mean	11.9	
SD	5.6	
Range	1–27	
Margin dose	12 Gy/50% isodose	
Coverage	100%	
Conformity index		
Mean	1.27	
SD	0.20	
Range	1.10–2.79	
Follow-up data		
No. of patients	204	
Duration		
Mean	2.67 years	
SD	1.75 years	

(Continued on page 92)

Table 12.1 (*Continued*) Results of Vestibular Schwannoma Radiosurgery at the Gamma Knife Center of Brussels, 2000–2007

Range	1–7 years	
Tumor size		
Decreased (> 10%)	108	53%
Stable	41	20%
Increased (> 10%)		
Follow-up < 2 y	47	23%
Follow-up ≥ 2 y	8	4%
Hearing outcome		
GR grade stable	126	61.8%
GR grade improved	5	2.5%
GR grade worsened	73	35.7%
Serviceable hearing maintained	129/168	76.8%
Loss of serviceable hearing	39/168	23.2%
Loss of testable hearing	10	4.9%
Facial paresis	0	0%

Abbreviations: GR, Gardner-Robertson; SD, standard deviation.

54 years (standard deviation [SD] 15 years; range 11–88 years). There were 147 women and 153 men. The tumor was located on the left side in 162 patients and on the right side in 138 patients. For 267 patients (89%), radiosurgery was the first treatment of their vestibular schwannoma; 33 patients (11%) were treated by Gamma Knife for a residual or recurrent tumor after microsurgery. Hearing status before radiosurgery was assessed the day before treatment for all patients, using the Gardner-Robertson classification:[12] 168 patients (56%) had serviceable hearing (100 patients in class 1 and 68 patients in class 2), and 132 patients (44%) had nonserviceable hearing (60 patients in class 3, 4 patients in class 4, and 68 patients in class 5).

Radiosurgical Procedure

All patients were treated in the Brussels Gamma Knife Center using the Leksell Gamma Knife C (January 2000–September 2005) or 4C (September 2005–December 2007). A standard radiosurgical procedure was used: the Leksell G stereotactic frame was placed on the patient's head under local anesthesia with mild intravenous sedation. We performed for all patients stereotactic axial gadolinium-enhanced T1-weighted three-dimensional MR volume acquisitions divided in 1 mm slices, axial T2-weighted three-dimensional MR volume acquisitions divided in 1 mm slices, and bone CT densitometric imaging acquisition divided in 1 mm slices (**Fig. 12.1**). Treatment planning was performed with Leksell GammaPlan 5.3X (Elekta Instruments). A target volume was drawn using multimodality images, based on tumor visualization using T1- and T2-weighted MRI sequences and the osseous limits of the acoustic canal as noted on CT scan. The mean tumor volume was 1520 mm^3 (range 11–8,300 mm^3; SD 1664 mm^3) (**Table 12.1**). A conformal plan was achieved using 1 to 27 isocenters (mean 11.9; SD 5.6) of different diameters to cover 100% of the target volume with the prescription isodose (**Fig. 12.1**). Isocenters of 4 mm were used in 59.3% of the total number of shots, 8 mm isocenters in 36.7%, 14 mm isocenters in 3.3%, and 18 mm isocenters in 0.8%. The dosimetric planning used only collimators of the same diameter in 82.7% of cases and a combination of two collimators in 17.3% of cases. For all patients a marginal dose of 12 Gy was prescribed at the 50% isodose, and tumor coverage by the prescription isodose was 100%. The mean conformity index, calculated as the ratio of prescription isodose volume to target volume, was 1.27 (range 1.10–2.79; SD 0.20).

When dosimetry was finished, the dose planning was transferred to the operating console of Leksell Gamma Knife C/4C, and the treatment was delivered using the Automatic Positioning System.[6] The stereotactic frame was removed at the end of the treatment, and patients were discharged the next day.

Results

A standardized follow-up is proposed to the patients after treatment, which consists of MRI, an audiologic examination, and a clinical evaluation at 6 months, 1 year, 2 years, 3 years, 4 years, 5 years, 7 years, and 10 years after radiosurgery. In our database, a follow-up of ≥ 1 year is available for 204 patients (**Table 12.1**). The mean follow-up period is 2.67 years (range 1–7 years; SD 1.75 years); 38 patients have a follow-up ≥ 5 years.

At the last follow-up, tumor volume has significantly (i.e., > 10% change) decreased for 108 patients (53%), has remained stable for 41 patients (20%), and has increased significantly for 55 patients (27%). However, 47 of these 55 patients had a radiologic follow-up ≤ 2 years, when a transient increase in volume after radiosurgery will typically occur,[13] and must therefore not be considered as a failure of Gamma Knife treatment. Eight patients had to be treated for tumor progression after the radiosurgical treatment; so the total radiologic tumor control at last follow-up in our series is 96.1% (196/204 patients).

The audiologic outcome was analyzed in three ways: the Gardner-Robertson classification,[12] serviceable/nonserviceable hearing, and testable hearing/cophosis. At last follow-up, 126 patients (61.8%) remained at the same Gardner-Robertson hearing grade, 5 patients (2.5%) improved their hearing by ≥ 1 grade and 73 patients (35.7%) worsened their hearing by ≥ 1 grade. On the basis of Gardner-Robertson classification, no hearing worsening occurred in 64.3% of our patients following Gamma Knife treatment. Of the 168 patients with serviceable hearing before radiosurgery, 39 patients (23.2%) worsened their audiologic status to nonserviceable hearing. Thus, 76.8% of our patients have maintained useful hearing following radiosurgery. Only 10 patients (4.9%) have lost any testable hearing in the follow-up course after Gamma Knife treatment.

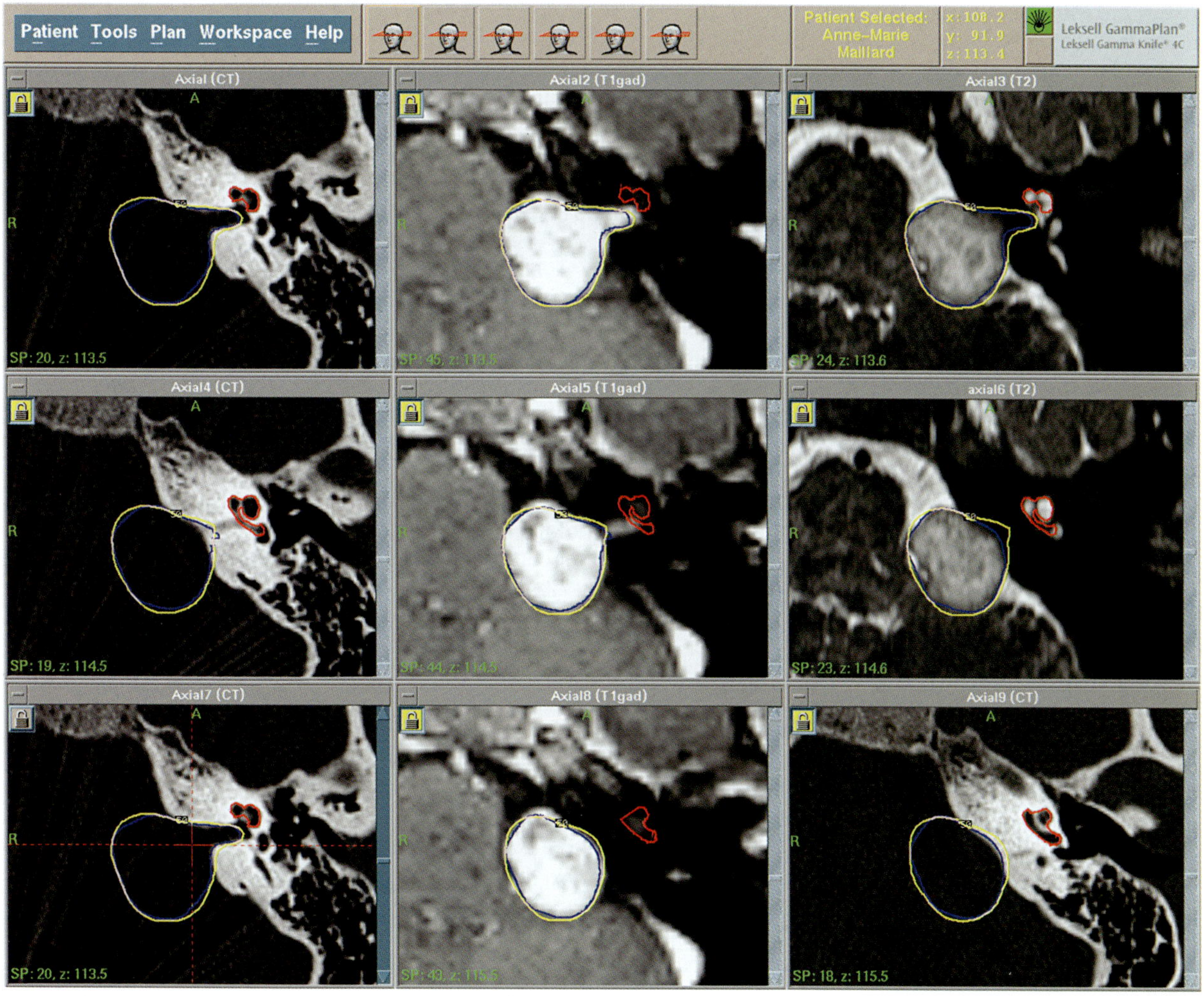

Fig. 12.1 Example of highly conformational dosimetric planning of a vestibular schwannoma using a combination of stereotactic axial bone computed tomography densitometric imaging acquisition divided in 1 mm slices, axial gadolinium-enhanced T1-weighted three-dimensional magnetic resonance (MR) volume acquisitions divided in 1 mm slices, and axial T2-weighted three-dimensional MR volume acquisitions divided in 1 mm slices. Blue line = tumor volume ; yellow line = 12 Gy isodose line ; red line = cochlea.

We have observed no new or increased facial paresis following Gamma Knife radiosurgery. We have had no secondary hydrocephalus and no other problem directly related to the Gamma Knife procedure.

Influence of Radiation Dose Distribution in Vestibular Schwannoma Radiosurgery

To analyze the role of radiation dose distribution in Gamma Knife radiosurgery for vestibular schwannomas, we made retrospective dosimetric studies in a group of 82 patients with testable hearing treated in our center.[14,15] Because one of the most accepted physiopathologic mechanisms of hearing deterioration after radiosurgery is an injury of the cochlear nerve inside the internal acoustic canal caused by enlargement of the intracanalicular part of the vestibular schwannoma during the inflammatory edema reaction after radiosurgery, we have focused our search for the influence of dose distribution in the intracanalicular portion of the vestibular schwannoma on hearing preservation after radiosurgery. We found that the integrated dose of radiation delivered to the intracanalicular portion of the vestibular schwannoma correlated with patients' hearing outcome.[14] We have analyzed two parameters that provide an assessment of dose homogeneity into the intracanalicular portion of the vestibular schwannoma: the maximum dose delivered to this volume, and the ratio between the integrated dose to this volume and the integrated dose to the total tumor volume. We have shown that in the group of patients with audiologic worsening after Gamma Knife radiosurgery a higher maximum dose and a higher percentage of the radiation energy were delivered on the intracanalicular portion of the tumor. These results suggest that the dosimetry of patients with hearing preservation after Gamma Knife radiosurgery is characterized by a higher homogeneity in dose distribution into the intracanalicular part of the vestibular schwannoma than the dosimetric planning of patients with audiologic worsening after the radiosurgical procedure.[14]

In the same group of 82 patients, we analyzed the relationship between the dose of radiation delivered to the cochlea during Gamma Knife treatment for vestibular schwannoma and the hearing outcome of these patients.[15] We found that a higher radiation dose received by cochlear structures was associated with a higher risk of hearing worsening after treatment.

These studies suggest that in vestibular schwannoma radiosurgery the audiologic outcome seems to be not only the consequence of the prescription dose used and the conformity of the dosimetric planning but also other dosimetric parameters such as the radiation energy delivered to some parts of the tumor, the homogeneity in dose distribution to some tumor areas, and the radiation dose delivered to some sensitive structures located outside the tumor volume.

◆ Experience of Other Radiosurgery Centers

No group has contributed scientifically more to the treatment of vestibular schwannoma by radiosurgery than Dr. L. D. Lunsford, D. Kondziolka, and J. Flickinger from the Pittsburgh Gamma Knife center. This group published their results of Gamma Knife treatment for vestibular schwannoma using a margin dose of 12 to 13 Gy[8] (**Table 12.2**). In a series of 216 patients treated with Gamma Knife using this low dose and followed up to 12 years after radiosurgery, they found a 10-year actuarial resection-free tumor control rate of 98.3% ± 1.0%. Among 121 hearing patients with > 3 years of follow-up, crude hearing preservation rates were 71% for keeping the same Gardner-Robertson hearing level, 74% for serviceable hearing, and 95% for any testable hearing. No patient developed new facial neuropathy after radiosurgery. The 10-year actuarial rate for preserving trigeminal nerve function was 94.9% ± 1.8%.

Other Gamma Knife centers have shown similar results (**Table 12.2**). Dr Régis and coworkers in Marseille is certainly the group with the largest experience in treating vestibular schwannomas with Gamma Knife. They reported their results on more than 1500 patients, including 1000 patients with more than a 3-year follow-up.[16] The group has used a 12 Gy margin dose for the treatment of vestibular schwannomas since 1992. Régis et al found a long-term tumor control rate of 97% and no facial palsy since the use of Gamma Knife model C with Automatic Positioning System;[16] the overall rate of hearing preservation was 60%.[9,17] Sheehan et al[18] and Litvack et al[19] reported comparable results.

More recently, other radiosurgical devices have been used for the treatment of vestibular schwannomas. The results of linear accelerator (linac)–based radiosurgical treatment for vestibular schwannomas are available in the literature. Foote et al[20] used a linac for the treatment of vestibular schwannomas in 149 patients; they prescribed a mean dose of 14 Gy at the 70 or 80% isodose. After a median duration of follow-up of 36 months (range 18–94 months), they found an overall radiologic tumor control rate of 93% and a 5-year actuarial tumor control rate of 87%. The overall actuarial incidences of facial and trigeminal neuropathies were 11.8 and 9.5%, respectively; in the 108 patients treated after 1994, these rates declined to 5 and 2%, respectively. A more recent publication by Friedman et al[21] confirmed these results.

Radiosurgery treatment with the CyberKnife (Accuray Inc., Sunnyvale, CA) has been used for single-fraction or fractionated radiosurgery for vestibular schwannomas. Ishihara et al[22] reported their results in a series of 38 patients treated with this device. Target irradiation was administered in 1 or 3 fractions (mean 2.5 fractions); the mean total margin dose was 17 Gy. After a mean follow-up period of 31.9 months, 94% of the tumors were controlled. The hearing preservation rate was 93%. Facial weakness and new trigeminal symptoms did not develop in any patients.

The efficacy of fractionated stereotactic radiotherapy (FSRT) in the management of vestibular schwannomas remains unclear. However, some authors have recently reported interesting results using this therapy.[11,23,24]

Proton beam therapy has also been used for the treatment of vestibular schwannomas. Weber et al[25] published their experience of a series of 88 patients with vestibular schwannomas irradiated with this radiosurgical tool

Table 12.2 Results of Series on Radiosurgery Treatment for Vestibular Schwannoma

Author	RS Device	No. of Cases	Dose-to-Tumor Margin	Median Isodose	Median Follow-Up	Tumor Control	Facial Preservation	Hearing Preservation
Chopra et al[8]	GK	216	12–13 Gy	50%	5.7 y	98.3%	100%	61.3%
Régis et al[16]	GK	1000	12 Gy	50%	NA	97%	100%	60%
Sheehan[18]	GK	> 400	NA	NA	NA	94%	98.5%	58%
Litvack et al[19]	GK	134	12 Gy	50%	31.7 m	96.7%	100%	61.7%
Foote et al[20]	linac	149	14 Gy	70–80%	36 m	93%	95%	NA
Friedman et al[21]	linac	296	12.5 Gy	70–80%	40 m	90%	99.3%	NA
Ishihara et al[22]	CyberKnife	38	17 Gy (1–3 fractions)	NA	31.9 m	94%	100%	93%
Weber et al[25]	Proton	88	12 Gy	70%	38.7 m	93.6%	91.1%	33.3%
Present study	GK	204	12 Gy	50%	2.67 y	96.1%	100%	64.2%

Abbreviations: GK, Gamma Knife; linac, linear accelerator; m, months; NA, not available; RS, radiosurgical; y, years.

using a dose of 12 cobalt gray equivalents prescribed at the median 70 isodose line and followed over a median period of 38.7 months. The actuarial 5-year tumor control rate was 93.6%. Of the 21 patients with functional hearing before radiosurgery, 7 patients (33%) retained serviceable hearing ability. Actuarial 5-year normal facial and trigeminal nerve function preservation rates were 91.1 and 89.4%, respectively.

Microsurgery after Radiosurgery

Several groups have reported their experience with microsurgery after failed radiosurgery for vestibular schwannomas. Debulking of these irradiated tumors is usually considered easy. Technical difficulties, such as thickening of the arachnoid, adherences with more complex dissection of the tumor from the facial nerve or the brainstem, and increased bleeding, have been described. The limitation in interpreting these studies is that they are, indeed, based on retrospective reviews of operation notes or neurosurgeons' comments of their operative findings, in a context in which the neurosurgeon is aware of the previous history of radiosurgery, which may have influenced the description of the surgery. Also, because the reported experience is short, it is difficult to conclude whether the number of cases with worsened functional outcome after microsurgery is higher than in patients who did not undergo radiosurgery before microsurgery. To avoid the risk of postoperative functional impairment, two recent articles advocate that microsurgery after radiosurgery should be performed only on the basis of new symptoms or clinical worsening, and not if the tumor volume increases, even after several years of follow-up.[26,27] Moreover, the same authors recommend that the surgical resection should be very cautious and conservative, limited to subtotal removal, in order preserve functions as much as possible.

Neurofibromatosis Type 2

Neurofibromatosis type 2 (NF2) is an autosomal dominant genetic disorder caused by mutations on chromosome 22. Patients will develop bilateral vestibular schwannomas as a hallmark of their disease. The natural history of NF2-associated vestibular schwannomas is progressive loss of hearing and eventually deafness. The traditional management of these tumors has been their microsurgical removal when they were growing and becoming symptomatic. More recently, as for sporadic vestibular schwannomas, radiosurgery has become a common management approach for these patients. The results of surgical resection of vestibular schwannomas in NF2 are associated with a high risk of complication, with deafness and a rate of facial palsy much higher than in their sporadic, unilateral counterpart. This may be because, in NF2, CN VII and VIII are located within the tumor and are sometimes even infiltrated by the tumor, whereas in sporadic cases, the nerves are usually displaced on the surface of the tumor. This difference in anatomopathology may also explain the poorer results of radiosurgery when compared with those reported in sporadic vestibular schwannomas. This is well illustrated in the 2007 study by the Pittsburgh group.[28] They reported on Gamma Knife radiosurgery in 74 vestibular schwannomas in 62 patients with NF2. The actuarial control rates were 85, 81, and 81% at 5, 10, and 15 years, respectively. The actuarial serviceable hearing preservation rates were 73, 59, and 48% at 1, 2, and 5 years, respectively, in a context where serviceable hearing was present in only 35% of the cases before radiosurgery. Facial neuropathy also occurred more frequently (8% of the cases). Although these results are not as good as the one reported in sporadic unilateral tumors, the Pittsburgh group did confirm that radiosurgery is an advantageous alternative to microsurgery in NF2-associated vestibular schwannomas, as it provides a high rate of tumor control, with higher hearing preservation and morbidity rates that are lower than with microsurgery.

Interestingly, in this study, no secondary malignancy was identified.[28] In contrast, based on their series of 118 patients with NF2 and 19 patients with von Hippel-Lindau disease who were treated with radiosurgery, Rowe et al reported two cases of gliomas that appeared, both in patients with NF2 (4%).[29] They concluded, however, that this may not represent an increased risk and that radiosurgery should be offered to these patients, in regards to the treatment options available and the natural history that these patients have to face.

Summary

Radiosurgery has become a common management approach for patients with vestibular schwannomas. Accumulated data show that it provides a high rate of tumor control, with higher hearing preservation and morbidity rates that are lower than with microsurgery. Thus, except when the tumor is too large or when symptoms are due to tumor compression, radiosurgery is often offered as the first choice of treatment or after previous subtotal resection. Our experience confirms these results and illustrates that this approach is reproducible among different centers.

References

1. Delbrouck C, Hassid S, Massager N, et al. Preservation of hearing in vestibular schwannomas treated by radiosurgery using Leksell Gamma Knife: preliminary report of a prospective Belgian clinical study. Acta Otorhinolaryngol Belg 2003;57:197–204
2. Leksell L. A note on the treatment of acoustic tumors. Acta Chir Scand 1971;137:763–765
3. Leksell L. The stereotaxic method and radiosurgery of the brain. Acta Chir Scand 1951;102:316–319
4. Noren G, Arndt J, Hindmarsh T. Stereotactic radiosurgery in cases of acoustic neuromas: further experiences. Neurosurgery 1983;13:12–22
5. Kamerer DB, Lunsford LD, Moller M. Gamma Knife: an alternative treatment for acoustic neuromas. Ann Otol Rhinol Laryngol 1988; 97:631–635
6. Levivier M, Lorenzoni J, Massager N, Ruiz S, Devriendt D, Brotchi J. Use of the Leksell Gamma Knife C with Automatic Positioning System for the treatment of meningioma and vestibular schwannoma. Neurosurg Focus 2003;14(5):8:1–5
7. Massager N, Abeloos L, Devriendt D, Op de Beeck M, Levivier M. Clinical evaluation of targeting accuracy of Gamma Knife radiosurgery in trigeminal neuralgia. Int J Radiat Oncol Biol Phys 2007;69:1514–1520

8. Chopra R, Kondziolka D, Niranjan A, Lunsford LD, Flickinger JC. Long-term follow-up of acoustic schwannoma radiosurgery with marginal tumor doses of 12 to 13 Gy. Int J Radiat Oncol Biol Phys 2007;68:845–851
9. Régis J, Delsanti C, Roche P-H, Thomassin J-M, Pellet W. Functional outcomes of radiosurgical treatment of vestibular schwannomas: 1000 successive cases and review of the literature. Neurochirurgie 2004;50(2–3):301–311
10. Yamamoto M, Hagiwara S, Ide M, et al. Conservative management of acoustic neurinomas: prospective study of long-term changes in tumor volume and auditory function. Minim Invasive Neurosurg 1998;41:86–92
11. Chan AW, Black P, Ojemann RG, et al. Stereotactic radiotherapy for vestibular schwannomas: favorable outcome with minimal toxicity. Neurosurgery 2005;57:60–70
12. Gardner G, Robertson JH. Hearing preservation in unilateral acoustic neuroma surgery. Ann Otol Rhinol Laryngol 1988;97:55–66
13. Delsanti C, Tamura M, Galanaud D, Régis J. Changing radiological results, pitfalls and criteria of failure. Neurochirurgie 2004;50(2–3, Pt 2): 312–319
14. Massager N, Nissim O, Delbrouck C, et al. Role of intracanalicular volumetric and dosimetric parameters on hearing preservation after vestibular schwannoma radiosurgery. Int J Radiat Oncol Biol Phys 2006;64:1331–1340
15. Massager N, Nissim O, Delbrouck C, et al. Irradiation of cochlear structures during vestibular schwannoma radiosurgery and associated hearing outcome. J Neurosurg 2007;107:733–739
16. Régis J, Roche PH, Delsanti C, et al. Modern management of vestibular schwannomas. Prog Neurol Surg 2007;20:129–141
17. Gabert K, Régis J, Delsanti C, et al. Preserving hearing function after Gamma Knife radiosurgery for unilateral vestibular schwannoma. Neurochirurgie 2004;50(2–3 Pt 2):350–357
18. Sheehan JP. Linear accelerator radiosurgery for vestibular schwannoma [Editorial]. J Neurosurg 2006;105:655–656
19. Litvack ZN, Noren G, Chougule PB, Zheng Z. Preservation of functional hearing after Gamma Knife surgery for vestibular schwannoma. Neurosurg Focus 2003;14(5):e3
20. Foote KD, Friedman WA, Buatti JM, Meeks SL, Bova FJ, Kubilis PS. Analysis of risk factors associated with radiosurgery for vestibular schwannoma. J Neurosurg 2001;95:440–449
21. Friedman WA, Bradshaw P, Myers A, Bova FJ. Linear accelerator radiosurgery for vestibular schwannomas. J Neurosurg 2006;105:657–661
22. Ishihara H, Saito K, Nishizaki T, et al. CyberKnife radiosurgery for vestibular schwannoma. Minim Invasive Neurosurg 2004;47:290–293
23. Fuss M, Debus J, Lohr F, et al. Conventionally fractionated stereotactic radiotherapy (FSRT) for acoustic neuromas. Int J Radiat Oncol Biol Phys 2000;48:1381–1387
24. Combs SE, Volk S, Schulz-Ertner D, et al. Management of acoustic neuromas with fractionated stereotactic radiotherapy (FSRT): long-term results in 106 patients treated in a single institution. Int J Radiat Oncol Biol Phys 2005;63:75–81
25. Weber DC, Chan AW, Bussiere MR, et al. Proton beam radiosurgery for vestibular schwannoma: tumor control and cranial nerve toxicity. Neurosurgery 2003;53:577–588
26. Iwai Y, Yamanaka K, Yamagata K, Yasui T. Surgery after radiosurgery for acoustic neuromas: surgical strategy and histological findings. Neurosurgery. Neurosurgery 2007;60(2, Suppl 1):75–82
27. Shuto T, Inomori S, Matsunaga S, Fujino H. Microsurgery for vestibular schwannoma after Gamma Knife radiosurgery. Acta Neurochir (Wien) 2008;150:229–234
28. Mathieu D, Kondziolka D, Flickinger JC, et al. Stereotactic radiosurgery for vestibular schwannomas in patients with neurofibromatosis type 2: an analysis of tumor control, complications and hearing preservation rates. Neurosurgery 2007;60:460–470
29. Rowe J, Grainger A, Walton L, et al. Safety of radiosurgery applied to conditions with abnormal tumor suppressor genes. Neurosurgery 2007;60:860–864

13

Stereotactic Radiosurgery for Nonvestibular Schwannomas

Ajay Niranjan, Hideyuki Kano, In-Young Kim, Douglas Kondziolka, and L. Dade Lunsford

Nonvestibular schwannomas are rare tumors of the brain, comprising < 0.5% of all intracranial tumors. Like vestibular schwannomas, most are histologically benign, and patients typically present with symptoms related to the affected cranial nerve. Accurate preoperative diagnosis is possible because of their characteristic features on magnetic resonance imaging (MRI).[1,2] Among nonvestibular schwannomas of the brain, trigeminal nerve schwannomas are the most common, comprising 0.8 to 8.0% of all intracranial schwannomas.[3–5] Other nonvestibular schwannomas of the brain are rare.

Schwannomas originating from oculomotor,[6,7] trochlear,[8–10] and abducens nerves[11–13] are extremely rare even when associated with neurofibromatosis. The majority of patients present with isolated cranial nerve (CN) deficits of the nerve harboring the tumor or symptoms of brainstem compression or hydrocephalus. When these tumors are localized to the cavernous sinus, they present with either cavernous sinus symptoms or an orbital apex syndrome (multiple deficits of CN III–VI). As of February 2008, only two case reports described the use of stereotactic radiosurgery (SRS) for trochlear and abducens schwannomas.[14,15]

Facial sensory dysfunction is the most common presenting symptom, although some patients present with trigeminal neuralgia. Despite advances in skull base surgery techniques, complete resection of trigeminal schwannomas remains a challenge for neurosurgeons. Surgical removal has been associated with a significant risk of new neurologic deficits and is not complete in most cases.[4,13,16–19] Based on its favorable response for other nerve sheath neoplasms, SRS has been applied to the management of trigeminal schwannomas to improve patient outcomes.

Facial nerve schwannomas arise from any segment of the nerve, from the cerebellopontine angle to the extracranial peripheral portion of the nerve. Facial weakness and hearing disturbances are the two principal symptoms of facial nerve schwannoma. Patients occasionally present with facial muscle spasms preceding the onset of facial weakness. Because facial palsy is a common sequela after attempted surgical resection, SRS was applied as a strategy to improve preservation of facial function.

Glossopharyngeal nerve schwannomas are the most common schwannomas in the region of the jugular bulb, followed by schwannomas of CN X, XI, and, rarely, XII. Tumors originating and expanding the jugular bulb result in progressive lower cranial nerve disorders. Larger jugular region tumors may extend from the intracranial to the extracranial compartment, leading to a dumbbell shape. Tumors expanding in the posterior fossa primarily present with deafness, vertigo, and ataxia, thereby mimicking vestibular schwannomas; involvement of lower cranial nerves is uncommon or late. Tumors arising in the jugular foramen and expanding extracranially present with hoarseness, a diminished gag reflex, and shoulder weakness, that is, a typical jugular foramen syndrome. Hypoglossal nerve schwannomas can be completely intracranial, intracranial/extracranial, or completely extracranial. Symptoms differ, depending on the location of the tumor. Tongue wasting is present for the majority of patients at the time of presentation. Suboccipital headaches, exacerbated by neck movements, are early symptoms of intracranial tumors. Patients with intracranial tumors may also exhibit jugular foramen cranial neuropathies or symptoms of brainstem compression.

◆ Materials and Methods

Between August 1987 and June 2007, 81 patients with nonvestibular schwannomas underwent Gamma Knife (Elekta Instruments AB, Stockholm, Sweden) SRS at our institution,

Table 13.1 Radiosurgical Parameters of 81 Patients with Nonvestibular Schwannoma at the University of Pittsburgh

Cranial Nerves Affected by Schwannomas	No. of Patients	Median Age (Years) (Range)	Median Tumor Volume (cc) (Range)	Median Margin Dose (Gy) (Range)
III, IV, VI	8	46 (19–59)	0.22 (0.03–7.40)	12.5 (11.0–13.0)
V	33	50 (15.1–83)	5.0 (0.5–18.0)	15 (12–18)
VII	6	39 (19–59)	1.75 (0.50–8.70)	12.5 (12.0–12.5)
IX, X	34	48 (21–74)	4.2 (0.6–10.4)	14 (12–18)

the Center for Image-Guided Neurosurgery at the University of Pittsburgh Medical Center Presbyterian (**Table 13.1**). Radiosurgery was performed with the model U, B, C, or 4-C Leksell Gamma Knife. Our radiosurgical technique has been described in detail in previous reports.[20] The procedure began with application of a model G Leksell stereotactic frame under conscious sedation and local scalp anesthesia, except in younger children, who underwent general anesthesia. After attaching a fiducial system to the frame, all patients underwent high-resolution MRI. A three-dimensional (3D) localizer sequence, which included axial, coronal, and sagittal images, was performed first. The tumor was then imaged using 3D gradient recalled sequence images. T2-weighted MRI using fast spin echo technique also was acquired to assess any suggestion of regional tumor infiltration. The images were exported to a computer workstation via the hospital Ethernet for dose planning. In all tumors the radiosurgery treatment volume was defined by the enhancing tumor volume. All patients received an intravenous dose of 20 to 40 mg of methylprednisolone after radiosurgery, and all were discharged from the hospital within 24 hours.

After SRS, the patients were instructed to have clinical and imaging follow-up every 6 months during the first year, then yearly for 2 years. If tumor growth was halted, additional imaging evaluations were requested at 4, 6, 8, and 12 years. If a new symptom or any existing cranial nerve function worsened, the patient was evaluated for tumor progression or an adverse radiation effect (ARE). A new MR image was then obtained to assess tumor status and the effect of SRS.

Oculomotor, Trochlear, and Abducens Schwannomas

From March 2000 to October 2007, eight patients with schwannomas originating from oculomotor nerves ($n = 2$), trochlear nerves, ($n = 5$), or abducens nerves ($n = 1$) underwent SRS. The mean age of the patients was 46.1 years (range 19 to 59). Two patients had a medical history of neurofibromatosis: one had an oculomotor schwannoma, which recurred after surgery, and the other patient had a trochlear schwannoma. This latter patient also had a small vestibular schwannoma in the ipsilateral cerebellopontine angle. Both tumors underwent SRS at the same procedure.

One patient (oculomotor schwannoma) underwent adjuvant radiosurgery for recurrence after prior surgery. For seven patients with tumors, SRS was used as a primary treatment. The diagnosis in these patients was based on (1) the individual patient's neuro-opthalmological signs that were compatible with the specific cranial nerve and (2) MRI findings of the tumors that confirmed a tumor with typical imaging characteristic of a schwannoma. The patients' chief complaints at the time of Gamma Knife radiosurgery were diplopia ($n = 5$), ptosis ($n = 1$), complete third nerve palsy ($n = 1$), and headache ($n = 1$). In patients with trochlear schwannomas, diplopia was due to impaired function of the ipsilateral superior oblique muscle. The symptom duration of diplopia ranged from 6 months to 4 years. Two patients had oculomotor schwannomas; one had complete ptosis after initial resection was attempted. The other patient exhibited periodic episodes of third nerve palsy and headache. The patient with abducens nerve schwannoma reported periodic headache. The median and mean tumor volumes were 0.22 and 1.32 cc, respectively (range 0.03 to 7.40). A median margin dose of 12.5 Gy (range 11.0 to 13.0) was prescribed to the tumor margin.

Trigeminal Schwannomas

We evaluated 33 patients with trigeminal schwannoma who had a minimum of 1-year follow-up. There were 17 men and 16 women, with a median age of 49.5 years (range 15.1–82.5 years). Eleven patients (33%) had undergone attempted resection, and one had prior stereotactic biopsy. Twenty-two patients (67%) underwent SRS as the primary procedure. The tumors were classified into root type (tumor predominantly located in the posterior fossa), ganglion type (tumor predominantly located in the middle fossa), and dumbbell type (tumor involving both the middle and posterior fossa).[21] The median tumor volume was 5.0 cc (range 0.5–18.0 cc). The median prescription dose delivered to the margins of the tumor was 15 Gy (range 12–22 Gy), and the maximum dose was 30 Gy (range 24 to 40 Gy).

Facial Nerve Schwannomas

Six patients had radiosurgery for facial nerve schwannomas and were eligible for evaluation at a minimum of 26 months (range12–64 months). The mean patient age was 39 years (range 19–59 years). Four patients were male, and two were female. No patient had neurofibromatosis. No patient received prior fractionated radiation therapy. Three had a prior resection, and in three the diagnosis was made based on imaging and clinical criteria. All patients had facial nerve symptoms (five with weakness and one with muscle twitching). Headache was noted by one patient. In the three patients with a prior resection, two had a reduction in hearing before surgery (speech discrimination scores of 80% and 30%). After surgery (and before SRS), two had a significant hearing decline to deafness on that side, and the other patient had a slight reduction from 80 to 72% speech discrimination at 85 dB. At the time of radiosurgery, House–Brackmann facial function grades were I ($n = 1$), II ($n = 3$), III ($n = 1$), and VI ($N = 1$). The radiosurgery margin dose was 12.0 to 12.5 Gy. The mean tumor volume was 1.75 mL. Five of six tumors had volumes < 1 mL, and one tumor was 8.7 mL. After radiosurgery, patients were evaluated with serial imaging and clinical assessments.

Jugular Foramen Schwannomas

Between August 1987 and December 2005, 34 patients (16 women, 18 men) with 35 jugular foramen schwannomas (unilateral tumors in 33 patients, bilateral tumors in 1 patient) underwent Gamma Knife SRS. Twenty-two patients had undergone one or more resections. For these 22 patients, radiosurgery was performed for tumors that recurred after complete resection ($n = 10$, median of 34 months after microsurgery), growth of a residual lesion thought to be initially stable ($n = 9$, median of 28 months after the last resection), and immediately after a first ($n = 1$) or second ($n = 2$) subtotal resection.

Thirteen patients underwent primary radiosurgery for jugular foramen schwannomas diagnosed by clinical and imaging criteria. Six patients had neurofibromatosis type 2 and had other intracranial tumors. Two patients had vestibular schwannomas, one had a contralateral jugular foramen tumor, two had trigeminal schwannomas, and three had meningiomas. One or more cranial nerve deficits were present in all 34 patients. Four patients had contralateral hemiparesis.

◆ Results

Oculomotor, Trochlear, and Abducens Schwannomas

All patients had tumor regression after SRS (**Fig. 13.1**). The progression-free periods ranged from 5 to 40 months (mean 20.1 months). Diplopia was improved in four of the five (80%) trochlear schwannoma patients at a mean follow-up of 22 months. Ptosis in an oculomotor schwannoma patient who had prior resection remained unchanged. Periodic ophthalmoplegia with headache in a patient with an oculomotor schwannoma remained unchanged. One patient with an abducens neuroma reported improvement in headache. No adverse radiation effects were observed.

Trigeminal Schwannomas

Follow-up imaging studies demonstrated tumor control in 29 of 33 (87.9%) tumors after SRS (**Fig. 13.2**). After radiosurgery, complete resolution of the tumor was identified in 2 tumors, and tumor regression was noted in 15 tumors. The appearance of 12 tumors remained unchanged after radiosurgery.

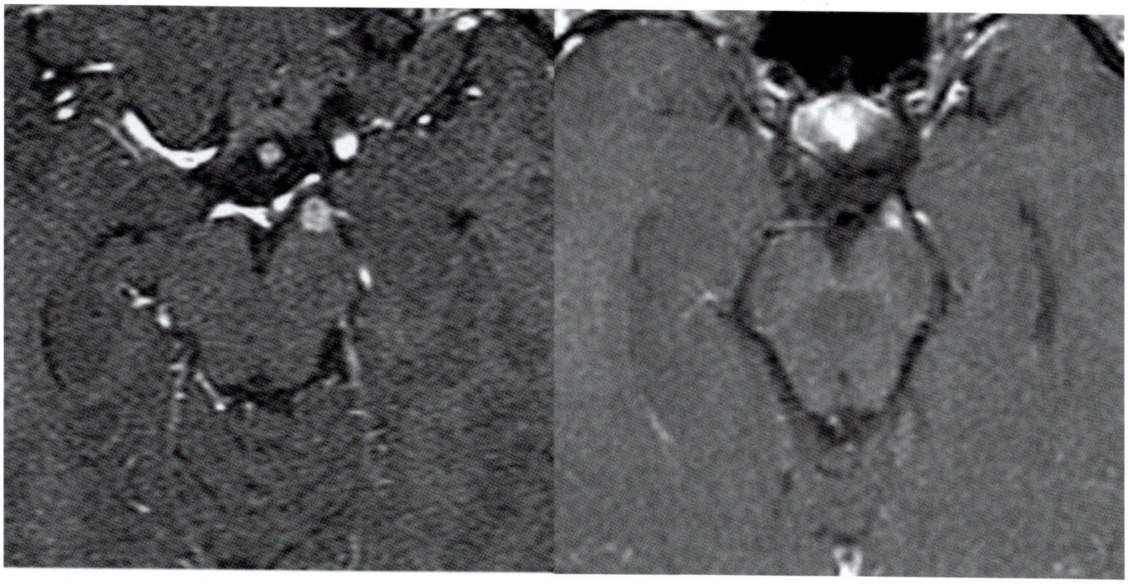

A B

Fig. 13.1 **(A)** Axial contrast-enhanced stereotactic magnetic resonance (MR) image of a 19-year-old woman at the time of radiosurgery shows an oculomotor nerve schwannoma on the left side. She underwent Gamma Knife radiosurgery using 12.5 Gy to tumor margin. **(B)** Axial T1-weighted contrast-enhanced MR image obtained 3 years after initial stereotactic radiosurgery documents tumor regression.

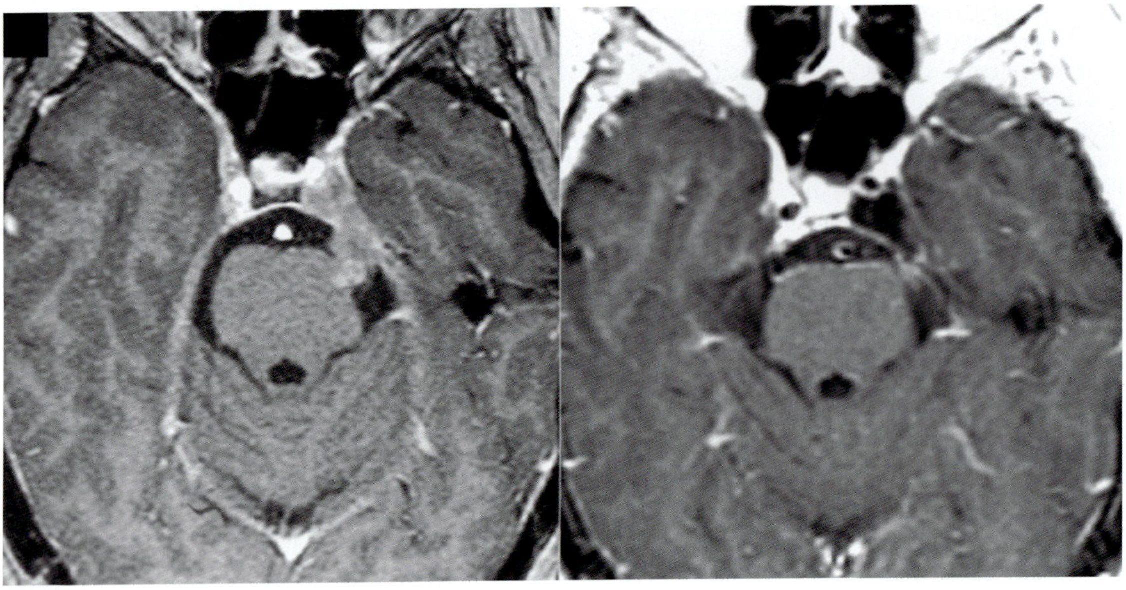

Fig. 13.2 A 49-year-old man presented with left-sided facial sensory loss. **(A)** Axial contrast-enhanced stereotactic magnetic resonance (MR) image obtained at the time of radiosurgery shows a left-sided dumbbell-shaped trigeminal schwannoma. The patient underwent radiosurgery using a margin dose of 13 Gy. **(B)** Follow-up MR image 8 years after initial radiosurgery shows tumor regression.

Localized in-field tumor progression was seen in four patients. The progression-free survival (PFS) rates after SRS were 97.0, 82.0, and 82.0% at 1, 5, and 10 years, respectively. In the entire series, 1 of 26 tumors (3.8%) with tumor volume of < 8.0 cc progressed in the SRS volume. The mean time to progression was 141.4 months. In contrast, three of seven lesions (42.9%) with tumor volume of > 8.0 cc exhibited local progression in the SRS volume. The median time to progression was 51.8 months. Kaplan–Meier plots generated for PFS showed that lesions with a volume of < 8.0 cc had 1-, 3-, and 5-year PFS rates of 100, 94.4, and 94.4%, respectively. Tumors with a target volume of > 8.0 cc had 1- and 3-year PFS rates of 85.7 and 64.3%, respectively. A target volume of < 8.0 cc was significantly associated with a better PFS rate ($p = 0.0007$).

Eleven of 33 symptomatic patients (33.3%) exhibited improvement in their neurologic symptoms or signs at a median of 9.5 months (range 2.7–88.5 months) after SRS. One of 11 patients (9.1%) who had prior surgical removal exhibited improvement in neurologic symptoms or signs, and 10 of 22 patients (45.5%) who had no prior surgical removal exhibited improvement. Patients without prior surgery had a significantly better chance of improvement (*t*-test: $p = .0367$). Eight of 11 improved patients exhibited tumor regression. Oculomotor nerve paresis improved in 1 of 2 patients, trochlear nerve impairment improved in 1 of 2 patients, trigeminal neuropathy improved in 7 of 23 patients, facial pain improved in 2 of 8 patients, and abducens nerve palsies improved in 5 of 9 patients. A facial palsy remained unchanged in one patient. Hearing loss did not improve (zero of three patients) (**Table 13.2**). Nineteen patients had no change in their pre-SRS neurologic deficits, whereas three patients had progression of their neurologic deficits. Two of three patients developed new cranial nerve deficits (facial anesthesia and facial pain) due to delayed tumor progression.

Two patients developed adverse radiation effects. Both patients developed increased peritumoral T2 signal changes without symptoms at 6-month and 2-year follow-up MRI, respectively. Both patients were successfully managed with oral corticosteroids.

Table 13.2 Results of Nonvestibular Schwannoma Radiosurgery at the University of Pittsburgh

Cranial Nerves Affected by Schwannomas	Follow-up (Months) Median (Range)	Tumor Control	Cranial Nerve Preservation
III, IV, VI	20 (5–40)	100%	100%
V	58 (7–148)	88%	91%
VII	26 (12–64)	100%	100%
IX, X	84 (18–170)	94%	98%

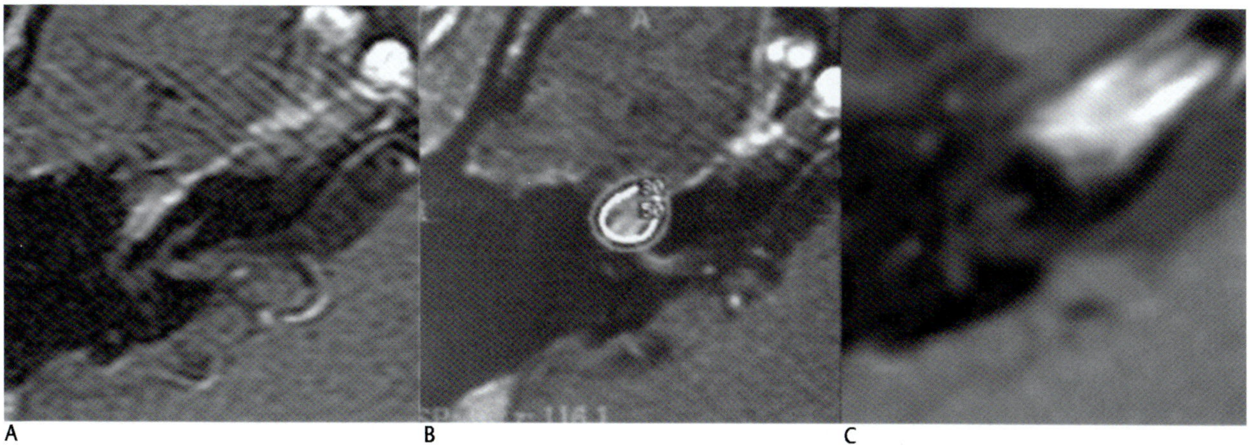

A B C

Fig. 13.3 **(A)** T1-weighted, contrast-enhanced axial magnetic resonance (MR) image of a 19-year-old man at the time of radiosurgery shows a right-sided facial nerve schwannoma. **(B)** Conformal radiosurgery was performed using 12 Gy at tumor margins. **(C)** Axial T1-weighted, contrast-enhanced MR image obtained 3 years after initial radiosurgery shows complete resolution of the enhancing tumor.

Facial Nerve Schwannomas

The mean follow-up in six patients who had radiosurgery for facial nerve schwannomas was 26 months (range 12–64 months). On later imaging, three tumors had regressed (with the longest follow-up), and three were unchanged (**Fig. 13.3**). All patients had preservation of their preradiosurgery facial function. No other effects were noted. In early follow-up, radiosurgery proved to be a safe and effective management approach for residual or newly diagnosed facial schwannomas.

Jugular Foramen Schwannomas

The follow-up period for patients with jugular schwannomas after stereotactic radiosurgery varied from 18 to 170 months (mean 83 months; median 84 months). An initial slight increase in tumor volume with central MRI contrast loss was observed in four patients. Two of these four patients required a 2-week course of oral corticosteroids, and two were followed without the need of further intervention. All four patients showed subsequent regression. Overall, 17 of 35 tumors showed tumor regression (minimal decrease of ≥ 25% of the tumor volume) at the time of the last follow-up MRI scan, and 16 remained stable (**Fig. 13.4**). One patient underwent surgery at another institution 7 months after stereotactic radiosurgery. He presented with increased glossopharyngeal and vagus nerve deficits, swallowing difficulty, and associated pneumonia. The tumor appeared enlarged with central necrosis seen on the MRI scan. A second patient underwent radiosurgery for a new lesion 9 years later. The PFS rate was 97 ± 2.7% at 5 years and 94 ± 5.9% at 10 years.

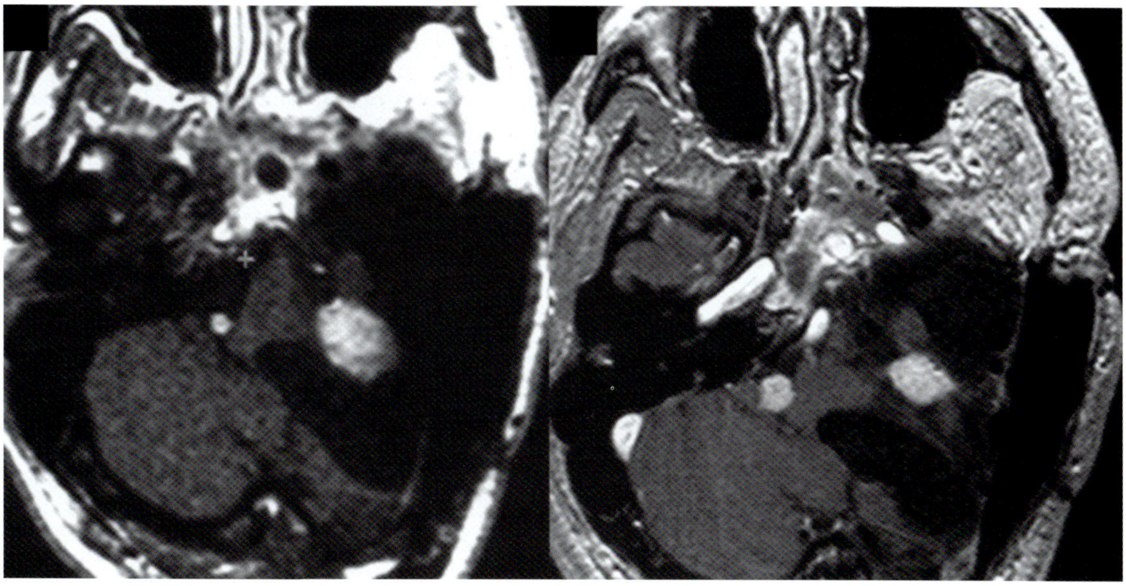

A B

Fig. 13.4 **(A)** T1-weighted, contrast-enhanced axial magnetic resonance (MR) image of a 44-year-old man at the time of radiosurgery showing a left-sided jugular foramen schwannoma. **(B)** Axial T1-weighted, contrast-enhanced MR image obtained 8 years after initial radiosurgery shows regressed tumor volume.

A total of 105 ipsilateral motor cranial nerves (glossopharyngeal, vagus, accessory, and hypoglossal nerves) were affected at the time of radiosurgery. Improvement of affected cranial nerves occurred in 22 (20%) nerves, whereas 81 (77%) remained stable, and only 2 (2%) worsened. This clinical worsening occurred in a single patient whose increase in tumor volume, perhaps transient, led to early surgical resection. All 35 unaffected nerves remained intact after radiosurgery. Overall preservation or improvement was noted in 138 of 140 (98%) motor cranial nerves. In patients without previous resection, 23 cranial nerves were originally affected, and 11 (47%) were improved at a median of 16 months after radiosurgery. We detected no additional cranial nerve morbidity. One patient showed distinct improvement in his ipsilateral speech discrimination score (from 35 to 87%) and in the pure tone average (from 55 to 30 dB) 19 months after radiosurgery. A second patient with a House-Brackmann grade IV facial neuropathy 4 years after microsurgery improved to grade II facial function 16 months after radiosurgery.

◆ Discussion

SRS has emerged as a primary management of patients with intracranial schwannomas. Such patients are excellent candidates for radiosurgery because of the noninfiltrative, well-delineated nature of their tumors. The success of nonvestibular schwannoma radiosurgery is similar to the outcomes of vestibular schwannoma radiosurgery. Longer follow-up is now available for vestibular schwannoma radiosurgery. This extensive experience confirmed high rates of tumor growth control (> 95%) at 10 to 15 years after the procedure. Consequently, radiosurgery is considered an effective alternative to surgical resection for patients with vestibular schwannomas. Our results confirm that nonvestibular schwannomas respond in a similar fashion.

Schwannomas of cranial nerves affecting ocular movement are rare. Microsurgical experience with these tumors also is limited.[7,10,11] There are no distinct reports of SRS for schwannomas originating from oculomotor, trochlear, or abducens nerves. Our literature search revealed only two cases that were included in a larger series of intracranial schwannomas.[14,15] Pollock et al[15] reported their experience of Gamma Knife SRS for a trochlear nerve schwannoma patient, and Chakrabarti et al[14] reported one abducens neuroma, which was treated with linear accelerator (linac)-based SRS. Our limited data suggest that SRS is effective for schwannomas of the nerves governing the ocular movement. We used relatively low marginal doses (11–13 Gy) to reduce the risk of brainstem or optic nerve injury. With these doses, none of our patients suffered adverse radiation effects after SRS. We believe that sensory nerves are more vulnerable to SRS risks than motor nerves. Because the oculomotor, trochlear, and abducens nerves are pure motor nerves, their radiation tolerance may be higher than that of sensory nerves.

Schwannomas of the trigeminal nerve comprise the largest segment of nonvestibular schwannomas. Pollock et al[15] reported outcomes after Gamma Knife radiosurgery in 24 patients with nonvestibular schwannomas, including 10 with trigeminal schwannomas. These authors reported a 96% tumor control rate (90% for trigeminal schwannomas). Three of 10 patients with trigeminal schwannomas suffered new or worsening trigeminal dysfunction after radiosurgery. Pan et al[22] treated 56 patients with trigeminal schwannoma using Gamma Knife radiosurgery. These authors reported a 93% tumor control rate at a mean follow-up duration of 68 months. Hasegawa et al[23] treated 37 patients with trigeminal schwannomas using Gamma Knife radiosurgery. These authors reported that the actuarial 5- and 10-year tumor control rates were both 84% at a mean follow-up duration of 54 months.

In our experience in Pittsburgh, the 5- and 10-year PFS rates after SRS were both 82%. The 3-year PFS rates based on tumor volumes of < 8.0 cc and > 8.0 cc were 94.4 and 64.3%, respectively. A target volume of < 8.0 cc was associated with a better PFS rate ($p = .0007$). Pan et al[22] ($n = 56$) reported complete relief of symptoms in 25%, improved symptoms in 44%, no change in symptoms in 14%, and slight worsening of symptoms in 9% of patients. Seven percent developed a mild worsening of symptoms related to tumor progression. Hasegawa et al[23] reported improvement in 40% of patients ($n = 37$) after trigeminal schwannoma Gamma Knife SRS. In our experience, 33.3% of patients with neurologic symptoms exhibited improvement, and 57.6% had no change in their pre-SRS neurologic deficits. Three patients (9.1%) had progression of their preexisting neurologic deficits. Two patients developed new cranial nerve deficits (facial anesthesia and facial pain) due to delayed tumor progression.

Schwannomas of the jugular foramen can arise from the glossopharyngeal, vagus, or spinal accessory nerves. The majority of patients present with a depressed gag reflex, dysphonia, palatal droop, hoarseness, swallowing difficulties, and shoulder weakness. Weakness of the sternocleidomastoid, trapezius, and long tract motor signs (Vernet syndrome) may also be detected. Other neurologic signs are the result of brainstem compression or hydrocephalus. With the widespread availability of MRI, patients are now being diagnosed earlier when lesions are confined to the jugular foramen.[7] Such tumors may affect the involved cranial nerves but have no brainstem compression. For large tumors associated with symptomatic brainstem compression, resection is considered the primary management modality. Patients without symptoms of brainstem mass effect are managed effectively by stereotactic radiosurgery. In our long-term experience, Gamma Knife radiosurgery has a high tumor control rate, excellent cranial nerve preservation rates, and no mortality.

Mabanta et al[24] managed nine patients with jugular foramen schwannomas using linac radiosurgery. The tumor control rate was 100% at a mean 32-month follow-up period. Five patients had improved neurologic symptoms, one patient had worsened facial nerve function, two developed hearing loss, and one had new onset of ataxia. Pollock et al[15] performed Gamma Knife radiosurgery in 10 patients with jugular foramen tumors. At an average of 43 months, the tumor control rate was 96%, and new lower cranial nerve deficits had not been detected. Zhang et al[25] treated 27 patients with jugular foramen schwannomas using the Gamma Knife. At an average of 38 months, the tumor control rate was 96%. They reported no complications, and 16 patients improved. One patient required a second radiosurgical procedure.

A total of 1267 patients with intracranial schwannomas underwent Gamma Knife radiosurgery at the University of Pittsburgh between 1987 and 2005. Only 35 (2.7%) had jugular foramen tumors. The median follow-up period was 81 months. The actuarial tumor control rate was 97% at 5 years and 94% at 10 years. After radiosurgery, two patients showed improvement in cranial nerve function. Lower cranial nerve function improvement was observed in 21% of the entire series, but 47% of patients without previous microsurgery improved. One patient showed worsening of his preexisting glossopharyngeal and vagus nerve deficits. Only one patient who underwent microsurgery 7 months after radiosurgery ostensibly had an increasing tumor volume associated with central necrosis on MRI. We now know that 5% of schwannomas may show temporary tumor volume enlargement between 6 and 18 months after radiosurgery. Because volume change is almost always temporary, surgical decompression, even in the presence of transient new symptoms, is rarely needed.

Nonvestibular schwannomas are uncommon tumors of the brain. An accurate preoperative clinical diagnosis supplemented by MRI is possible in most cases. Patients with small to moderate-sized tumors with intact cranial nerve function are optimal candidates for radiosurgery. Current radiosurgery techniques (multiisocenter, highly conformal, and selective dose planning based on stereotactic MRI and 11–13 Gy tumor marginal doses) are associated with a high tumor control rate and minimal risk of adverse radiation effects. For larger tumors, initial resection followed by delayed radiosurgery for residual tumor is an effective option.

References

1. Ikushima I, Korogi Y, Kuratsu J, et al. Dynamic MRI of meningiomas and schwannomas: is differential diagnosis possible? Neuroradiology 1997;39:633–638
2. Majoie CB, Hulsmans FJ, Castelijns JA, et al. Primary nerve-sheath tumours of the trigeminal nerve: clinical and MRI findings. Neuroradiology 1999;41:100–108
3. Konovalov AN, Spallone A, Mukhamedjanov DJ, Tcherekajev VA, Makhmudov UB. Trigeminal neurinomas: a series of 111 surgical cases from a single institution. Acta Neurochir (Wien) 1996;138: 1027–1035
4. McCormick PC, Bello JA, Post KD. Trigeminal schwannoma: surgical series of 14 cases with review of the literature. J Neurosurg 1988;69: 850–860
5. Tancioni F, Gaetani P, Villani L, Zappoli F, Rodriguez Y, Baena R. Neurinoma of the trigeminal root and atypical trigeminal neuralgia: case report and review of the literature. Surg Neurol 1995;44:36–42
6. Leunda G, Vaquero J, Cabezudo J, Garcia-Uria J, Bravo G. Schwannoma of the oculomotor nerves: report of four cases. J Neurosurg 1982;57: 563–565
7. Ohata K, Takami T, Goto T, Ishibashi K. Schwannoma of the oculomotor nerve. Neurol India 2006;54:437–439
8. Gerganov V, Amir S, Koerbel A, Brandes A, Stan A, Madjid S. Cystic trochlear nerve schwannoma: case report. Surg Neurol 2007;68:221–225
9. Ho KL. Schwannoma of the trochlear nerve: case report. J Neurosurg 1981;55:132–135
10. Ohba S, Miwa T, Kawase T. Trochlear nerve schwannoma with intratumoral hemorrhage: case report. Neurosurgery 2006;58:E791
11. Acharya R, Husain S, Chhabra SS, Patir R, Bhalla S, Seghal AD. Sixth nerve schwannoma: a case report with literature review. Neurol Sci 2003;24:74–79
12. Ginsberg F, Peyster RG, Rose WS, Drapkin AJ. Sixth nerve schwannoma: MR and CT demonstration. J Comput Assist Tomogr 1988;12: 482–484
13. Nakamura M, Carvalho GA, Samii M. Abducens nerve schwannoma: a case report and review of the literature. Surg Neurol 2002;57:183–188, discussion 188–189
14. Chakrabarti KB, Doughty D, Plowman PN. Stereotactic multiple arc radiotherapy, II: Cranial neuroma. Br J Neurosurg 1996;10:577–583
15. Pollock BE, Foote RL, Stafford SL. Stereotactic radiosurgery: the preferred management for patients with nonvestibular schwannomas? Int J Radiat Oncol Biol Phys 2002;52:1002–1007
16. Al-Mefty O, Ayoubi S, Gaber E. Trigeminal schwannomas: removal of dumbbell-shaped tumors through the expanded Meckel cave and outcomes of cranial nerve function. J Neurosurg 2002;96:453–463
17. Goel A, Muzumdar D, Raman C. Trigeminal neuroma: analysis of surgical experience with 73 cases. Neurosurgery 2003;52:783–790, discussion 790
18. Sarma S, Sekhar LN, Schessel DA. Nonvestibular schwannomas of the brain: a 7-year experience. Neurosurgery 2002;50:437–438, discussion 438–439
19. Taha JM, Tew JM Jr, van Loveren HR, Keller JT, el-Kalliny M. Comparison of conventional and skull base surgical approaches for the excision of trigeminal neurinomas. J Neurosurg 1995;82:719–725
20. Nettel B, Niranjan A, Martin JJ, et al. Gamma Knife radiosurgery for trigeminal schwannomas. Surg Neurol 2004;62:435–444, discussion 444–436
21. Lesoin F, Rousseaux M, Villette L, et al. Neurinomas of the trigeminal nerve. Acta Neurochir (Wien) 1986;82:118–122
22. Pan L, Wang EM, Zhang N, et al. Long-term results of Leksell Gamma Knife surgery for trigeminal schwannomas. J Neurosurg 2005; 102(Suppl):220–224
23. Hasegawa T, Kida Y, Yoshimoto M, Koike J. Trigeminal schwannomas: results of Gamma Knife surgery in 37 cases. J Neurosurg 2007;106:18–23
24. Mabanta SR, Buatti JM, Friedman WA, Meeks SL, Mendenhall WM, Bova FJ. Linear accelerator radiosurgery for nonacoustic schwannomas. Int J Radiat Oncol Biol Phys 1999;43:545–548
25. Zhang N, Pan L, Dai JZ, Wang BJ, Wang EM, Cai PW. Gamma Knife radiosurgery for jugular foramen schwannomas. J Neurosurg 2002;97: 456–458

14

Stereotactic Radiosurgery for Trigeminal Neuralgia

Jean Régis, Noriko Murata, Shoji Yomo, Yasser Arkha, Philippe Roussel, and Anne Donnet

Trigeminal neuralgia, also known as tic douloureux, is a serious health problem, with a prevalence rate of 4 to 5 per 100,000 people.[1] Patients typically describe a severe and sudden pain in the face, like an electric shock.[2] There is growing evidence that, in most patients, one of the causal factors is compression of the trigeminal nerve root, close to its entry into the pons, by an aberrant arterial or venous loop.[3] Microvascular decompression (MVD), first described in the 1950s by Taarnhoj,[4] treats the putative cause by separating the loop from the trigeminal nerve. The pain may be effectively treated by a series of percutaneous techniques (thermocoagulation, microcompression, and glycerol injection) that produce a partial lesion of the trigeminal nerve.[5–12]

The concept of stereotactic radiosurgery was introduced by Lars Leksell, who, in 1951, first began performing clinical radiosurgery with a stereotactic x-ray beam on patients suffering from essential trigeminal neuralgia.[13–15] The use of the Gamma Knife (Elekta Instruments AB, Stockholm, Sweden) with 201-source cobalt 60 was finally adopted in 1968. However, because of the efficacy of this tool in the treatment of other diseases, the introduction of the glycerol technique and later of effective drugs for the treatment of trigeminal neuralgia, and, primarily, the absence of high-quality neuroimaging for targeting, at this time the Gamma Knife was temporarily abandoned for this indication. The availability of high-quality three-dimensional magnetic resonance imaging (MRI) for precise targeting of normal structures and evidence of certain limitations of other techniques prompted a reappraisal of Gamma Knife surgery for trigeminal neuralgia in the 1990s.[16]

The evidence for safety and efficacy is based on retrospective case studies and one recent prospective trial.[17] The evidence supporting the use of other modalities of surgical treatment for trigeminal neuralgia is based only on retrospective case studies.[1] Additionally, the numerous studies published to date have not used uniform outcome measures, making a comparison between techniques difficult.[18] It must be acknowledged that none of the currently available techniques are perfect (**Table 14.1**), thus explaining the continuing effort of neurosurgeons to develop new treatment methods. All these treatments must be rigorously evaluated to know how best to help these patients.

Table 14.2 compares published studies according to the device used, either Gamma Knife, CyberKnife, Novalis, or adapted linear accelerator (linac); the percentage of patients treated, with the maximum dose <70 Gy, between 70 and 80 Gy, and >80 Gy; the distance between the center of the shot and the emergence of the nerve; the median follow-up

Table 14.1 Summary of the Average Results Found in the Literature for Each Neurosurgical Approach

	Radiofrequency Rhizotomy (%) (*n* = 6205)	Glycerol Injection (%) (*n* = 1217)	Balloon Compression (%) (*n* = 759)	MVD (%) (*n* = 1417)	GKS (%) (*n* = 1280)
Initial pain relief	98.0%	91.0	93.0	98.0	90.0
Pain recurrence	23.0	54.0	21.0	15.0	18.0
Facial numbness	98.0	60.0	72.0	2.0	13.0
Perioperative morbidity	1.2	1.0	1.7	10.0	0
Mortality	0	0	0	0.6	0

Note: The letter *n* refers to the cumulative number of patients given in the literature for each of these approaches.

Abbreviations: GKS, Gamma Knife surgery; MVD, microvascular decompression.

Table 14.2 Summary of the Main Series in the Literature

Study	No. of Patients	Male/ Female Ratio	Age (years)	Device	% Patients Maximum Dose			Distance to Emergence (mm)	Median F-up (months)	% Patients with					Median Dose BS (Gy)	Output Factor
					< 70 Gy	70 to 80 Gy	> 80 Gy			Previous Procedure	Pain Free	Pain Relief	Side Effects (B/NB)	Recurrence		
Arkha et al[19]	262	128/ 134	68.0	GK	0	33.2	66.8	8.5	37.5 (12–147)	42.0	88.9	60.0	12.9 (12.5/0.4)	21.0–34.0	< 12 Gy/ 10 mm³	0.80/0.87
Longhi et al[48]	160	73/87	63.4	GK	0	Mean 85	75 to 95	2 to 5	37.4	42.5	61.0 (free without meds)	90.0	9.5	18.0	< 15 Gy/ 20 mm³	0.87
Fountas et al[37]	106	38/68	72.3	GK	0	94.4	5.6	0	36 (12–72)	46.2	82.5/69.4	91.3/77.6	16.0	NA	30% line	
Pusztaszeri et al[58]	17	9/08	71.0	linac	17	0	0	0	12 (2–60)	58.8	35.0	70.0	5.8	29.4	30%	
Régis et al[17]	110	15/57	68.2	GK	0	med 85, 70 to 90		7.84	> 12	44.5	83.0	97.0	10.0 (5.0–5.0)	17.0	< 12 Gy/ 10 mm³	0.8
Yomo et al[67]	86	36/64	76.0	GK	0	97.0	3	REZ in 27 cases, RG in 58 cases	40	52.0	64.0	87.0	15.0	8.0	NA	
Urgosik et al[65]	107	46/61	75.0	GK	0	100.0	0	0	60 (6–94)	60.0	80.4	96.3	20.0	25.0	14	
Sheehan et al[29]	136	66/70	68.0	GK	1.4	98.0	0.7	2 to 4	19	54.0	44.0	70.0	19.0	24.0	NA	
Lim et al[82]	41	18/23	68.0	CyberKnife	0	70.7	29.3	2 to 3	11 (6–15)	31.7	87.8	92.7	51.2 (28.6–32.6)	15.8	< 50% line	
McNatt et al[52]	49	20/29	68.0	GK	0	100.0	0	0	49 (12–70)	36.0	46.0	61.0	52	23.0	12 or less	0.8/0.84
Richards et al[60]	28	9/19	74.0	linac	0	100.0	0	0	12 (1–40)	46.0	57.0	75.0	14.2	46.0 (11.0–24.0)	< 20 Gy	
Massager et al[51]	47	31/16	69.0	GK	0	0	100	9.5/10.2/ 11.3	16 (6–42)	38.0	59.0	71.0	4.0–38.0	4.0	10.6/9.3/ 7.3	0.86
Brisman[31,32]	293	117/176	70.0	GK	0	100.0	0	few mm from BS	23 (5–55)	43.3	21.8	68.3	10.5–11.1	23.9	40–50% line	0.85/0.87
Shaya et al[62]	40	7/33	64.3	GK (model B)	0	90.0	10	2 to 4	14.1 (3–31)	25.0	40.0	70.0	17.5	17.0	NA	
Chen et al[34]	32	15/17	67.0	linac	37.0	0	67	NA	8	10.0	78.0	87.0	0–9.3	NA	20–30% line	
Cheuk et al[35]	112	34/62	62.02	GK	60.0–80.0 (med 75)		0	2 to 4	NA	31.3	80.2	89.6	5.2–10.4	NA	10–20% line	
Frighetto et al[38]	22	6/16	22.0	linac	5.0 (70.0–85.0)		17	NA (8.0–52.0)	21.2	22.0	68.1	95.3	0–36.3	23.8	30% line	
Goss et al[39]	25	32/68	65.0	linac	0	0	25	0	18 (8–52)	32.0	76.0	100.0	32.0	0–44.0	30% line	0.68
Petit et al[55]	112	42/70	64.0	GK	0	100.0	0	2 to 4	30 (8–66)	46.5	77.0	86.0	3.1–4.2	29.0	20% line	
Kondziolka et al[45]	220	94/126	70.0	GK	2.07	94.6	2.7	2 to 4	24 (6–78)	61.4	40.0	69.1	0.4–10.0	13.6	20–30% line	
Pollock et al[58]	117	54/63	67.8	GK	0	56.0	44	5.9	26 (1–48)	58.0	58.0	85.0	37 (12.0–25.0)	16.0	20–40% line	0.8
Maesawa et al[50]	220	94/126	70.0	GK	2.7	94.6	2.7	2 to 4	22 (6–78)	61.4	40.0	69.1	0.4–10.0	13.6	20–30% line	
Rogers et al[72]	54	21/33	67.0	GK	0	100	0	0	12 (3–28)	46.0	41.0	71.0	0–14.0	21.0	NA	
Kannan et al[41]	6	5/01	56.0	GK	0	100	0	2 to 4	10 (5–16)	16.6	66.0	100.0	0	0	12,6	
Young et al[70]	110	NA	64.7	GK	7	93	0		19.8 (4.0–49.0)	34.0	76.4	88.0	0–2.7	34.0		
Kondziolka et al[44]	106	NA	67.0	GK	0	94	6	2 to 4	18 (6–48)	78.0	60.0	77.0	10.0	0–10.0	< 30% line	

Abbreviations: BS, brainstem; GK, Gamma Knife; f-up, follow-up; linac, linear accelerator; NA, not available; NB, non bothersome; REZ, root entry zone; GY, gray.

and extreme values of follow-up (given in parentheses); the percentage of patients previously operated (for ipsilateral trigeminal neuralgia); the percentage of patients pain free at the time of the last follow-up; the percentage of patients with pain relief and side effects (B/NB bothersome vs non bothersome); the dose delivered to the brainstem (evaluated differently by the different authors); and the output factor used for the 4 mm helmet. Note that the worst results in terms of pain control are seen in the study using the lowest dose as the maximum (<70 Gy). The highest rates of toxicity are seen in those studies using the more posterior shot with a very short distance between the center of the shot and the emergence of the nerve, especially when high doses are used.

The heterogeneity of clinical results after radiosurgery is suggestive of the strong impact of pre- and perioperative parameters. To better define the role of Gamma Knife surgery in the treatment of drug-resistant trigeminal neuralgia, a clear understanding of the impact of these parameters is mandatory. In 2006, we published the only prospective trial in line with the strict criteria proposed by Zackrzewska and Lopez[18] and with a minimum follow-up of 1 year.[17] More recently, we analyzed the long-term outcome in our overall experience.[19] In this chapter, we will critically analyze these results and those from the literature.

Materials and Methods

Since 1993 our trigeminal neuralgia radiosurgery cases have been evaluated prospectively, with the primary objective to investigate if single Gamma Knife surgery treatment of the cisternal part of the trigeminal nerve root for trigeminal neuralgia resulted in a decrease and/or cessation of pain attacks for each patient compared with before Gamma Knife surgery. The secondary objectives were to estimate changes in the intensity of pain attacks per day, the mean number of pain attacks, and the neurologic examination and search for the influence of the pre- and perioperative parameters on the safety efficacy variables. The diagnosis of trigeminal neuralgia was made according to the International Headache Society definition; its definitions of primary or secondary cases and typical versus atypical were also employed.[2] Prior to treatment, each patient underwent the same routine diagnostic procedures, including MRI.

We included patients with a clear clinical profile corresponding to trigeminal neuralgia[2] and with a persistent pain level during the previous month of mean intensity superior to 5/10 on the visual analogue scale (VAS), despite optimized drug therapy (or drug therapy limited by dose-related side effects). None of the patients had a lesion adjacent to the trigeminal pathways, as shown using MRI.[2] We excluded those patients who were pregnant and women who were breastfeeding. The procedure on the day of Gamma Knife surgery treatment was started with application of the Leksell stereotactic frame (Elekta) to the patient's head, under local anesthesia. After the frame fixation, MRI and computed tomography (CT) were used for the dose planning with the Leksell GammaPlan (Elekta). The MR images were calibrated before examination and verified by comparison to the CT images to minimize magnetic distortion errors. One single exposure with the 4 mm collimator was placed on the anterior part of the cisternal portion of the trigeminal nerve (**Fig. 14.1**). The theoretical aim was to deliver a dose of 90 Gy as the maximum. However, the maximum dose was determined integrating the measured dose to the brainstem and the age of the patient. Multiple sclerosis was also considered to necessitate a lower dosage (**Fig. 14.2**). Leksell Gamma Knife (Model B, Elekta) treatment proceeded according to routines of the department, and the patients were discharged within 12 hours after radiosurgery. All the procedures were performed by the same neurosurgeon (JR). Clinical examination was performed before and > 1 year after Gamma Knife surgery, including corneal reflex, eye examination, skin examination, pinprick test, and sensitivity examination (search for hypoesthesia). MRI was systematically performed in all patients before radiosurgery but was not routinely repeated during the follow-up.

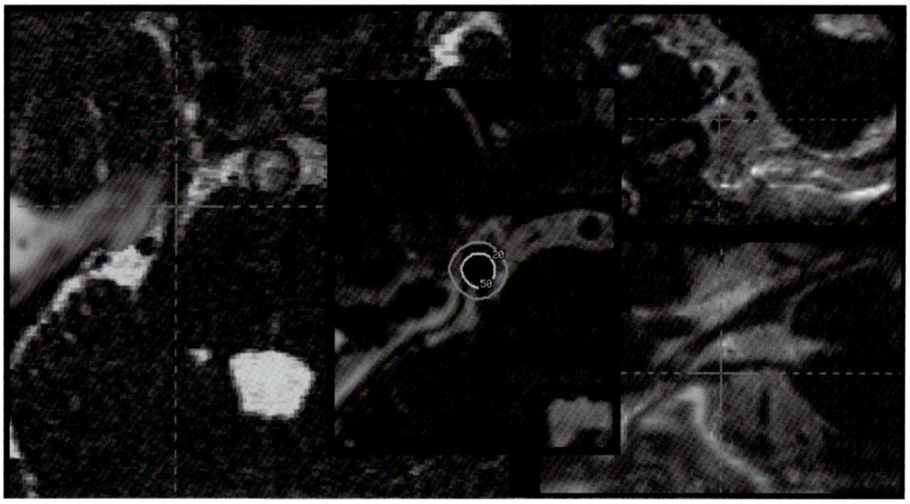

Fig. 14.1 Dose planning displayed in axial view. On high-resolution stereotactic magnetic resonance imaging (MRI; constructive interference steady state [CISS] sequence, Siemens 1.5 T) fused with the bony window of the high-resolution computed tomography (CT) scan, a single 4 mm isocenter is positioned on the anterior portion of the nerve around 7.5 mm from its emergence at the level of the brainstem. Note the spatial relationship between the trigeminal incisura of the petrous bone apex and the plexus triangularis of the trigeminal nerve. Based on this landmark visible on a nonenhanced CT scan, radiosurgery can be performed safely and efficiently in a patient presenting with a pacemaker, contraindicating MR examination.

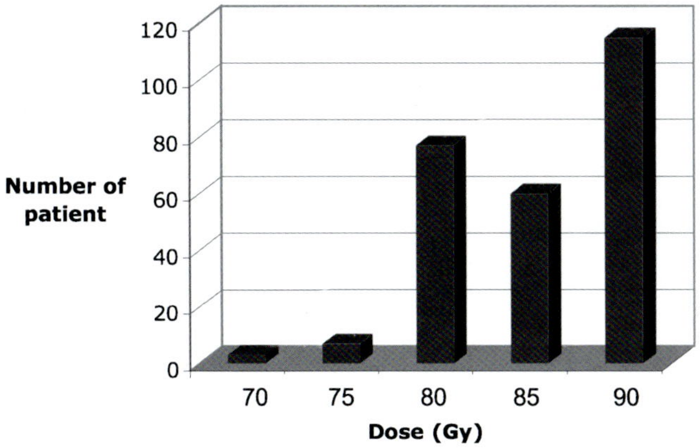

Fig. 14.2 Graph displaying the number of patients for each regimen of maximum doses between 70 and 90 Gy. Note that a significant percentage of the patients are receiving maximum doses < 90 Gy due to their special cisternal anatomy associated with a higher risk of damage to the brainstem.

Outcome measures used here are defined as follows:[17]

Class I: Pain free without medication

Class II: Pain free with medication

Class III: Pain frequency reduction superior to 90%

Class IV: Pain frequency reduction between 50 and 90%

Class V: No significant reduction in pain frequency

Class VI: Pain worsening

A recurrence was defined as the change from class I to a lower outcome class. Thus, the situation of a patient who had been pain free without medication (class I) and who then restarted taking specific drugs but who remained pain free on medication (class II) was considered as a "recurrence." A minor recurrence was defined as well tolerated by the patient (lower frequency and intensity of pain) and not requiring the proposal of a new surgical therapy. A major recurrence was defined as requiring consideration of a further surgical procedure.

◆ Results

Included in the study were 334 patients, 262 of whom were assessable for more than 1 year of follow-up.[2] The median follow-up was 37.5 months (range 12–147 months). Our published results and those from the main literature series are summarized in **Table 14.2.** Two hundred and sixty-two patients were treated (128 males and 134 females), with an age range from 29 to 90 years (median age 68 years). The median duration of the disease was 74 months (mean 111.7 months; range 10–529 months). The side affected was the left in 128 cases and the right in 134. Twenty-one patients had multiple sclerosis. Eighty-one of 110 patients (73.6%) reported severe side effects from the drug therapy. A vascular conflict with the trigeminal nerve was clearly demonstrated by preoperative MRI in 167 patients (64%). Before radiosurgery, 110 patients had already been operated, with thermocoagulation (1–3 times) in 64 patients, balloon microcompression (1–3 times) in 53, surgical MVD in 27, glycerol rhizolysis in 7, pars major microsurgical partial section in 1, and Gamma Knife surgery in 1. Gamma Knife surgery was performed as the first surgical operation in 152 patients.

The median maximum dose was 85.0 Gy (minimum 70.0 Gy; maximum 90.0 Gy). The median dose rate was 1.45 Gy (range 1.25–1.65 Gy). The output factor for dose calculation at this time was 0.80. The median of the distance between the center of the isocenter and the emergence was 8.5 mm. The median of the maximum dose to the brainstem (calculated as the point of the dose–volume histogram corresponding to the 10 mm^3 receiving the highest dose; in other words, the maximum dose received by > 10 mm^3 of the brainstem) was 10.8 Gy (0–16 Gy). No technical failure was encountered.

Initial pain relief occurred in 88.9% of the patients after a median delay of 15 days (range 0–72 weeks) after Gamma Knife surgery (**Table 14.2**). Ninety patients (34%) reported pain recurrence 1 to 72 months after initial relief (**Fig. 14.2**), with a median delay of 10 months. An actuarial curve describing the pain-free probability according to time[19] demonstrates a plateau at 5 years with a rate of pain freedom of 60%.

Due to treatment failure or insufficient pain relief, 55 patients (21%) received additional surgical treatment, namely, a microcompression in 9 patients and a thermocoagulation in 11 patients, including 4 who received both. One patient underwent MVD. All these patients have been followed for > 1 year after this new surgery. Seven of these 17 patients (42%) had received surgical treatment between 1 and 4 times prior to inclusion in the study.[19] Not infrequently, patients who were pain free were reluctant to stop their medication completely, due to anxiety about the risk of recurrence.

A new functional disturbance of the V nerve was reported in 34 patients (12.9%) in the long term, with a median onset delay of 12 months.[2–64] This disturbance was described as not disabling in 8 patients (3.05%), a minor discomfort in 21 (8%), bothersome in 5 (1.9%), and very bothersome in 1 (0.4%). The median delay for hypoesthesia onset was 10 months (range 1–72 months). An actuarial curve describing the hypoesthesia-free probability according to time[19] demonstrates a plateau at 5 years with a rate of hypoesthesia freedom of 83%.

There was no significant change in corneal reflex, eye examination, or skin examination during the study. None of the patients experienced dry eyes, keratitis, masseter weakness, neuropathic pain, or anesthesia dolorosa.

The statistical analysis of our overall series[19] demonstrated that a past history of surgical treatment of the trigeminal neuralgia on the same side was a predictor of toxicity in both univariate analyses (p = 0.0026) and multivariate analyses (p = .006). A small diameter of the ipsilateral trigeminal nerve (p = .0201) and a low ratio of diameters reflecting an important difference in size, with an ipsilateral nerve smaller than the contralateral nerve (p = .0218), are predictors of toxicity only in univariate analyses.

Positive predictors of success were found to be a higher dose delivered to the plexus triangularis ($p = .0498$), maximum dose to the brainstem, does delivered to the emergence of the nerve ($p = .0016$), minimum dose delivered to the nerve ($p = .0199$), smaller volume of the ipsilateral trigeminal nerve ($p = .0073$), and smaller distance between the center of the shot and the anatomical emergence of the nerve ($p = .049$). A history of multiple sclerosis was clearly a predictor of failure. In our prospective trial,[17] we found that the probability of pain freedom at the time of the last follow-up was lower in patients younger than age 60 (66.7% instead of 90.9%; $p = .01$) or with a "trigeminal cistern surface" >39 mm^2 (72.0% instead of 89.5%; $p = .05$. There was an almost significant ($p = .059$) difference in the change in the number of attacks when patients with previous surgical treatment were compared with those without. The rate of failure at the last follow-up was 11.7% in patients never operated on as compared with 19.5% in patients previously operated.

Discussion

In the early 1990s, the availability of high-resolution MRI and the discovery of the limits of the other surgical alternatives promoted the reappraisal of Gamma Knife surgery in essential trigeminal neuralgia.[20] Rand and colleagues suggested the target shift from the gasserian ganglion to the cisternal nerve.[16] Hakanson and Lindquist[21] promoted the concept of the dorsal root entry zone (DREZ). In 1993, Alexander and Lindquist[21] defined the anatomical DREZ from a dose-planning point of view as follows: "a 4 mm collimator centered on the trigeminal root entry zone treated with a dose of 70 Gy to the center, including the nerve root and the adjacent brainstem within the 50% isodose surface (35 Gy)."[21]

I met Bob Rand in Paris in 1992, and he told me that, in his experience, the cisternal posterior target was not safe and recommended that high dosages ~90 Gy be used on the anterior cisternal portion. Since this discussion, the custom at the Timone University Hospital in Marseille has been to use a more anterior cisternal target that we call the retrogasserian or plexus triangularis target (**Fig. 14.1**). The plexus triangularis made sense because of the work of Sindou et al demonstrating that when the tip of the probe in thermocoagulations was located at the level of the plexus, the rate of pain cessation was high and the risk of toxicity much lower.[10] Similarly, groups using balloon microcompression have found converging results (when the balloon extends into the posterior fossa, with a strong compression of the plexus triangularis, which displays a pear or diabolo shape).[22,23] Finally, retrogasserian sections were historically performed at the location of the plexus triangularis.[25] Reviewing our experience, the optimum distance from the emergence of the nerve has in fact turned out to be 7.5 to 8.0 mm.[20] In Tokyo, we reported on our first series of trigeminal neuralgia treated with Gamma Knife surgery using 90 Gy and the plexus triangularis target.[25] Interestingly, Doug Kondziolka mentioned on this occasion that he quite systematically obtained failures using much lower dosages and proposed to evaluate the impact of the maximum dose on the probability of pain cessation. Kondziolka and colleagues at the University of Pittsburgh,[22] later aggregated the first cases from Los Angeles, Marseille, Pittsburgh, Rhode Island, and Seattle. Their study, based on the assumption that the target was the same in all cases, demonstrated that the maximum dose played a major role in the efficacy of the treatment, with no effect on its safety.[26] Specifically, patients treated with a maximum dose <70 Gy very rarely experienced pain alleviation. Thus, 70 Gy as the maximum became a standard dose for those using the "Pittsburgh way." Since this time the position of our team has been to insist on the fact that this pioneering study carried an important bias in the heterogeneity of the anatomical targets used.[17,20,27] Thus, we considered that further trials were mandatory to elucidate the best treatment parameters for the best safety/efficacy, before defining the role of Gamma Knife surgery among the other surgical alternatives.[17,28–30] Two articles published in the *Journal of Neurosurgery* in 2005 in the same issue (associated with a negative editorial) reported very poor middle/long-term results of Gamma Knife surgery in trigeminal neuralgia, with 71 and 21% excellent/good results at 6 months and 2 years, respectively, in Tawk et al[30] and 47, 45, and 34% excellent/good results at 1, 2, and 3 years, respectively, in Sheehan et al.[29] Importantly, the maximum dose in these series was heterogeneous (50–90 Gy in Sheehan et al[30]), with a low rate of 9% of facial numbness.[28–30]

Predictors of Pain Cessation, Pain Recurrence, and Toxicity in Radiosurgery for Trigeminal Neuralgia

There are huge discrepancies between treatment centers in terms of the results reported (**Table 14.2**). The range of these results has been reported as 35 to 100% for initial pain cessation, 0 to 42% for pain recurrence, and 0 to 57% for trigeminal nerve injury.[26,29,31–70] These differences may reflect the lack of homogeneity in the methodology of evaluation and the scoring techniques used. Frequently, the rates of complete pain freedom and of drug cessation are not explicitly indicated. The reported follow-up is often heterogeneous, with some studies including very short-term follow-up in the final analysis. However, several retrospective studies have identified some pre- and perioperative parameters that appear to significantly influence the outcome. A diagnosis of multiple sclerosis[71,72] and a past history of surgery for the treatment of trigeminal neuralgia on the same side[50,57] have both been linked to a lower rate of pain control. On several occasions we have found inconsistencies between our series and series from the literature, but each time we have finally found behind these differences clear explanations in technical nuances (**Fig. 14.3**). However, these discrepancies were superficial, and a schematic figure of the influence of some dose-planning parameters is rising.

The maximum dose is clearly related to the probability of pain cessation in our series and the literature (**Fig. 14.3**). In secondary trigeminal neuralgia,[68] it is worth noting that a marginal dose ~14 to 15 Gy seems to result in a high rate of

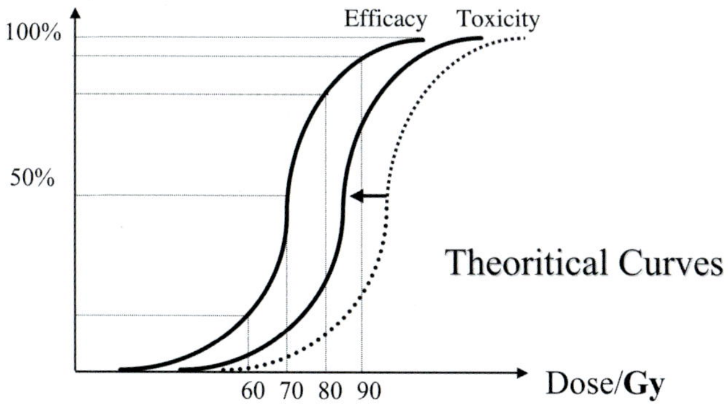

Fig. 14.3 The relationship between the maximum dose and the safety/efficacy of the treatment may be modeled as a double sigmoid curve. Both the probability of prolonged pain freedom (*left curve*) and the risk of hypoesthesia are increased with the increased maximum dose (*two right curves*). Under 70 Gy, the safety rate is excellent, but the efficacy rate regarding pain alleviation is very poor. Beyond 90 Gy, the rate of pain relief is very good, but any increase of the maximum dose can lead to a very significant increase in the risk of trigeminal nerve injury. Our hypothesis is that the choice of a target at the level of the emergence of the nerve dramatically narrows the "safety space" between the two sigmoid curves compared with our cisternal target (7–8 mm from the emergence). When using the dorsal root entry zone (DREZ) target, dose escalation allows dramatic improvement of the results, although with a heavy price to pay in terms of trigeminal nerve injury (*dotted line*). With the retrogasserian target (*continuous line*), a highly efficient dosage (90 Gy) can be delivered safely.

pain cessation when applied to cerebellopontine angle tumors (**Fig. 14.4**). In essential trigeminal neuralgia, following our publication discussing the high rate of pain freedom using 90 Gy, Pollock et al published a study comparing the 70 Gy maximum dose in 27 patients and the 90 Gy maximum dose in 41 patients.[56] In this study, high-dose radiosurgery is associated not only with a higher chance of pain relief (61% instead of 41%) but also with a higher chance of trigeminal nerve injury (54% instead of 15%).[56] Although Pollock et al's study demonstrated the influence of the maximum dose on the probability of complete pain relief, it did not confirm the very low rate of hypoesthesia we observed in our population. Between our two series there is one major difference: the anatomical location of the target.[27] We hypothesized on the occasion of a comment published in the *Journal of Neurosurgery*[27] that this lower toxicity in our series was due to the longer distance between the center of the isocenter and the anatomical emergence of the fifth nerve (**Fig. 14.3**). At this time, Pollock responded by saying, "I doubt that any dosimetric manipulation (e.g., dose, target, length of irradiated nerve) would have provided a qualitative change in the results published during the past several years with regards to trigeminal radiosurgery. . . ."[27]

The location of the dose application on the nerve is turning out to be a crucial predictor, especially for toxicity (**Fig. 14.3**). What accounts for the difference between the two anatomical targets? The dose to the DREZ and the dose to the brainstem, or more precisely to the trigeminal nerve pathways in the brainstem (**Fig. 14.5**), are dramatically increased with the so-called DREZ target. The dorsal root entry zone is histologically defined as the zone where the peripheral myelination (Schwann cells) leaves place to the central type of myelination (oligodendroglia). In 2002 De Ridder et al demonstrated the fact that the location of this zone is highly variable and can spread more distally in some patients.[73] Conversely, McLaughlin et al emphasized the fact that the dorsal root entry or exit zone can be variable in length, particularly in the case of the trigeminal nerve, and it may extend to a more distal portion of the nerve than previously described.[74] The variability of the limit between the Schwann cells and the glial environment of the nerve as it exits the brainstem, classically located 3 mm from the nerve's emergence, must be borne in mind.[73] Of course, there is no in vivo possibility to evaluate individually the extent of the DREZ on the nerve, which makes the term *DREZ target* inappropriate. The term *emergence target* is preferred. Another clinical discrepancy has been mentioned by Noren. In essential trigeminal neuralgia using very high doses, the rate of hypoesthesia is, in our experience, much lower than in the historical experience of cerebellopontine angle tumors.[75,76] Here, again, the doses to the pathway of the trigeminal nerve in the brainstem are much higher in the second group of patients.[75,76] This is an additional argument

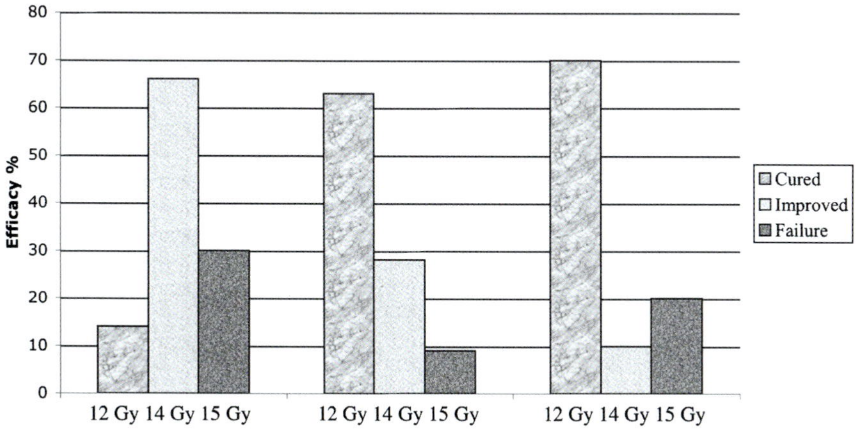

Fig. 14.4 A population of patients presenting with cerebellopontine angle tumors associated with secondary trigeminal neuralgia displayed the influence of the marginal dose on the probability of pain cessation. When the dose at the periphery is increased from 12 to 15 Gy, the probability of pain cessation increases from 15 to 70%. Foote et al 79 demonstrated that this effect was related to the dose delivered to the brainstem and not correlated to the dose delivered to the trigeminal nerve.

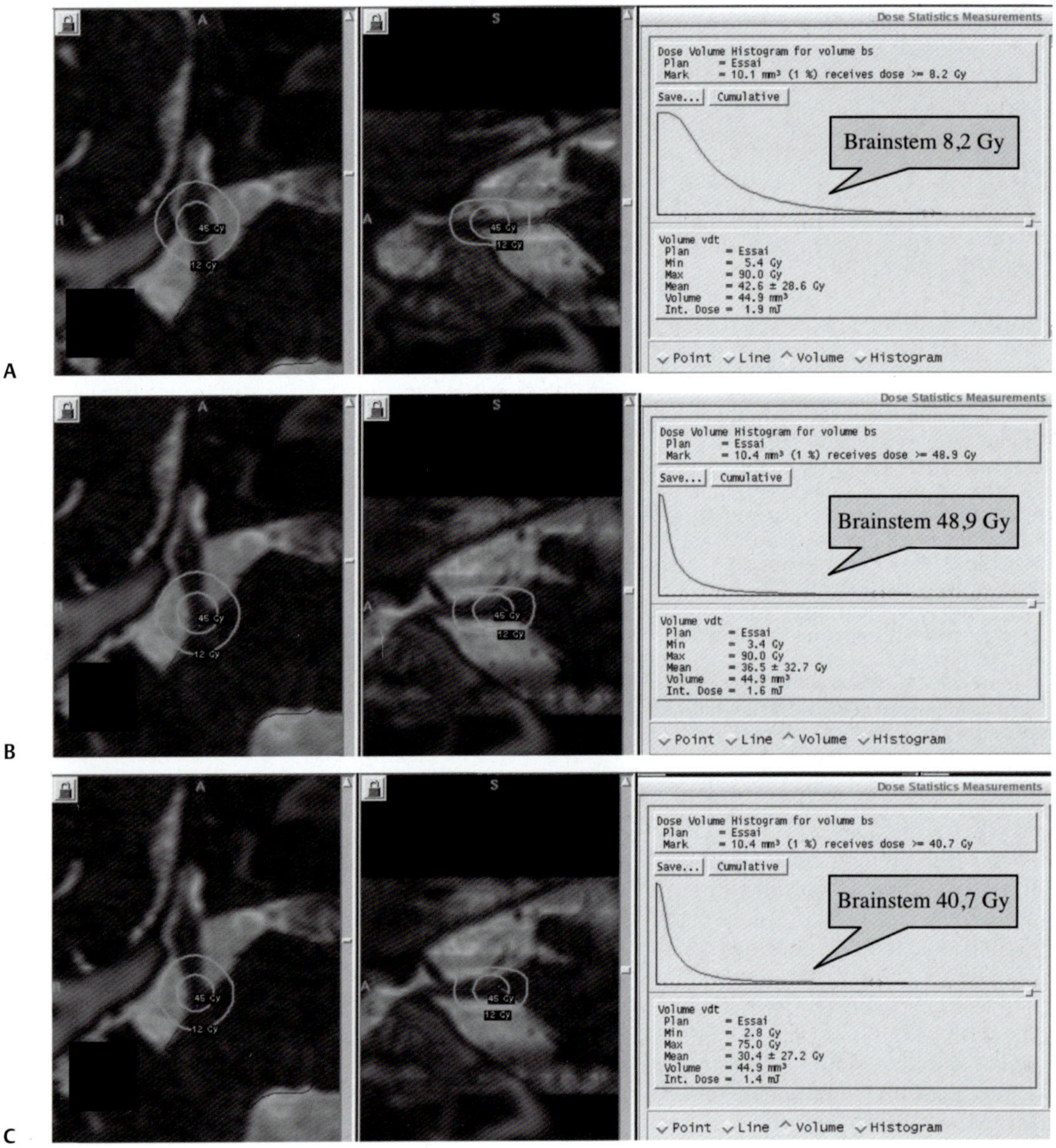

Fig. 14.5 Comparison of **(A)** the cisternal retrogasserian target and **(B)** the so-called dorsal root entry zone (DREZ) target. When the cistern is large, 90 Gy can be delivered very safely 7 to 8 mm anteriorly on the cisternal portion of the trigeminal nerve while very modest doses are delivered to the brainstem, much lower than in the DREZ target if the same dose is used or **(C)** if a lower dose (75 Gy) is used.

for the role of the central trigeminal pathways in radiosurgically induced hypoesthesia (**Fig. 14.6**). Conversely, Foote et al,[77] in a series of vestibular schwannomas treated by linac radiosurgery, demonstrated the direct relationship between the risk of trigeminal nerve function disturbance and the dose to the brainstem (but the absence of a relationship to the dose delivered to the nerve itself). Finally, the complication of dry eye syndrome reported by Matsuda et al[78] never occurred in our series.[19] These authors used a posterior target and correlated this complication with the delivery of high doses to the brainstem.[39,78]

The integrated dose to the nerve (the volume of the nerve irradiated and/or the average dose) has been reported to correlate to the risk of trigeminal nerve function disturbance. Flickinger et al, in a trial comparing two 4 mm isocenters to one, found a dramatic increase in the rate of toxicity.[36] Kanner et al,[79] using a 4 and an 8 mm isocenter superimposed, observed similar toxicity. Interestingly, these two teams found no benefit in terms of the rate of pain relief. Massager et al,[51] published results comparable to ours in terms of pain cessation but with a much higher incidence of hypoesthesia: 43% instead of 15% in our overall series.[19] After a cautious analysis, we discovered that in cases of a narrow cistern with too high of a dosage delivered to the brainstem, the attitudes of the two teams diverged (**Fig. 14.7**). In these cases, our attitude was to lower the maximum dose, but the Brussels team's attitude was to keep the 90 Gy maximum dose and rely on shielding for reducing the dose to the brainstem. At this

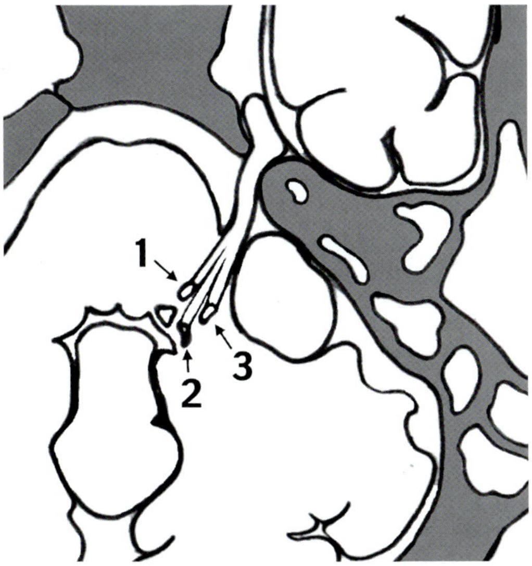

Fig. 14.6 Drawing illustrating the role of the central trigeminal pathways in radiosurgically induced hypoesthesia. This demonstrates the topological relationship between a lesion in the cerebellopontine angle (i.e., acoustic nerve) and the trigeminal nuclei and pathways in the brainstem. 1, nucleus motorius nervi trigemini; 2, nucleus mesencephalicus nervi trigemini; 3, nucleus sensorius principalis nervi trigemini.

time, we maintain that this plugging strategy accounted for the different rates of toxicity (**Fig. 14.7**). To confirm this hypothesis, we shared with the Brussels team our material to allow them to test for the influence of this parameter in our two series. Massager et al found that in patients with a large cistern, our methods were similar and results homogeneous with ~20% of trigeminal nerve disturbance.[80] In patients with narrow cisterns, the Brussels shielding strategy led to a dramatic increase ($p < .05$) of the mean dose (42.86 Gy instead of 38.01) and integrated dose (3.28 instead of 2.76), with, consequently, a rate of hypoesthesia rising from 15% with no bothersome hypoesthesia to 50% including 10% bothersome hypoesthesia ($p < .05$). In this study, as in the Flickinger and Kanner studies, no significant benefit was associated with the increased volume of nerve treated.[36,79,80] Thus, the dose/volume to the nerve can account for huge differences in the hypoesthesia rate. The study by Massager et al confirms both our results in term of efficacy and safety and the influence of the integrated dose, showing how much technical nuances can influence the results.[80] Thus, the mean dose to the nerve is linked to two other parameters. Of course, the average dose to the nerve is influenced by the volume of the nerve, and we must keep in mind that both the toxicity and the safety rates turn out to be influenced by the atrophy of the nerve. This also indicates how much the variability of cisternal anatomy can influence the clinical outcome, especially for those who are not aware of these technical nuances.

The predictions in the literature results based on this factor are turning out to be quite efficient. The team at the University of California at Los Angeles (UCLA) reported the results of 196 patients, with follow-up among 126 patients treated between 1996 and 2006.[81] A 4 mm shot was placed on the nerve emergence, with 90 Gy at the center (**Fig. 14.8**).[25] As predicted, the short-term successful pain outcome was high (90–95%), with a 10 to 35% recurrence rate and a long-term pain relief rate of 70%. Because of the location of the shot, not surprisingly, the rate of numbness was very high (58.3%), including 19.4% severely bothersome numbness, 30.5% subjective dry eyes, and 30.5% decreased corneal reflex. The toxicity to the brainstem is well illustrated by the 46 patients investigated with postoperative MRIs demonstrating high signal and contrast enhancement in the brainstem. The Stanford University team reported the results of 83 patients treated between 2002 and 2006.[82] The maximum dose was between 71.4 and 86.4 Gy, with a special strategy (**Fig. 14.8**) covering all the nerve (important integrated dose).[83] As predicted, due to the volume of nerve treated, the rate of hypoesthesia was high (74% numbness, with 39% severe numbness). Moreover, the Stanford authors demonstrated that a longer length of treatment resulted in higher rates of numbness. Patients treated with a maximum dose > 75 Gy had a much higher chance of being pain free. Spencer et al[84] reported on 350 patients, with follow-up available for 320; they tested the role of the anatomical position of the shot (separating the types of shots as brainstem, touching, and not touching). They found that the location had no influence on the quality of the results, but that the more often the shot was located close to the brainstem, the more likely the patient was to experience numbness (16.7–40%), confirming our hypothesis that the major role of the central trigeminal nerve pathway is in the incidence of radiosurgically induced hypoesthesia.

Two clinical strategies are possible. The conservative approach tends to obtain better results in terms of pain control with rare hypoesthesia but required high doses to be delivered anteriorly. A more radical approach is to use a similar dosage posteriorly at the level of the nerve emergence,[85,86] based on the argument that hypoesthesia increases the chance of pain relief.[87] Opposite to this attitude is our position, which argues that radiosurgery, unlike percutaneous treatment, offers very good pain control without any hypoesthesia for the majority of patients. Nothing is worse and more difficult to treat than a neuropathic pain or an anesthesia dolorosa. Consequently, we prefer to take the risk of proposing a new procedure rather than inducing severe hypoesthesia.

Our recommendation is to place a single 4 mm shot on the cisternal portion of the nerve 7.5 to 8.0 mm from the emergence of the brainstem, with a maximum dose of 90 Gy (**Fig. 14.5**). In cases where the dose to the brainstem is too high, start by decreasing the maximum dose; if insufficient, plugging (shielding) is possible (**Fig. 14.7**).

A correlation between hypoesthesia and pain response does, however, exist.[72] Rogers et al reported a higher probability of pain cessation in patients experiencing trigeminal injury after radiosurgery.[87] We failed to find this significant correlation, but it is of interest to note that 100% of the patients experiencing hypoesthesia after Gamma Knife surgery in our series were cured. A study by Maesawa et al found that the absence of preoperative sensory disturbance or previous surgery correlated significantly with complete or partial pain relief over time.[50]

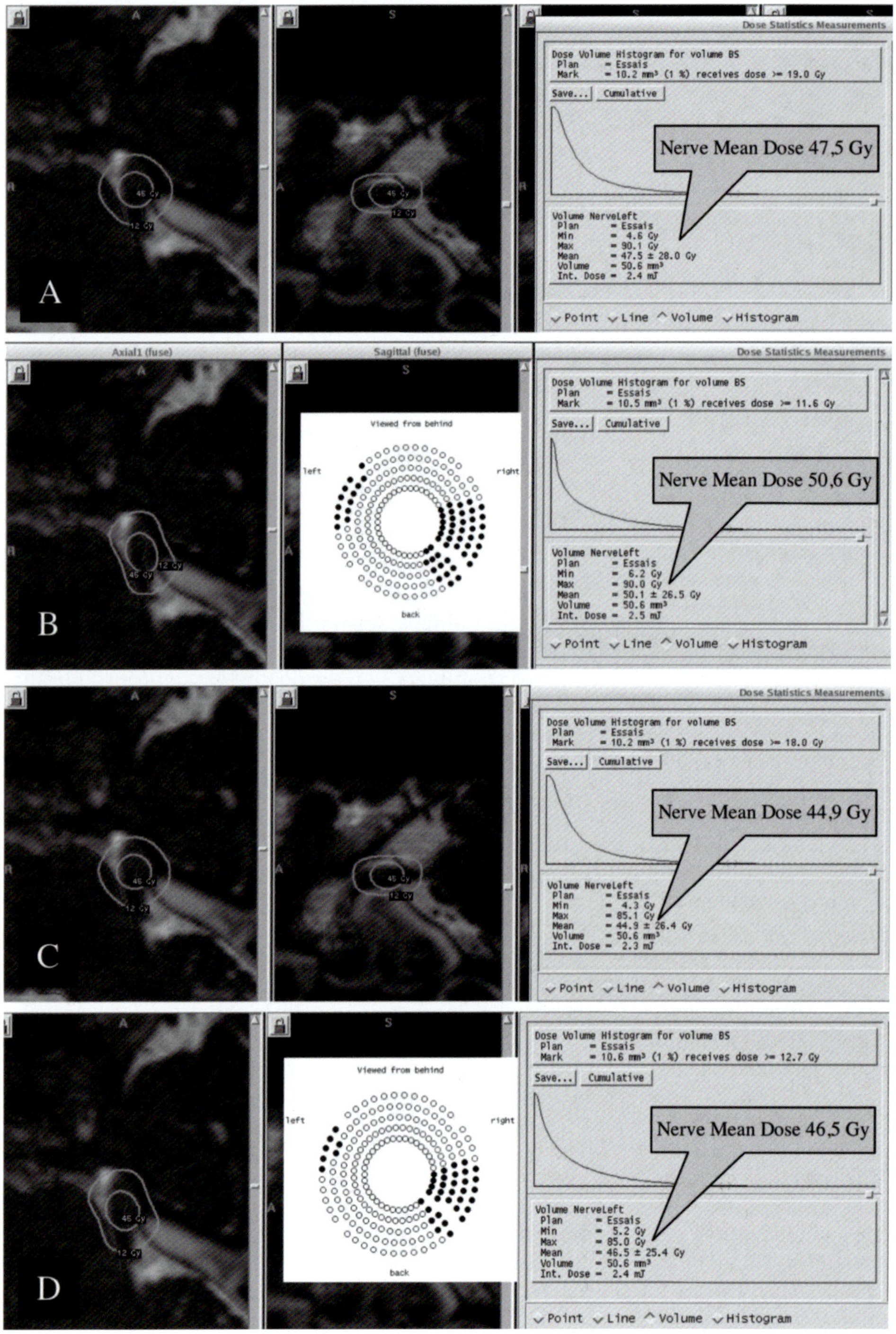

Fig. 14.7 Influence of the trigeminal nerve cistern morphology. **(A)** In cases of patients with very narrow cisterns, with the usual dose planning, the dose to the brainstem may be too high. **(B)** It is important not to increase the volume of nerve treated when using plugging to avoid the "Flickinger effect" (a dramatic increase in toxicity on the trigeminal nerve when the volume of nerve treated is increased). For the same reason, beam blocking is always preceded by a decrease in the maximum dose. **(C)** Thus, the maximum dose is first decreased to spare the brainstem. **(D)** If the dose is still too high, in a second step, the use of beam blocking on a moderate number of beams improves this sparing.

Surgical methods for the treatment of trigeminal neuralgia can be separated into two groups (**Table 14.1**). Ablative techniques (thermocoagulation, balloon microcompression, and glycerol injection) are usually performed percutaneously under brief general anesthesia. They have in common a very high rate of trigeminal nerve dysfunction (including keratitis for V1 territory) but are simple techniques that are easy to repeat and readily suitable for the elderly.[88] MVD is established as the technique of choice and has the major advantage of treating the probable cause of the disease as

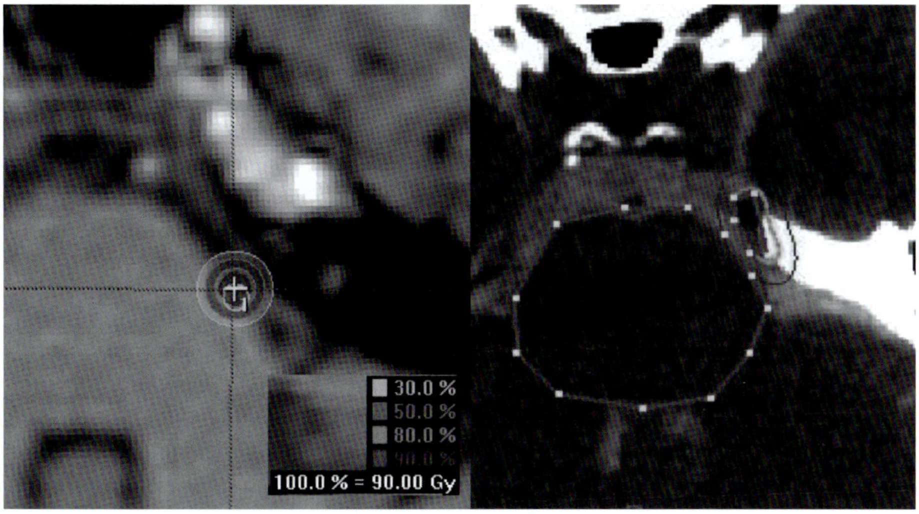

A B

Fig. 14.8 Typical dose planning for trigeminal neuralgia with **(A)** the Novalis stereotactic system (BrainLAB Ag, Feldkirchen, Germany) and **(B)** the CyberKnife (Accuray Inc., Sunnyvale, CA) according to the dosimetric approaches developed, respectively, by Antonio DeSalles and John Adler. The UCLA strategy consisted of delivering a high dose (90 Gy) centered on the emergence of the nerve, which means generously overlapping the pathway of the fifth cranial nerve in the brainstem. The rate of success is good (70% on the middle term) thanks to the high dose, but the rate of hypoesthesia is very high (58.3% numbness, 19.4% severe bothersome numbness, 30.5% subjective dry eyes, and 30.5% decreased corneal reflex). The idea behind the UCLA strategy is to favor the cure rate more than the sparing of the nerve function. The Stanford University strategy is more original, with the targeting of a large volume of nerve on 6.75 mm of its length with a moderate dose of 76 Gy (range 71.4–86.4 Gy). Due to the "Flickinger effect," the hypoesthesia rate is high despite the moderate dose, with 74% reported numbness (61% mild to moderate numbness and 39% severe numbness). Conversely, our model has demonstrated a higher rate of numbness with a longer treated length of nerve and both a higher rate of success (92% vs 71%) and an increased risk of hypoesthesia (42% vs 25%) with a higher dose ($<$75 Gy vs $>$75 Gy).

well as offering a very low risk of subsequent trigeminal nerve dysfunction.[89–91] This procedure is, of course, performed under general anesthesia with a craniotomy. Perioperative mortality is rare, oculomotor deficits are usually transient, and the incidence of facial palsy and deafness is reasonably low in experienced hands.[89–91] Radiosurgery has the advantage of being the least invasive available procedure and is performed under local anesthesia. Additionally, the rate of trigeminal dysfunction is remarkably low and comparable to that occurring with MVD. It is intriguing to consider the rarity of clinical injury to the trigeminal nerve, in spite of a high rate of pain cessation. With percutaneous treatment, particularly with thermocoagulation, the induction of hypoesthesia is essentially mandatory for prolonged pain cessation.[92] With radiosurgery, the majority of patients experience the disappearance of trigeminal neuralgia without sustaining any trigeminal nerve dysfunction (even if the appearance of posttreatment hypoesthesia does increase the probability of pain cessation).[87] This evidence is rather surprising in terms of the physiopathology of the effect, but it clearly constitutes an advantage of radiosurgery over percutaneous techniques.

Multiple sclerosis in patients presenting with trigeminal neuralgia has been reported as being associated with a lower rate of successful treatment.[71] However, due to the particular difficulties related to this condition when using other surgical techniques, several authors have reported radiosurgery to be a technique that provides an acceptable safety–efficacy ratio in such patients. In line with this, and based on the assumption that patients with multiple sclerosis are often more sensitive to any surgical intervention, any patient with the condition in our series was systematically subjected to use of a lower dose (median of the maximum dose 80 Gy), which perhaps explains the lower incidence of pain cessation for this specific group.[73]

◆ Indications of Radiosurgery

According to the literature, Gamma Knife surgery is frequently proposed in everyday practice, including in good candidates for MVD.[57] Even if some authors use the very good safety–efficacy ratio of radiosurgery as an argument for promoting this treatment as a first-line alternative to conventional methods,[70] we still recommend MVD in young patients, as this remains, in our opinion, the gold standard treatment for this group. In young patients declining MVD, radiosurgery may be offered on the grounds that it results in a very low rate of numbness for a similar rate of efficacy as compared with percutaneous methods. However, the exact indications for radiosurgery are still a matter of controversy. Only prospective randomized controlled trials comparing each of the alternative methods to the gold standard (MVD) are likely to clarify this issue.

A cautious review of the literature shows a huge heterogeneity in surgical practice. Clearly, local practice, skills, and technical availability greatly influence the form of treatment

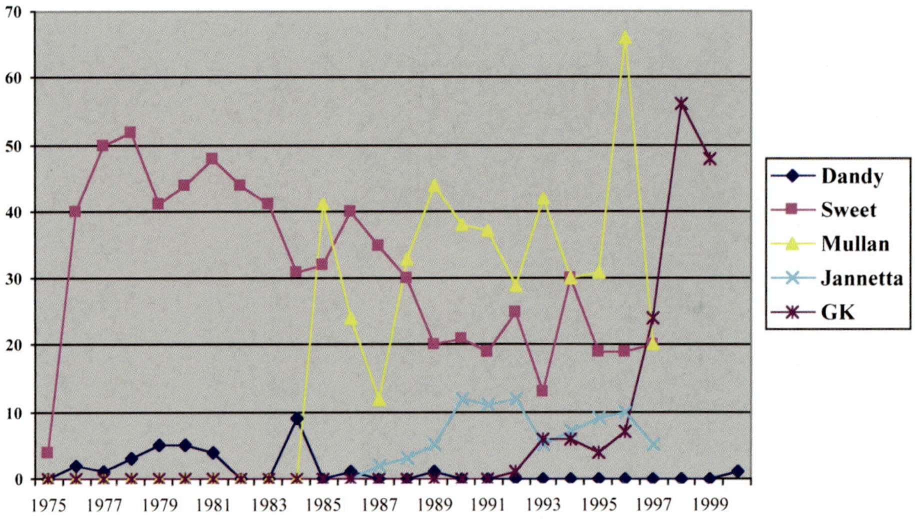

Fig. 14.9 Summary of 25 years of trigeminal neuralgia surgical management in the functional neurosurgery department of the Timone University Hospital. This graph demonstrates the continued use of all treatment options to afford relief to trigeminal neuralgia patients.

offered. In our center, all the main techniques—MVD, thermocoagulation, balloon microcompression, and radiosurgery—are available and currently practiced (**Fig. 14.9**). We believe that this diminishes the bias in terms of optimal treatment choice for an individual patient at a particular moment in his or her medical history.

◆ Summary

Radiosurgery has been suggested as the least invasive surgical technique for the treatment of trigeminal neuralgia. Our prospective trial, which fulfilled the Zakrzewska criterion, has established Gamma Knife surgery as a safe and effective treatment of trigeminal neuralgia. However, a wide range of results exists in the literature in terms of both pain control and toxicity. If the methodology of evaluation can account for the differences between some series found in the literature, a comparison of the main large series seriously evaluated demonstrates the important differences in the results. Our hypothesis is that technical nuances can explain these differences. In our experience, high-dose (80–90 Gy) retrogasserian (7–8 mm from the brainstem) Gamma Knife surgery offers patients a greater chance of long-term pain relief and a lower risk of trigeminal nerve functional disturbance. Possibly radiosurgery directed to a more anterior portion of the cisternal nerve may allow the safe use of higher doses by reduction of the risk of sensory loss.

Our results and the results from the literature demonstrate that radiosurgery applied to the cisternal anterior trigeminal nerve using high doses is a safe and effective treatment for trigeminal neuralgia in the long term, offering a low, rarely troublesome rate of hypoesthesia.

To further refine the role of Gamma Knife surgery, a randomized controlled comparative study fulfilling stringent quality criteria is required.[93]

Acknowledgments Supported by Timone University Hospital (Assistance Publique des Hôpitaux de Marseille).

References

1. Merrison AF, Fuller G. Treatment options for trigeminal neuralgia. BMJ 2003;327:1360–1361
2. Classification and diagnostic criteria for headache disorders, cranial neuralgia and facial pain. Cephalalgia 1988;8(Suppl 7):1–96
3. Love S, Coakham HB. Trigeminal neuralgia: pathology and pathogenesis. Brain 2001;124:2347–2360
4. Taarnhoj P. Decompression of the trigeminal root and the posterior part of the ganglion as treatment in trigeminal neuralgia. J Neurosurg 1952;9:288–290
5. Brown JA, McDaniel MD, Weaver MT. Percutaneous trigeminal nerve compression for treatment of trigeminal neuralgia: results in 50 patients. Neurosurgery 1993;32:570–573
6. Kanpolat Y, Savas A, Bekar A, Berk C. Percutaneous controlled radiofrequency trigeminal rhizotomy for the treatment of idiopathic trigeminal neuralgia: 25-year experience with 1,600 patients. Neurosurgery 2001;48:524–532
7. Latchaw JP Jr., Hardy RW Jr., Forsythe SB, Cook AF. Trigeminal neuralgia treated by radiofrequency coagulation. J Neurosurg 1983;59:479–484
8. North RB, Kidd DH, Piantadosi S, Carson BS. Percutaneous retrogasserian glycerol rhizotomy: predictors of success and failure in treatment of trigeminal neuralgia. J Neurosurg 1990;72:851–856
9. Oturai AB, Jensen K, Eriksen J, Madsen F. Neurosurgery for trigeminal neuralgia: comparison of alcohol block, neurectomy, and radiofrequency coagulation. Clin J Pain 1996;12:311–315
10. Sindou M, Keravel Y, Abdennebi B, Szapiro J. Traitement neurochirurgical de la névralgie trigéminale. Neurochirurgie 1987;33:89–111
11. Slettebo H, Hirschberg H, Lindegaard KF. Long-term results after percutaneous retrogasserian glycerol rhizotomy in patients with trigeminal neuralgia. Acta Neurochir (Wien) 1993;122:231–235
12. Zakrzewska JM, Jassim S, Bulman JS. A prospective, longitudinal study on patients with trigeminal neuralgia who underwent radiofrequency thermocoagulation of the gasserian ganglion. Pain 1999;79:51–58
13. Leksell L. Stereotaxis and radiosurgery: an operative system. In: Thomas CC, ed. Springfield; 1971
14. Leksell L. Sterotaxic radiosurgery in trigeminal neuralgia. Acta Chir Scand 1971;137:311–314
15. Lindquist C, Kihlstrom L, Hellstrand E. Functional neurosurgery: a future for the Gamma Knife? Stereotact Funct Neurosurg 1991;57:72–81
16. Rand RW, Jacques DB, Melbye RW, Copcutt BG, Levenick MN, Fisher MR. Leksell Gamma Knife treatment of tic douloureux. Stereotact Funct Neurosurg 1993;61(Suppl 1):93–102
17. Régis J, Metellus P, Hayashi M, Roussel P, Donnet A, Bille-Turc F. Prospective controlled trial of Gamma Knife surgery for essential trigeminal neuralgia. J Neurosurg 2006;104:913–924

18. Zakrzewska JM, Lopez BC. Quality of reporting in evaluations of surgical treatment of trigeminal neuralgia: recommendations for future reports. Neurosurgery 2003;53:110–120
19. Arkha Y, Murata N, Yomo S, Roussel P, Donnet A, Régis J. Gamma Knife surgery for essential trigeminal neuralgia: long-term results in a series of 262 patients. Journal of Neurosurgery 2008 (Submitted)
20. Régis J, Bartolomei F, Metellus P, et al. Radiosurgery for trigeminal neuralgia and epilepsy. Neurosurg Clin N Am 1999;10:359–377
21. Alexander E, Lindquist C. Special indications: radiosurgery for functional neurosurgery and epilepsy. In: Alexander E III, Loeffler J, Lunsford L, eds. Stereotactic Radiosurgery. New York: Mc Graw-Hill; 1993:221–225
22. Lichtor T, Mullan JF. A 10-year follow-up review of percutaneous microcompression of the trigeminal ganglion. J Neurosurg 1990;72:49–54
23. Mullan S, Lichtor T. Percutaneous microcompression of the trigeminal ganglion for trigeminal neuralgia. J Neurosurg 1983;59:1007–1012
24. Frazier CH. Operation for the radical cure of trigeminal neuralgia: analysis of five hundred cases. Ann Surg 1928;88:534–547
25. Régis J, Manera L, Dufour H, Porcheron D, Sedan R, Peragut JC. Effect of the Gamma Knife on trigeminal neuralgia. Stereotact Funct Neurosurg 1995;64(Suppl 1):182–192
26. Kondziolka D, Lunsford LD, Flickinger JC, et al. Stereotactic radiosurgery for trigeminal neuralgia: a multiinstitutional study using the Gamma unit. J Neurosurg 1996;84:940–945
27. Régis J. High-dose trigeminal neuralgia radiosurgery associated with increased risk of trigeminal nerve dysfunction. Neurosurgery 2002;50:1401–1403
28. Burchiel KJ. Gamma Knife and trigeminal neuralgia. J Neurosurg 2005; 102:431–432
29. Sheehan J, Pan HC, Stroila M, Steiner L. Gamma Knife surgery for trigeminal neuralgia: outcomes and prognostic factors. J Neurosurg 2005;102:434–441
30. Tawk RG, Duffy-Fronckowiak M, Scott BE, et al. Stereotactic Gamma Knife surgery for trigeminal neuralgia: detailed analysis of treatment response. J Neurosurg 2005;102:442–449
31. Brisman R. Gamma Knife radiosurgery for primary management for trigeminal neuralgia. J Neurosurg 2000;93(Suppl 3):159–161
32. Brisman R. Gamma Knife surgery with a dose of 75 to 76.8 gray for trigeminal neuralgia. J Neurosurg 2004;100:848–854
33. Chang JW, Chang JH, Park YG, Chung SS. Gamma Knife radiosurgery for idiopathic and secondary trigeminal neuralgia. J Neurosurg 2000; 93(Suppl 3):147–151
34. Chen JC, Girvigian M, Greathouse H, Miller M, Rahimian J. Treatment of trigeminal neuralgia with linear accelerator radiosurgery: initial results. J Neurosurg 2004;101(Suppl 3):346–350
35. Cheuk AV, Chin LS, Petit JH, Herman JM, Fang HB, Regine WF. Gamma Knife surgery for trigeminal neuralgia: outcome, imaging, and brainstem correlates. Int J Radiat Oncol Biol Phys 2004;60:537–541
36. Flickinger JC, Pollock BE, Kondziolka D, et al. Does increased nerve length within the treatment volume improve trigeminal neuralgia radiosurgery? A prospective double-blind, randomized study. Int J Radiat Oncol Biol Phys 2001;51:449–454
37. Fountas KN, Smith JR, Lee GP, Jenkins PD, Cantrell RR, Sheils WC. Gamma Knife stereotactic radiosurgical treatment of idiopathic trigeminal neuralgia: long-term outcome and complications. Neurosurg Focus 2007;23:E8:1–7
38. Frighetto L, De Salles AA, Smith ZA, Goss B, Selch M, Solberg T. Noninvasive linear accelerator radiosurgery as the primary treatment for trigeminal neuralgia. Neurology 2004;62:660–662
39. Goss BW, Frighetto L, DeSalles AA, Smith Z, Solberg T, Selch M. Linear accelerator radiosurgery using 90 gray for essential trigeminal neuralgia: results and dose volume histogram analysis. Neurosurgery 2003; 53:823–830
40. Han PP, Shetter AG, Smith KA, et al. Gamma Knife radiosurgery for trigeminal neuralgia: experience at the Barrow Neurological Institute. Stereotact Funct Neurosurg 1999;73:131–133
41. Kannan V, Deopujari CE, Misra BK, Shetty PG, Shroff MM, Pendse AM. Gamma Knife radiosurgery for trigeminal neuralgia. Australas Radiol 1999;43:339–341
42. Kondziolka D, Flickinger JC, Lunsford LD, Habeck M. Trigeminal neuralgia radiosurgery: the University of Pittsburgh experience. Stereotact Funct Neurosurg 1996;66(Suppl 1):343–348
43. Kondziolka D, Lunsford L, Flickinger J. Gamma Knife radiosurgery as the first surgery for trigeminal neuralgia. Stereotact Funct Neurosurg 1998;70(Suppl 1):187–191
44. Kondziolka D, Lunsford L, Habeck M, Flickinger J. Gamma Knife radiosurgery for trigeminal neuralgia. Neurosurg Clin N Am 1997;8:79–85
45. Kondziolka D, Lunsford LD, Flickinger JC. Stereotactic radiosurgery for the treatment of trigeminal neuralgia. Clin J Pain 2002;18:42–47
46. Kondziolka D, Perez B, Flickinger JC, Habeck M, Lunsford LD. Gamma Knife radiosurgery for trigeminal neuralgia: results and expectations. Arch Neurol 1998;55:1524–1529
47. Kondziolka D, Perez B, Flickinger JC, Lunsford LD. Radiosurgery for trigeminal neuralgia. Prog Neurol Surg 1998;14:2121–2221
48. Longhi M, Rizzo P, Nicolato A, Foroni R, Reggio M, Gerosa M. Gamma Knife radiosurgery for trigeminal neuralgia: results and potentially predictive parameters: 1. Idiopathic trigeminal neuralgia. Neurosurgery 2007;61:1254–1260
49. Lunsford LD, Young RF. Radiosurgery for trigeminal neuralgia. Surg Neurol 2000;54:285–287
50. Maesawa S, Salame C, Flickinger JC, Pirris S, Kondziolka D, Lunsford LD. Clinical outcomes after stereotactic radiosurgery for idiopathic trigeminal neuralgia. J Neurosurg 2001;94:14–20
51. Massager N, Lorenzoni J, Devriendt D, Desmedt F, Brotchi J, Levivier M. Gamma Knife surgery for idiopathic trigeminal neuralgia performed using a far-anterior cisternal target and a high dose of radiation. J Neurosurg 2004;100:597–605
52. McNatt SA, Yu C, Giannotta SL, Zee CS, Apuzzo ML, Petrovich Z. Gamma Knife radiosurgery for trigeminal neuralgia. Neurosurgery 2005;56:1295–1301
53. Mehta V, Meier R, Gilrein J, Vermeulen S, Young R. Gamma Knife radiosurgery for treatment of trigeminal neuralgia. Int J Radiat Oncol Biol Phys 2003;57:S136
54. Nicol B, Regine WF, Courtney C, Meigooni A, Sanders M, Young B. Gamma Knife radiosurgery using 90 Gy for trigeminal neuralgia. J Neurosurg 2000;93(Suppl 3):152–154
55. Petit JH, Herman JM, Nagda S, DiBiase SJ, Chin LS. Radiosurgical treatment of trigeminal neuralgia: evaluating quality of life and treatment outcomes. Int J Radiat Oncol Biol Phys 2003;56:1147–1153
56. Pollock BE, Phuong LK, Foote RL, Stafford SL, Gorman DA. High-dose trigeminal neuralgia radiosurgery associated with increased risk of trigeminal nerve dysfunction. Neurosurgery 2001;49:58–62
57. Pollock BE, Phuong LK, Gorman DA, Foote RL, Stafford SL. Stereotactic radiosurgery for idiopathic trigeminal neuralgia. J Neurosurg 2002; 97:347–353
58. Pusztaszeri M, Villemure JG, Regli L, Do HP, Pica A. Radiosurgery for trigeminal neuralgia using a linear accelerator with BrainLab system: report on initial experience in Lausanne, Switzerland. Swiss Med Wkly 2007;137:682–686
59. Rand RW. Leksell Gamma Knife treatment of tic douloureux. Neurosurg Clin N Am 1997;8:75–78
60. Richards GM, Bradley KA, Tome WA, Bentzen SM, Resnick DK, Mehta MP. Linear accelerator radiosurgery for trigeminal neuralgia. Neurosurgery 2005;57:1193–1200
61. Romanelli P, Heit G, Chang SD, Martin D, Pham C, Adler J. CyberKnife radiosurgery for trigeminal neuralgia. Stereotact Funct Neurosurg 2003;81:105–109
62. Shaya M, Jawahar A, Caldito G, Sin A, Willis BK, Nanda A. Gamma Knife radiosurgery for trigeminal neuralgia: a study of predictors of success, efficacy, safety, and outcome at LSUHSC. Surg Neurol 2004;61: 529–534
63. Shetter AG, Rogers CL, Ponce F, Fiedler JA, Smith K, Speiser BL. Gamma Knife radiosurgery for recurrent trigeminal neuralgia. J Neurosurg 2002;97:536–538
64. Smith ZA, De Salles AA, Frighetto L, et al. Dedicated linear accelerator radiosurgery for the treatment of trigeminal neuralgia. J Neurosurg 2003;99:511–516
65. Urgosik D, Liscak R, Novotny J Jr., Vymazal J, Vladyka V. Treatment of essential trigeminal neuralgia with Gamma Knife surgery. J Neurosurg 2005;102(Suppl):29–33
66. Urgosik D, Vymazal J, Vladyka V, Liscak R. Gamma Knife treatment of trigeminal neuralgia: clinical and electrophysiological study. Stereotact Funct Neurosurg 1998;70(Suppl 1):200–209
67. Yomo S, Takihana T, Hatano M, Hirai T. Gamma Knife surgery for trigeminal neuralgia. No Shinkei Geka Sokuho 2006;16:501–509
68. Young RF. Functional neurosurgery with the Leksell Gamma Knife. Stereotact Funct Neurosurg 1996;66:19–23
69. Young RF, Vermeulen SS, Grimm P, Blasko J, Posewitz A. Gamma Knife radiosurgery for treatment of trigeminal neuralgia: idiopathic and tumor related. Neurology 1997;48:608–614

70. Young RF, Vermulen S, Posewitz A. Gamma Knife radiosurgery for the treatment of trigeminal neuralgia. Stereotact Funct Neurosurg 1998; 70(Suppl 1):192–199

71. Huang E, Teh BS, Zeck O, et al. Gamma Knife radiosurgery for treatment of trigeminal neuralgia in multiple sclerosis patients. Stereotact Funct Neurosurg 2002;79:44–50

72. Rogers CL, Shetter AG, Ponce FA, Fiedler JA, Smith KA, Speiser BL. Gamma Knife radiosurgery for trigeminal neuralgia associated with multiple sclerosis. J Neurosurg 2002;97:529–532

73. De Ridder D, Moller A, Verlooy J, Cornelissen M, De Ridder L. Is the root entry/exit zone important in microvascular compression syndromes? Neurosurgery 2002;51:427–433

74. McLaughlin MR, Jannetta PJ, Clyde BL, Subach BR, Comey CH, Resnick DK. Microvascular decompression of cranial nerves: lessons learned after 4400 operations. J Neurosurg 1999;90:1–8

75. Régis J, Metellus P, Dufour H, et al. Long-term outcome after Gamma Knife surgery for secondary trigeminal neuralgia. J Neurosurg 2001;95:199–205

76. Régis J, Metellus P, Lazorthes Y, Porcheron D, Peragut JC. Effect of Gamma Knife on secondary trigeminal neuralgia. Stereotact Funct Neurosurg 1998;70(Suppl 1):210–217

77. Foote KD, Friedman WA, Buatti JM, Meeks SL, Bova FJ, Kubilis PS. Analysis of risk factors associated with radiosurgery for vestibular schwannoma. J Neurosurg 2001;95:440–449

78. Matsuda S, Serizawa T, Sato M, Ono J. Gamma Knife radiosurgery for trigeminal neuralgia: the dry-eye complication. J Neurosurg 2002;97: 525–528

79. Kanner AA, Neyman G, Suh JH, Weinhous MS, Lee SY, Barnett GH. Gamma Knife radiosurgery for trigeminal neuralgia: comparing the use of a 4-mm versus concentric 4- and 8-mm collimators. Stereotact Funct Neurosurg 2004;82:49–57

80. Massager N, Murata N, Tamura M, Devriendt D, Levivier M, Régis J. Influence of nerve radiation dose in the incidence of trigeminal dysfunction after trigeminal neuralgia radiosurgery. Neurosurgery 2007;60:681–687

81. Gorgulho A, Mitchell E, De Salles A, et al. Stereotactic radiosurgery (SRS) for trigeminal neuralgia: clinical, radiological and dosimetric characteristics of patients presenting immediate pain relief. Paper presented at: Eighth International Stereotactic Radiosurgery Society Congress; San Francisco; June 23–27, 2007

82. Lim M, Bower R, Soltys S, et al. Treating trigeminal neuralgia with the CyberKnife: single center experience. Paper presented at: Eighth International Stereotactic Radiosurgery Society Congress; San Francisco; June 23–27, 2007

83. Lim M, Villavicencio AT, Burneikiene S, et al. CyberKnife radiosurgery for idiopathic trigeminal neuralgia. Neurosurg Focus 2005;18:E9

84. Spencer S, Swaid S, Young P, Guthrie B, et al. The impact of dose rate on outcomes of Gamma Knife radiosurgery in patients with face pain. Paper presented at: Eighth International Stereotactic Radiosurgery Society Congress; San Francisco; June 23–27, 2007

85. Gorgulho A, De Salles AA, McArthur D, et al. Brainstem and trigeminal nerve changes after radiosurgery for trigeminal pain. Surg Neurol 2006;66:127–135

86. Gorgulho AA, De Salles AA. Impact of radiosurgery on the surgical treatment of trigeminal neuralgia. Surg Neurol 2006;66:350–356

87. Rogers CL, Shetter AG, Fiedler JA, Smith KA, Han PP, Speiser BL. Gamma Knife radiosurgery for trigeminal neuralgia: the initial experience of the Barrow Neurological Institute. Int J Radiat Oncol Biol Phys 2000;47:1013–1019

88. Lopez BC, Hamlyn PJ, Zakrzewska JM. Systematic review of ablative neurosurgical techniques for the treatment of trigeminal neuralgia. Neurosurgery 2004;54:973–982

89. Barker FG II, Jannetta PJ, Bissonette DJ, Jho HD. Trigeminal numbness and tic relief after microvascular decompression for typical trigeminal neuralgia. Neurosurgery 1997;40:39–45

90. Barker FG II, Jannetta PJ, Bissonette DJ, Larkins MV, Jho HD. The long-term outcome of microvascular decompression for trigeminal neuralgia. N Engl J Med 1996;334:1077–1083

91. Broggi G, Ferroli P, Franzini A, Servello D, Dones I. Microvascular decompression for trigeminal neuralgia: comments on a series of 250 cases, including 10 patients with multiple sclerosis. J Neurol Neurosurg Psychiatry 2000;68:59–64

92. Siegfried J. 500 Percutaneous thermocoagulations of the gasserian ganglion for trigeminal pain. Surg Neurol 1977;8:126–131

93. Lopez BC, Hamlyn PJ, Zakrzewska JM. Stereotactic radiosurgery for primary trigeminal neuralgia: state of the evidence and recommendations for future reports. J Neurol Neurosurg Psychiatry 2004;75: 1019–1024

15

Stereotactic Radiosurgery for Movement Disorders

Joel Bauman and John Y. K. Lee

The field of movement disorder functional neurosurgery has undergone a renaissance over the past 15 years. In large part, this is due to the rise of deep brain stimulation (DBS) in the treatment of medically refractory movement disorders. Within this setting, permanently destructive neuroablative procedures have become less popular. However, Gamma Knife (Elekta Instruments AB, Stockholm, Sweden) and occasionally linear accelerator (linac)–based radiosurgical units to perform thalamotomies and pallidotomies may still have some role in the neurosurgeon's ability to treat movement disorders. Neuroablation with high-dose radiation is the least invasive method, eliminating complications such as hemorrhage, infection, and hardware breakage. It can thus be performed on patients with significantly higher surgical risk factors for open procedures, such as medical comorbidities and intolerance of an awake procedure. Here we review the evidence for radiosurgical lesioning in the treatment of patients with medically refractory movement disorders. For comparison and context, we also briefly review the evidence for radiofrequency ablation as well as DBS.

Surgical Thalamotomy and Thalamic Deep Brain Stimulation

Until Benabid introduced DBS in 1987, radiofrequency (RF) lesioning of the ventral intermediate nucleus (Vim) of the thalamus was the primary method for treatment of medically intractable tremor-predominant Parkinson disease and essential tremor.[1–3] Before considering the merits of radiosurgical thalamotomy, it is worthwhile to review the role of conventional RF thalamotomy in the treatment of tremor, particularly as it compares with DBS. In patients with essential tremor, Schuurman et al compared DBS to RF lesioning and found results slightly favoring DBS.[4] Tremor suppression was achieved in 79% of patients who had had a thalamotomy, compared with 90% of patients who underwent DBS. More patients who underwent DBS achieved functional improvement. In addition, Tasker compared data from patients who had undergone RF thalamotomy and thalamic stimulation and found clearly superior results with DBS.[5] He found tremor recurrence in 15% of patients who had had a thalamotomy, as opposed to 5% of patients who underwent DBS. Of the patients who had a thalamotomy, 23% required repeat procedures for tremor control. Only half of the thalamotomy cohort obtained 50% improvement in dexterity, writing, and drinking, whereas all of the DBS subgroup achieved improvement. Furthermore, thalamotomy resulted in a decline in writing performance in 23% of patients, as opposed to no patient in the DBS group, whereas all of the patients who underwent DBS achieved better than 50% improvement in dexterity, writing, and drinking ability.

Complications of thalamotomy can be significant, especially when performed bilaterally. Common complications of bilateral thalamotomy include dysarthria and ataxia,[5–7] which have resulted in a desire to avoid bilateral ablation procedures. Schuurman et al found that patients who had RF thalamotomy were more likely to develop somnolence, cognitive deterioration, dysarthria, and ataxia compared with a randomized prospective cohort of patients who underwent DBS, although both groups had excellent symptomatic control of tremor.[8] When these complications occur in patients who undergo DBS, an adjustment of the stimulation parameters can usually correct these problems.[5] These studies highlight the factors behind the shift away from ablative procedures: efficacy, safety, and reversibility of adverse effects. Unlike thalamotomy, the therapeutic index of DBS (e.g., the difference between beneficial effect and adverse effect) can be navigated through careful programming.[9] It is in this context that the use of radiosurgical thalamotomy must be considered.

Radiosurgical Thalamotomy

Gamma Knife thalamotomy differs from RF thalamotomy in several key aspects. Gamma Knife thalamotomy is minimally invasive: there is no incision, bur hole, or physical penetration of any brain parenchyma. Thus, the risk of hemorrhagic or infectious complications is potentially lower than RF thalamotomy. In contrast, targeting for a Gamma Knife thalamotomy relies solely on imaging-defined anatomy. Physiologic macrostimulation and microelectrode recording are not available to assist the operator. Additionally, lesion generation is delayed and can be variable in size, as suggested by some recent publications.[10] Thus, Gamma Knife thalamotomy has both advantages and disadvantages that may shape its role in the treatment of movement disorders.

The current technique for targeting the Vim thalamus is similar to conventional stereotactic procedures. The Leksell model G stereotactic frame (Elekta) is attached to the patient's head, and high-resolution magnetic resonance (MR) images are obtained with a 1.5 tesla scanner. Contrast-enhanced images are acquired, including through the basal ganglia, midbrain, third ventricle, and anterior and posterior commissures (AC, PC). Axial fast inversion recovery sequences are performed for optimal gray-white differentiation and identification of the internal capsule. The Vim contralateral to the predominant tremor extremity is targeted as follows: anterior-posterior is one quarter the AC distance plus 1 mm anterior to PC; laterality is one half the third ventricle width plus 11 mm; superior-inferior is 2.5 mm superior to the AC–PC line. The 20% isodose line of the 4 mm collimator shot is placed medial to the internal capsule. A gamma angle of 110 degrees sometimes allows for better conformity to Vim in anterior-posterior and superior-inferior planes. On the model U Gamma Knife, beam blocking is not necessary, and a gamma angle of 60 to 70 degrees is used. The maximum dose of 130 to 140 Gy is delivered with one 4 mm isocenter.

There are several case series of Gamma Knife thalamotomy patients in the literature, documenting the success of this technique for the treatment of tremor. Friehs et al first examined thalamic radiosurgical lesioning in patients who had a contralateral RF lesion or a previously mapped lesion.[11] To date, Ohye et al have reported radiosurgical thalamotomy in 70 patients with Parkinson disease.[10] Tremor was suppressed by at least two thirds in over 80% of patients, with continued effect even after 10 years in some patients.[10,12] However, a significant subset of these patients had undergone a prior contralateral stereotactic procedure or ipsilateral procedure and were thus receiving a radiosurgical "boost." In this respect, the anatomical targeting was assisted. Duma et al reported a series of 38 radiosurgical thalamotomies over a 5-year period. In this series of patients, 24% had complete relief of tremor, 55% had "excellent or good" improvement in their tremor, and 21% of patients had only "mild" or no relief of tremor. Median follow-up was 28 months.[13,14] Importantly, only four of these patients underwent bilateral procedures.

Young et al published the largest series of patients undergoing Gamma Knife thalamotomy. The authors retrospectively reviewed records of 158 patients who had undergone radiosurgical thalamotomy for tremor, including 102 patients with Parkinson disease and 52 with essential tremor (ET).[15] Four-year follow-up data were available for 48% of the patients, including 74 patients with Parkinson disease and 16 with ET. Fifty-nine of the patients with Parkinson disease (79.7%) and 14 of the patients with ET (87.5%) were still tremor free or nearly tremor free at this interval. Two patients experienced permanent neurologic deficits, including hemiparesis and mild facial paresthesias. One patient sustained a transient deficit. No cognitive changes were reported. Young et al's finding of 88% of patients tremor free or nearly tremor free at 4 years following Gamma Knife thalamotomy is remarkable; however, the results for ET should be interpreted with caution, as follow-up involved less than one third of the treatment group. Similarly, Niranjan et al found that Fahn-Tolosa-Marin grades of tremor, handwriting, and drawing showed marked improvement after radiosurgical thalamotomy, including complete tremor arrest in 75% of patients with ET.[16] In an update of the Pittsburgh series, Kondziolka et al demonstrated significant improvement in action tremor in 88% of patients with Gamma Knife thalamotomy.[17] Typically, the response time was 1 to 4 months; however, three patients improved significantly within 2 days. Tremor and handwriting scores were both improved in 69% of patients. Three patients (12%) had no change in their tremor and writing scores. One patient experienced a mild right hemiparesis and speech impairment following radiosurgery. Another patient had a transient mild right hemiparesis and dysphagia. No other complications were noted. The overall complication rate was 7.7% (2/26). Both patients eventually maintained only mild neurologic deficits.

One difference between Gamma Knife radiosurgical thalamotomy and RF thalamotomy is the time for radiosurgical lesioning to take effect. Benefits and complications from radiosurgery occur between 1 and 12 months after the procedure.[10,13,16] This delay is due to the time needed for radiation to functionally damage or destroy the targeted tissue. The lesion effect can be accelerated with increased doses;[18] however, the optimal dose for Gamma Knife radiosurgical lesioning has not been established. Peak central doses can range from 120 to 200 Gy. Duma et al reported an improved clinical outcome with higher doses, suggesting a dose–response curve.[14] However, Okun et al reported a high percentage of complications in a series of eight patients, seven of whom were treated with a maximum dose of 200 Gy.[19] To date, a systematic study of dose–response–complication rate has not been performed. Nonetheless, most neurosurgeons perform radiosurgical lesioning for functional disorders at lower doses (e.g., 140 Gy).[16]

Because of the delay in effect after Gamma Knife thalamotomy, an accurate documentation of complications requires vigilant follow-up. In Young et al's series, 3 of 74 patients developed a complication.[15] Other reports consist of single events without mention of the total number of procedures or patients undergoing treatment. Siderowf et al reported one case of a complex, involuntary movement after Gamma Knife radiosurgical thalamotomy.[20] Unfortunately, particular dose parameters were not specified in that case report. Okun et al reported a series of eight patients who developed multiple complications, including hemiplegia, homonymous visual field deficit, hand weakness, dysarthria, hypophonia, aphasia, arm and face numbness, and pseudobulbar laughter.[19] These complications all occurred after treatment at one Gamma Knife center, and the same rate of complications has not been reported elsewhere. Thus, the true incidence of complications after radiosurgical thalamotomy is not well known, owing to poor long-term follow-up and lack of uniform dosing.

Variability in lesion size may relate to complications associated with radiosurgical thalamotomy. Animal studies in rodents and nonhuman primates have demonstrated the ability to create necrotic lesions in animal brain parenchyma.[18,21,22] Dose, volume, and time are the key components that determine the nature of functional ablation.[3,11,18] In general, the typical post–Gamma Knife thalamotomy MRI demonstrates a well-demarcated, peripherally enhancing lesion of 4 to 5 mm in size, surrounding a low-signal central region. On T2-weighted studies, localized adjacent high-signal areas may indicate the peripheral neuronal effect, appearing as an increase in intra- or extracellular water (**Figs. 15.1** and **15.2**). Two patients with complications had different MRI findings, consisting of a larger ring-enhancing lesion on T1-weighted (**Fig. 15.3**) and extensive high-signal change peripherally on T2-weighted imaging. The eventual radiographic resolution suggested that the effects were not due to radiation necrosis, but rather vasogenic edema. Ohye et al reported similar findings of two distinct lesion types, using a single 4 mm collimator isocenter with central doses of 130 Gy: one lesion is ~7 to 8 mm in diameter, well circumscribed, surrounding a low-signal area; the other is irregular, consists of high signal, and extends into the medial thalamic area and/or internal capsule with streaking along the thalamocapsular border.[10,14] The lesion types could not be associated with the patient's age, cortical atrophy, or symptom type (e.g., tremor, rigidity, or dystonia).

Gamma Knife radiosurgical thalamotomy remains a useful technique for unilateral ET. Its role in Parkinson disease is less well established, primarily because unilateral thalamotomy is

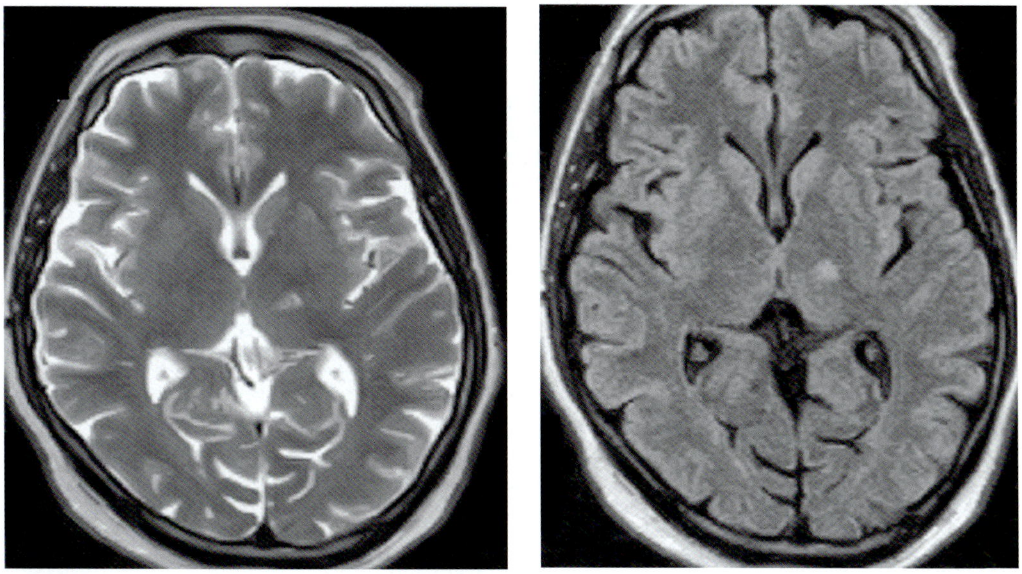

A

B

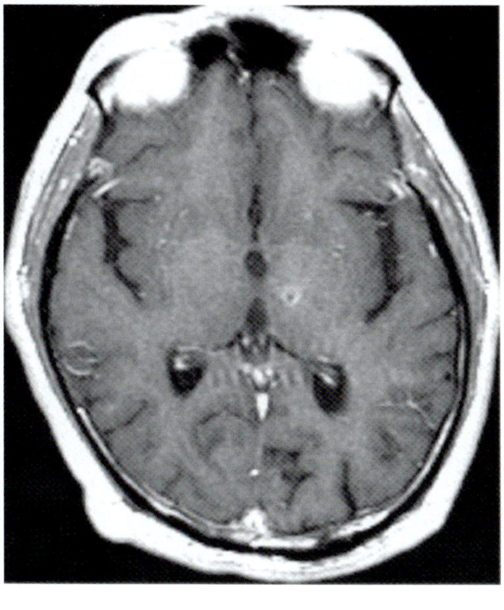

C

Fig. 15.1 **(A)** T2-weighted axial image demonstrating magnetic resonance signal changes in the left ventral intermediate nucleus of the thalamus 6 months after Gamma Knife thalamotomy. **(B)** Fluid-attenuated inversion recovery (FLAIR) image of the same lesion. **(C)** T1-weighted gadolinium enhanced image demonstrates peripheral of the lesion.

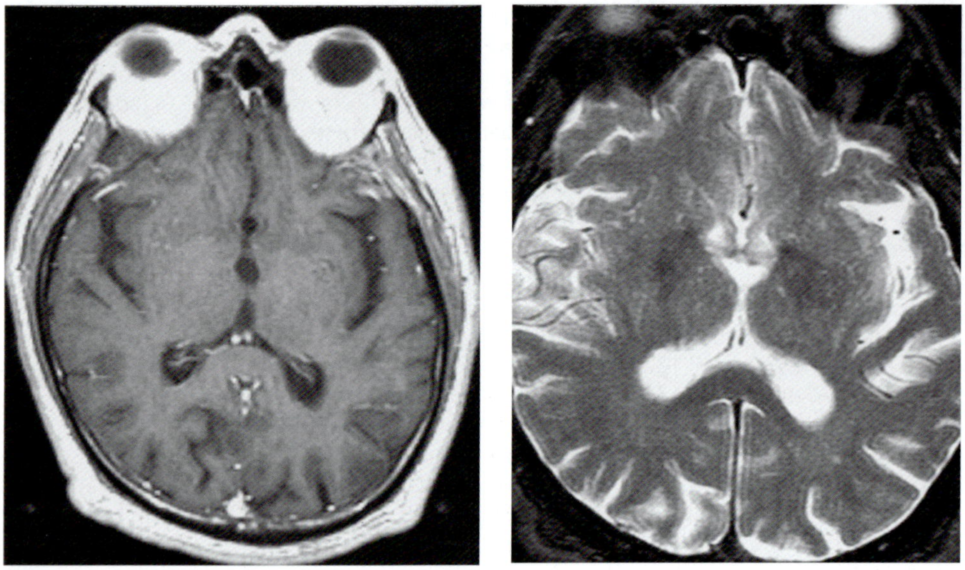

Fig. 15.2 **(A)** T1-weighted gadolinium enhanced axial image demonstrating resolution of enhancement pattern after 1 year. **(B)** T2-weighted image also demonstrates resolution of signal change.

currently not commonly used to treat patients with Parkinson disease. Pallidotomy is typically considered more effective in this regard. The follow-up evidence for Gamma Knife thalamotomy has typically been retrospective, nonblind, and single-centered. Hence, it lacks a multicenter, double-blind study, thus making it difficult to accurately compare radiosurgical thalamotomy to DBS or even RF thalamotomy. Nevertheless, Gamma Knife thalamotomy can successfully reduce tremor in patients with ET, and it remains a valuable tool in a subset of patients who are not candidates for open surgery.

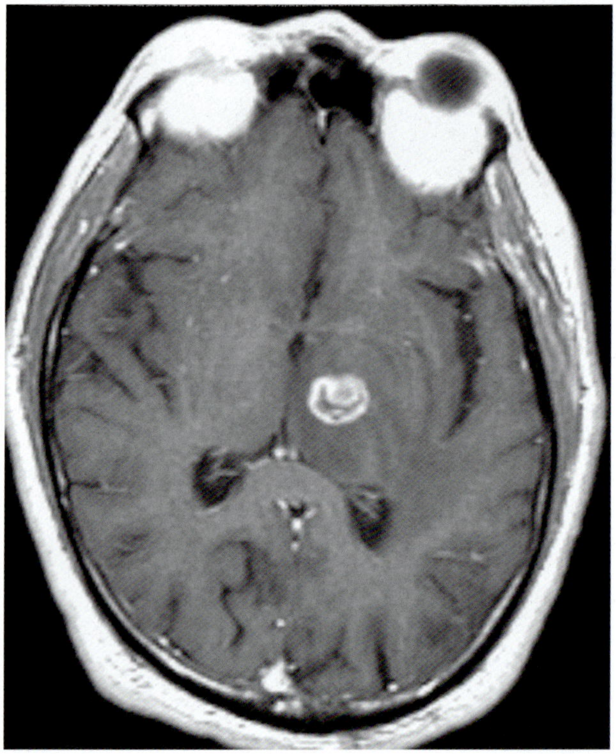

Fig. 15.3 T1-weighted gadolinium axial image demonstrating a lesion in the left ventral intermediate nucleus of the thalamus larger than anticipated and extending into the internal capsule.

In conclusion, lesioning of the thalamus is an alternative treatment for tremor, and Gamma Knife ablation may be effective when properly performed. Gamma Knife thalamotomy remains an option for patients who cannot undergo an open surgical procedure. For example, patients with severe disabling ET and coexisting medical conditions such as a mechanical mitral valve necessitating anticoagulation may be candidates for Gamma Knife radiosurgical thalamotomy. Gamma Knife radiosurgery of the Vim thalamus, however, should be performed only by neurosurgeons who have experience in both DBS and RF thalamic procedures because targeting the thalamus without neurophysiologic mapping can be very challenging.

◆ Surgical Pallidotomy and Pallidal Deep Brain Stimulation

Since the reintroduction by Laitinen and colleagues in 1992, many successful pallidotomies have been performed throughout the world in the treatment of Parkinson disease.[23] The most consistent effect of pallidal ablation appears to be the relief of contralateral levodopa (L-dopa)–induced dyskinesias, whereas the amount of improvement in contralateral bradykinesia, rigidity, and tremor differs among the many studies.[24] In contrast to ablation, stimulation of the globus pallidus internus (GPi) is primarily used to treat dystonia, rather than dyskinesia. GPi DBS for dystonia typically results in gradual improvement over several months. Current data suggest that more mobile, fluid abnormal posturing may respond more quickly, whereas fixed, tonic abnormal posturing may be slower to improve.[25–27] Bilateral GPi DBS has been used for both primary and secondary dystonias.

The pallidotomy is a time-honored surgical procedure that was performed in the 1950s by many surgeons, including Guiot, Spiegel and Wycis, Talairach, Riechert, and Leksell. The reintroduction of Leksell's posteroventral pallidotomy by Laitinen in 1992 (after its disappearance, which coincided with the benefits of L-dopa therapy) initiated a resurgence of interest in the surgical treatment of movement disorders. One of the most consistent benefits of RF pallidotomy is improvement in contralateral drug-induced dyskinesias. Nearly every study has documented improvement in L-dopa dyskinesias, with ranges from 61 to 82%.[28–36] Tremor appears to respond by 33 to 90% at 6 months, although tremor alone is not an indication for pallidotomy. The results for the symptoms of parkinsonian rigidity, bradykinesia, and gait are not as consistent, demonstrating mild benefit at best. Given these results, conventional pallidotomy is recommended only for patients who are severely disabled by asymmetric L-dopa dyskinesias and who are also ineligible for implanted hardware systems. Bilateral pallidotomies are not considered a good option for most patients, given the high rates of cognitive complications after bilateral destructive lesions in the globus pallidus.[37]

◆ Radiosurgical Pallidotomy

Gamma Knife radiosurgical pallidotomy is less invasive than conventional RF pallidotomy. It can theoretically provide excellent relief of L-dopa-induced dyskinesias and tremor with potentially fewer complications than conventional pallidotomies. However, Gamma Knife pallidotomy is even less commonly performed than Gamma Knife thalamotomy. Only case reports and limited case series are available for review. Indeed, the last published case series of patients treated with Gamma Knife pallidotomy is from 1998,[38] which most likely reflects both the established success of subthalamic nucleus DBS in the treatment of Parkinson disease and the higher complication rates of Gamma Knife pallidotomy.

Friedman et al reported four patients in 1995 who were treated with 180 Gy to the right posteroventral pallidum for advanced disease.[39] One patient had improvement in dyskinesias but also experienced a transient psychosis. The three other patients neither improved nor suffered a complication. In a later publication, Friedman et al reported two patients who underwent radiosurgical pallidotomy with lower doses of 120 to 140 Gy.[40] The procedure was performed only in those patients who had undergone a prior contralateral RF pallidotomy with physiologic mapping. A mirror-image lesion was created, assuming symmetry between the two sides. Both of these patients, however, developed significant complications: hemiparesis in one patient and hypophonia and swallowing difficulties in the other. In addition, Friedman et al reported a stroke in another patient undergoing Gamma Knife pallidotomy.[41] This outcome was attributed to vascular hyalinization and thrombosis.

Young et al have reported the largest series of Gamma Knife pallidotomies consisting of 29 patients.[42] Rigidity and bradykinesias improved in approximately two thirds of the patients; however, Unified Parkinson Disease Rating Scale (UPDRS) scores were not consistently evaluated by blinded observers in this study. Only 1 of these 29 patients developed a complication: hemianopsia 9 months after the procedure. Okun et al reported other complications after Gamma Knife pallidotomy performed in one center.[19] The patients had been treated with varying doses of 200, 150, and 100 Gy. Each experienced a visual field loss and either a hemiparesis or dysarthria. Duma theorized that the pallidum may be particularly susceptible to radiation treatment effect complications, given its small vessel blood supply and its high levels of iron.[43]

Compared with Gamma Knife thalamotomy, there is a relative dearth of published Gamma Knife pallidotomy series in the treatment of Parkinson disease. This low number most likely represents a lack of enthusiasm on the part of the treating surgeons and referring neurologists. There are few studies that truly document the benefit of Gamma Knife pallidotomy in a blinded and unbiased fashion, and there are several reports of complications after Gamma Knife pallidotomy. Hence, Gamma Knife pallidotomy cannot be recommended as a viable method of lesioning in the treatment of Parkinson disease without further careful study.

◆ Surgical Subthalamotomy and Subthalamic Deep Brain Stimulation

At the present time, DBS of the subthalamic nucleus is the most widely practiced surgical treatment for patients with idiopathic Parkinson disease. Benabid et al were the first group to demonstrate the efficacy of subthalamic nucleus DBS in the treatment of Parkinson disease in the mid-1990s.[44] One-year follow-up of 24 patients implanted with bilateral subthalamic nucleus DBS demonstrated that UPDRS activities of daily living (ADL) and motor scores improved by 60% in the off-medication state.[45] The UPDRS subscores for akinesia (56%), tremor (80%), rigidity (68%), and gait (55%) also improved, in contrast to the results seen with Vim stimulation.[46]

Subthalamotomy in the form of ischemic strokes or hemorrhages has classically been described as causing hemiballism. However, there are case reports of parkinsonian patients with spontaneous subthalamic nucleus hemorrhage who have experienced motor improvement without the occurrence of hemiballism.[47,48] In addition, there are centers outside the United States that have reported on the benefits of therapeutic subthalamic nucleus ablative surgery using traditional RF lesioning techniques. The Cuban group reported their results in 18 patients following bilateral dorsal subthalamotomy.[49] After a 16-month average follow-up period, there was a 58% improvement in UPDRS motor scores in the "off" period. Three patients developed severe generalized chorea, dysarthria, and balance instability that lasted 6 months from which they spontaneously recovered. Similarly, the Bristol group reported their results on 50 subthalamotomies in 39 patients.[50] Following unilateral subthalamic nucleus lesions, patients demonstrated a 46% improvement in the motor UPDRS score at 24 months. In addition, average L-dopa doses were reduced by 50%. In terms of complications, one patient developed an intracerebral hemorrhage, and one developed postoperative hemiballism on the side contralateral to the subthalamic nucleus lesion, lasting for 3 weeks, with spontaneous resolution. Hence, subthalamotomy via RF lesioning is a procedure in its infancy, with ~50 patients in the reported literature. The results are promising, but safety and efficacy remain to be proven.

◆ Radiosurgical Subthalamotomy

There is only a single case report in the literature of a patient treated with Gamma Knife subthalamotomy for Parkinson disease.[51] The patient had undergone a prior RF pallidotomy, then underwent Gamma Knife radiosurgery with a single 120 Gy 4 mm shot to the subthalamic nucleus. Forty-two months after the procedure, her postoperative UPDRS score had decreased from 28 to 11. She had no side effects. Although this is a promising case report, Gamma Knife subthalamotomy remains in its infancy.

◆ Summary

Although DBS of basal ganglia targets is currently the preferred method in the surgical treatment of patients with movement disorders such as Parkinson disease, ET, and dystonia, Gamma Knife radiosurgical lesioning continues to remain a useful alternative in a small subset of patients. For example, Gamma Knife thalamotomy may be a treatment option for patients with ET who have surgical contraindications, such as a coagulopathy, or anatomical risk factors, such as multiple cavernous malformations. Gamma Knife radiosurgical lesioning for movement disorders should ideally be performed by neurosurgeons who are involved with DBS and who have an intimate understanding of the basal ganglia neuroanatomy. In contrast to Gamma Knife thalamotomy, Gamma Knife pallidotomy and subthalamotomy currently play only a limited role in the treatment of patients with movement disorders.

References

1. Benabid AL, Chirossel JP, Mercier C, et al. Removable, adjustable and reusable implants for stereotactic interstitial radiosurgery of brain tumors. Appl Neurophysiol 1987;50:278–280
2. Tasker RR, Siqueira J, Hawrylyshyn P, Organ LW. What happened to Vim thalamotomy for Parkinson's disease? Appl Neurophysiol 1983; 46(1–4):68–83
3. Miles J, Redfern RM. The place of thalamotomy in the treatment of parkinsonism. Br J Neurosurg 1987;1(3):311–315
4. Schuurman PR, Bosch DA, Bossuyt PM, et al. A comparison of continuous thalamic stimulation and thalamotomy for suppression of severe tremor [comment]. N Engl J Med 2000;342(7):461–468
5. Tasker RR. Deep brain stimulation is preferable to thalamotomy for tremor suppression. Surg Neurol 1998;49(2):145–153, discussion 153–154
6. Matsumoto K, Asano T, Baba T, Miyamoto T, Ohmoto T. Long-term follow-up results of bilateral thalamotomy for parkinsonism. Appl Neurophysiol 1976;39(3–4):257–260
7. Hirai T, Miyazaki M, Nakajima H, Shibazaki T, Ohye C. The correlation between tremor characteristics and the predicted volume of effective lesions in stereotaxic nucleus ventralis intermedius thalamotomy. Brain 1983;106(Pt 4):1001–1018
8. Schuurman P, Bruins J, Merkus M, Bosch D, Speelman J. A comparison of neuropsychological effects of thalamotomy and thalamic stimulation. Neurology 2002;59(8):1232–1239
9. Volkmann J, Herzog J, Kopper F, Deuschl G. Introduction to the programming of deep brain stimulators. Mov Disord 2002;17(Suppl 3): S181–S187
10. Ohye C, Shibazaki T, Sato S. Gamma Knife thalamotomy for movement disorders: evaluation of the thalamic lesion and clinical results. J Neurosurg 2005;102(Suppl):234–240
11. Friehs GM, Noren G, Ohye C, et al. Lesion size following Gamma Knife treatment for functional disorders. Stereotact Funct Neurosurg 1996; 66(Suppl 1):320–328
12. Ohye C. Use of selective thalamotomy for various kinds of movement disorder, based on basic studies. Stereotact Funct Neurosurg 2000; 75(2–3):54–65
13. Duma CM, Jacques D, Kopyov OV. The treatment of movement disorders using Gamma Knife stereotactic radiosurgery. Neurosurg Clin N Am 1999;10(2):379–389
14. Duma CM, Jacques DB, Kopyov OV, Mark RJ, Copcutt B, Farokhi HK. Gamma Knife radiosurgery for thalamotomy in parkinsonian tremor: a five-year experience. J Neurosurg 1998;88(6):1044–1049
15. Young RF, Jacques S, Mark R, et al. Gamma Knife thalamotomy for treatment of tremor: long-term results. J Neurosurg 2000;93(Suppl 3): 128–135
16. Niranjan A, Kondziolka D, Baser S, Heyman R, Lunsford LD. Functional outcomes after Gamma Knife thalamotomy for essential tremor and MS-related tremor. Neurology 2000;55(3):443–446
17. Kondziolka D, Ong JG, Lee JY, Moore RY, Flickinger JC, Lunsford LD. Gamma Knife thalamotomy for essential tremor. J Neurosurg 2008; 108(1):111–117
18. Kondziolka D, Lunsford LD, Claassen D, Maitz AH, Flickinger JC. Radiobiology of radiosurgery, I: The normal rat brain model. Neurosurgery 1992;31(2):271–279
19. Okun MS, Stover NP, Subramanian T, et al. Complications of Gamma Knife surgery for Parkinson disease. Arch Neurol 2001;58(12): 1995–2002
20. Siderowf A, Gollump SM, Stern MB, Baltuch GH, Riina HA. Emergence of complex, involuntary movements after Gamma Knife radiosurgery for essential tremor. Mov Disord 2001;16(5):965–967
21. Andersson B, Larsson B, Leksell L, et al. Histopathology of late local radiolesions in the goat brain. Acta Radiol Ther Phys Biol 1970;9(5):385–394
22. Larsson B, Leksell L, Rexed B, Sourander P, Mair W, Andersson B. The high-energy proton beam as a neurosurgical tool. Nature 1958;182(4644): 1222–1223
23. Laitinen LV, Bergenheim AT, Hariz MI. Leksell's posteroventral pallidotomy in the treatment of Parkinson's disease. J Neurosurg 1992; 76(1):53–61
24. Lang AE, Duff J, Saint-Cyr JA, et al. Posteroventral medial pallidotomy in Parkinson's disease. J Neurol 1999;246(Suppl 2):1128–1141
25. Coubes P, Cif L, El Fertit H, et al. Electrical stimulation of the globus pallidus internus in patients with primary generalized dystonia: long-term results. J Neurosurg 2004;101(2):189–194
26. Coubes P, Roubertie A, Vayssiere N, Hemm S, Echenne B. Treatment of DYT1-generalised dystonia by stimulation of the internal globus pallidus. Lancet 2000;355(9222):2220–2221
27. Kumar R, Dagher A, Hutchison WD, Lang AE, Lozano AM. Globus pallidus deep brain stimulation for generalized dystonia: clinical and PET investigation. Neurology 1999;53(4):871–874
28. Johansson F, Malm J, Nordh E, Hariz M. Usefulness of pallidotomy in advanced Parkinson's disease. J Neurol Neurosurg Psychiatry 1997; 62(2):125–132
29. Kishore A, Turnbull IM, Snow BJ, et al. Efficacy, stability and predictors of outcome of pallidotomy for Parkinson's disease: six-month follow-up with additional 1-year observations. Brain 1997;120(Pt 5): 729–737
30. Kondziolka D, Bonaroti E, Baser S, Brandt F, Kim YS, Lunsford LD. Outcomes after stereotactically guided pallidotomy for advanced Parkinson's disease. J Neurosurg 1999;90(2):197–202

31. Masterman D, DeSalles A, Baloh RW, et al. Motor, cognitive, and behavioral performance following unilateral ventroposterior pallidotomy for Parkinson disease. Arch Neurol 1998;55(9):1201–1208
32. Lang AE, Lozano A, Tasker R, Duff J, Saint-Cyr J, Trepanier L. Neuropsychological and behavioral changes and weight gain after medial pallidotomy. Ann Neurol 1997;41(6):834–836
33. Vitek JL, Bakay RA. The role of pallidotomy in Parkinson's disease and dystonia. Curr Opin Neurol 1997;10(4):332–339
34. Iacono RP, Lonser RR, Mandybur G, Yamada S. Stimulation of the globus pallidus in Parkinson's disease. Br J Neurosurg 1995;9(4): 505–510
35. Baron MS, Vitek JL, Bakay RA, et al. Treatment of advanced Parkinson's disease by posterior GPi pallidotomy: 1-year results of a pilot study. Ann Neurol 1996;40(3):355–366
36. Baron MS, Vitek JL, Bakay RA, et al. Treatment of advanced Parkinson's disease by unilateral posterior GPi pallidotomy: 4-year results of a pilot study. Mov Disord 2000;15(2):230–237
37. Ghika J, Villemure JG, Fankhauser H, Favre J, Assal G, Ghika-Schmid F. Efficiency and safety of bilateral contemporaneous pallidal stimulation (deep brain stimulation) in levodopa-responsive patients with Parkinson's disease with severe motor fluctuations: a 2-year follow-up review. J Neurosurg 1998;89(5):713–718
38. Young RF, Shumway-Cook A, Vermeulen SS, et al. Gamma Knife radiosurgery as a lesioning technique in movement disorder surgery. J Neurosurg 1998;89(2):183–193
39. Friedman JH, Epstein M, Sanes JN, et al. Gamma Knife pallidotomy in advanced Parkinson's disease. Ann Neurol 1996;39(4):535–538
40. Friedman DP, Goldman HW, Flanders AE, Gollomp SM, Curran WJ Jr. Stereotactic radiosurgical pallidotomy and thalamotomy with the Gamma Knife: MR imaging findings with clinical correlation–preliminary experience. Radiology 1999;212(1):143–150
41. Friedman JH, Fernandez HH, Sikirica M, Stopa E, Friehs G. Stroke induced by Gamma Knife pallidotomy: autopsy result. Neurology 2002;58(11):1695–1697
42. Young RF, Shumway-Cook A, Vermeulen SS, et al. Gamma Knife radiosurgery as a lesioning technique in movement disorder surgery. J Neurosurg 1998;89(2):183–193
43. Duma CM. Movement disorder radiosurgery—planning, physics and complication avoidance. Prog Neurol Surg 2007;20:249–266
44. Benabid AL, Pollak P, Gross C, et al. Acute and long-term effects of subthalamic nucleus stimulation in Parkinson's disease. Stereotact Funct Neurosurg 1994;62(1–4):76–84
45. Limousin P, Krack P, Pollak P, et al. Electrical stimulation of the subthalamic nucleus in advanced Parkinson's disease. N Engl J Med 1998; 339(16):1105–1111
46. Benabid AL, Pollak P, Gao D, et al. Chronic electrical stimulation of the ventralis intermedius nucleus of the thalamus as a treatment of movement disorders [see comment]. J Neurosurg 1996;84(2):203–214
47. Sellal F, Hirsch E, Lisovoski F, Mutschler V, Collard M, Marescaux C. Contralateral disappearance of parkinsonian signs after subthalamic hematoma. Neurology 1992;42(1):255–256
48. Vidakovic A, Dragasevic N, Kostic VS. Hemiballism: report of 25 cases. J Neurol Neurosurg Psychiatry 1994;57(8):945–949
49. Alvarez L, Macias R, Lopez G, et al. Bilateral subthalamotomy in Parkinson's disease: initial and long-term response. Brain 2005;128 (Pt 3):570–583
50. Gill SS, Heywood P. Bilateral dorsolateral subthalamotomy for advanced Parkinson's disease. Lancet 1997;350(9086):1224
51. Keep MF, Mastrofrancesco L, Erdman D, Murphy B, Ashby LS. Gamma Knife subthalamotomy for Parkinson disease: the subthalamic nucleus as a new radiosurgical target. Case report. J Neurosurg 2002 97(5, Suppl): 592–599

16

Stereotactic Radiosurgery for Epilepsy

Mark Quigg and Nicholas M. Barbaro

In association with epilepsy, radiosurgery is most often used in the treatment of symptomatic lesions, such as tumors or vascular malformations; epilepsy in these cases is often one of several presenting symptoms and often improves as a benefit of the treatment of the lesion. Recently, the use of radiosurgery has expanded to the treatment of physiologic lesions, such as those seen in mesial temporal lobe epilepsy, and previously inoperable epileptic lesions, such as hypothalamic hamartomas. This review will outline the radiosurgical treatment of epilepsy with special attention to mesial temporal lobe epilepsy.

◆ Experimental Models for and Effects of Radiation on Epilepsy

Investigations on the effects of focal irradiation on epileptic lesions in experimental animal models of partial epilepsy carry some common findings that are important when evaluating trials of radiosurgery in human epilepsy. First, experimental models of focal epilepsy demonstrate that destruction of neuronal tissue through radionecrosis is not required. Instead, application of sufficient radiation to the epileptogenic penumbra surrounding a lesion appears to be the critical variable. Second, seizure response, either in successful remission or in a paradoxical worsening, varies with target, dose, and postoperative duration. Third, the treatment target, dose, and volume remain empirically determined, and scaling up from experimental models to humans is not straightforward.

It is not known how radiation produces an antiepileptic effect. Sensitivity to ionizing radiation is largely dependent on mitotic rate; therefore, neurons are relatively radioresistant. In kindled mice, although total brain radiation terminates seizure-induced mitotic activity in hippocampal dentate gyri, treated mice have no changes in seizure threshold or clinical seizure phenotype. Therefore, radiation-induced changes in mitotic activity may not underlie the antiepileptic effect.[1] Tissue necrosis is not necessary.[2–5] Histology of radiosurgery-treated rat hippocampi shows changes of experimental hippocampal sclerosis rather than changes typical of acute or chronic severe radiation injury.[2–5] Similarly, after radiosurgery of human hippocampi, histopathology of resected tissue following "rescue" temporal lobectomy reveals hippocampal cell loss and fibrillary astrocytosis consistent with epilepsy-related sclerosis. No radiation-induced histopathologic changes are seen.[6]

Although neurons are resistant to radionecrosis, mitotically active structures—vasculature and glia—are not. One hypothesis, therefore, is that neuronal damage results from ischemia caused by radiation vasculitis. Accordingly, the major pathologic findings following focal radiation consist of endothelial damage.[7] Other hypotheses suggest that radiated neuronal circuits undergo neuromodulation that renders an anticonvulsant (or, sometimes, a paradoxically proconvulsant) effect. Differential susceptibility to irradiation or ischemia among different neuronal populations within epileptogenic circuits may account for this phenomenon.[8]

Given these possible mechanisms, studies with the use of models of partial epilepsy address some of the questions regarding target, administration, time course, and clinical sequelae. These models include electrically kindled rats[2,9] studied through seizure surrogates of afterdischarge threshold or severity as well as rat models that experience spontaneous seizures.[3–5] The earliest of these series established that there might be a pro- or anticonvulsant effect of radiosurgery that varies with postoperative duration or dose. Kindled rats with doses $\leq$ 25 Gy to the amygdala experience clinically more intense seizures.[9] Kindled rats treated with 40 Gy to the hippocampus initially experience a transient decrease in seizure threshold that later increases.[2]

Other experiments established relationships between dose and latency with experimental limbic seizures. In animals monitored for 6 weeks, doses of 80 and 100 Gy cause seizure reductions within 2 to 4 weeks postoperatively, whereas lesser doses cause reductions of slower onset. Increasing doses of radiosurgery correlate with higher percentages of rats that became seizure free.[5] Other studies indicate that there is a threshold effect, with single treatments of 30 Gy being equally effective as 60 Gy.[4] Therefore, "overdosing" beyond a tissue-damaging level carries little advantage. Long-term electroencephalogram (EEG) monitoring for periods of up to 10 months in epileptic rats establishes that the anticonvulsant effects of radiosurgery are durable.[3]

In summary, preclinical literature suggests that single-fraction focal radiosurgery has a dose-dependent effect on epileptic lesions. These experiments help define a therapeutic window of treatment dose bounded by ineffectiveness, paradoxical exacerbation, or delayed remission at the lower doses and by tissue necrosis at higher doses. Evaluation of human studies, therefore, requires particular attention to treatment dose, volume, and target.

◆ Treatment of Lesional Epilepsy

Epileptogenic Tumors

Given the variety of types, pathology, and locations of central nervous system (CNS) tumors, the studies on the effects of radiosurgery on tumor-associated epilepsy are few. Schrottner et al, however, concentrated on the dose absorbed by tissue in tumor penumbra, dividing patients in two groups according to the volume of tissue outside the tumor that had received 10 Gy or more.[10] Outcome was retrospectively ranked at mean duration of ~2 years as "excellent" (Engel class I and II) or not. High-volume patients achieved a 66% improvement rate compared with 42% for the low-volume group. Because all patients achieved tumor control with radiosurgery (thus removing tumor response as a confounder), the differing rates of seizure improvement suggest that higher radiosurgery volumes delivered to tumor penumbra are important in modifying tumor-associated epilepsy.

Arteriovenous Malformations

The potential efficacy of radiosurgery in the treatment of symptomatic localization-related epilepsies is most evident in the treatment of arteriovenous malformations (AVMs), with an across-study mean seizure-remission rate of 70%.[11–15] Representative is the large series accumulated by Steiner et al, who reported that seizures remit after radiosurgery in 69% of patients with AVMs and epilepsy.[12] A later study[15] described dose–volume effects on epileptogenic AVMs opposite that reported for epileptogenic tumors, in that seizure remission is better with smaller AVMs.[15] The amount of radiation to the margin had no clear effect. Neither study found a relationship between obliteration of the AVM and seizure remission.[12,15]

Cavernous Malformations

Rebleeding[16] and epilepsy,[17] with independent incidences of ~2.5% per patient per year for either, form the bulk of morbidity associated with cavernous malformations (CMs). The across-study proportion of seizure remission reported in retrospective case series is 50%,[18–22] but the radiation dose may account for the broad range of remission, with greater doses associated with increased remission. For example, representing the two extremes in efficacy, Kim et al[19] used a mean marginal dose of 15 Gy and a center dose of 26 Gy for a remission rate of 70%, whereas Shih and Pan[22] reported mean doses of 13 Gy marginal and 21 Gy central for a remission rate of 25%. The volume or marginal dose applied to the brain surrounding CMs, thought important in epileptogenic tumors[10] and possibly AVMs,[12] has not been systematically studied in terms of seizure control. Retrospective studies of open resection suggest that removal of the hemosiderin-stained tissue surrounding CMs is associated with better outcomes;[23] therefore, variable outcomes following radiosurgery may also stem from targeting of epileptogenic tissue surrounding CMs.

Unfortunately, excess morbidity in terms of radiotoxicity with higher doses and postoperative hemorrhage with lower doses remains a concern. For example, the early Swedish experience determined that radiosurgery did not appreciably alter the natural course of CMs while exposing patients to radiation-induced complications that exceeded by 7 times those expected for the same dose for AVMs.[24] A case of a patient treated with radiosurgery for a bilateral CM and intractable epilepsy reported delayed (>2 years postoperative) radionecrosis and intractable edema, requiring craniotomy and hyperbaric oxygen treatments.[25] A more recent retrospective comparison concluded that open resection resulted in better seizure control and rebleeding avoidance than radiosurgery.[22] This study, as well as comparisons to the ~70 to 80% seizure remission rate seen after open surgery for CMs,[26,27] suggests that any benefits of noninvasive radiosurgery over open surgery for CMs must be weighed against risks of less efficacy and possibly increased toxicities. From the viewpoint of an epileptologist, the thorough presurgical localization of the epileptic network in the region of CMs should guide resection, whether performed with open surgery or radiosurgery.

Hypothalamic Hamartomas

Hypothalamic hamartomas are an important cause of an epileptic encephalopathy marked by medically intractable gelastic and other seizures usually accompanied by behavioral and cognitive decline. Although hypothalamic hamartomas are difficult to excise with the use of standard surgical techniques, radiosurgery has the advantage of noninvasive access. Series of radiosurgery treatment of hypothalamic hamartomas[28–33] demonstrate a seizure remission rate of 27% across studies. Although this rate appears low, seizure remission alone underestimates the benefits on morbidity and custodial care required in these cases of severe epilepsy. Behavioral outcomes have not been rigorously quantified, but most reports cited above note that the majority of patients undergoes anecdotal improvements in behavior, sleep quality, and learning.

A European multicenter, prospective trial of radiosurgery for hypothalamic hamartomas has enrolled 60 patients, 27 of whom exceeded 3 years follow-up.[32] This study emphasizes the evolution of seizure changes during the postoperative period. Within the first 2 months a slight improvement in seizure rate typically occurs. Seizures transiently worsen in frequency before reduction and remission occur. Behavioral improvements, along with EEG normalization, tend to occur in a more linear fashion. Morbidity is low, with no ill effects except for one instance of poikilothermia noted among the above reports. Some data emphasize the importance of the marginal dose of radiation[32] as noted in tumors and AVMs. Patients treated with doses >17 Gy to the margin of hypothalamic hamartomas have greater rates of seizure remission than those receiving <13 Gy.[28] Radiosurgery may be one of several nontraditional surgical approaches that can improve what is otherwise a devastating epileptic encephalopathy.

Treatment of Physiologic Epilepsies

Mesial Temporal Lobe Epilepsy

Mesial temporal lobe epilepsy (MTLE) consists of atrophy, gliosis, and selective neuronal loss within the hippocampus and associated limbic system. It is the most frequent cause of medically intractable epilepsy in adults. Radiosurgery may have several potential benefits that drive its consideration despite the well-established efficacy of open surgery for MTLE.[34] First, open surgery has a small but real risk of surgical complications, such as bleeding, infection, and postoperative pain. Second, open surgery is expensive. The average cost per patient for open microsurgery is nearly 50% more than that for radiosurgery for treatment of similar disorders;[35] admittedly, no cost comparisons have confined their scope to epilepsy surgery. Third, some of the adverse events of open surgery involve changes in neuropsychological testing. Fourth, some patients, as well as physicians, hold persistent biases against open surgery despite proven efficacy; noninvasive techniques may facilitate appropriate consideration of epilepsy surgery.

The first surgical series employing radiosurgery in a systematic fashion in the treatment of physiologic focal epilepsy was reported by Talairach et al,[36] who treated 44 patients between 1959 and 1973 with the use of yitrium,[90] yielding a 75% rate of seizure remission over mean follow-up duration of 5.7 years. Unfortunately, initial attempts in Sweden with Gamma Knife (Elekta Instruments AB, Stockholm, Sweden) surgery[37] and elsewhere with the use of fractionated radiotherapy and other techniques[38] were not encouraging. Many of these patients, however, were treated before uniform definitions of MTLE existed.

Régis and colleagues revived interest in radiosurgery of MTLE in 1995, when their pilot studies with the use of the Gamma Knife for clearly defined MTLE showed high rates of seizure remission.[39] Since their initial publication, seven studies treating a total of 49 patients reported a wide range of efficacies of seizure remission[6,40–45] with an across-study average of 45%. The largest study to date is by Regis et al, who treated 21 patients with 24 Gy, yielding a 62% rate of seizure remission at 2-years' follow-up.[44] A recent report on longer term follow-up (≥ 5 years; mean follow-up ~8 years) of 15 patients from this same practice (although not necessarily from the same cohort) shows that seizure remission remains durable, with 60% of patients experiencing either seizure remission or nondisabling auras.[46] Because long-term follow-up was not conducted with intent-to-treat criteria, the results may be susceptible to sampling bias.

The variability in results of radiosurgery therapy for MTLE underscores the difficulties in the determination of basic parameters of anatomical target, dose, and target volume. The anatomical targets in radiosurgery of MTLE are the least variable factor, with all studies[6,40–44] specifying that the 50% isodose volume contains regions thought most important in the generation of mesial seizures: the amygdala, the head and anterior body of the hippocampus, and the parahippocampal gyrus. Dose and target volume are more variable. Comparison of the above studies suggests that low-dose protocols (≤ 20 Gy)[6,41,42] are less successful than higher dose protocols (24 Gy).[40,44,45]

Regis et al outlined the typical postoperative course, and in many respects it follows the polyphasic course described after radiosurgery of hypothalamic hamartomas.[32] Most clinical or neuroimaging changes occur between 9 and 12 months.[39,40,44,47] Nearly all patients experience exacerbations in auras before seizures decrease or remit.[44] The most dramatic drop in seizure rate occurs between 12 and 18 months, coinciding with the development and resolution of maximal magnetic resonance imaging (MRI) changes.

Other morbidities reported by Régis et al[44] in their prospective study are visual field deficits in 52% of patients, mostly quadrantanopia, as would be seen after standard temporal lobectomy. One subject had a hemianopia (indicating direct involvement of the optic tract), and another had mixed deficits. Other morbidities were headache, nausea, vomiting, and depression. Headache requires special comment, as it coincides in some subjects with postoperative edema. Steroids, in response to headache, visual field changes, or MRI changes, were used in 62% of patients, but no evidence guides their initiation or effectiveness.

One potential problem of radiosurgery compared with open surgery is that the latency between radiosurgery and remission may expose patients to continued seizures. Two deaths occurred during the latency period in a case series of five patients treated with "low-dose" radiation.[42] Allowing enough time for maturation of the radiosurgical lesion may have allowed some patients treated with lower doses to demonstrate remission, given that animal models treated with lower doses demonstrated improvements at a slower rate than those treated with higher doses.[4,5] Future trials of radiosurgery may need to consider anticonvulsant prophylaxis during the latency period.

Beyond seizure efficacy, studies have begun to evaluate secondary outcome measures such as cognition. In fact, radiosurgery of MTLE may serve as an interesting model of the effects of focal radiation on cognition, especially because controversies over the cognitive sequelae of focal or fractionated radiation therapy are often engendered by

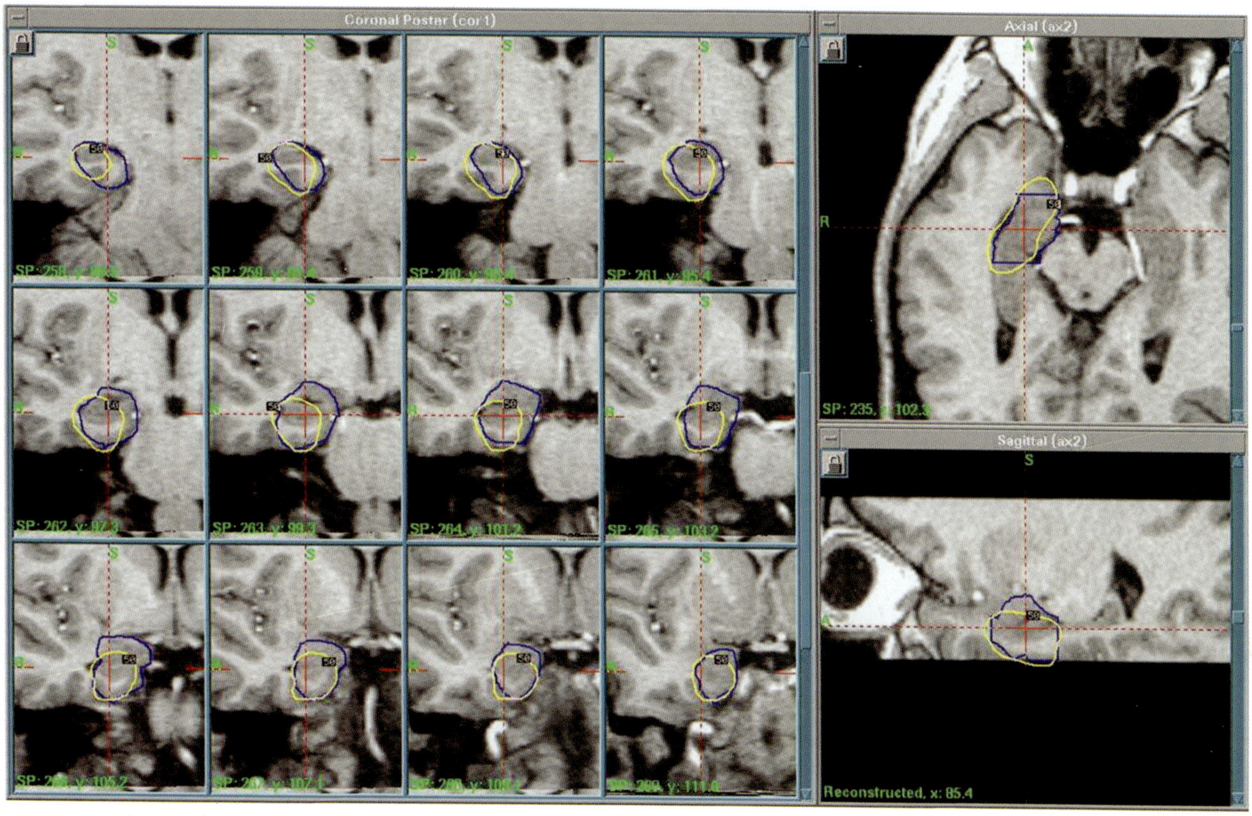

Fig. 16.1 A typical Gamma Knife dose plan for a patient with right-sided temporal lobe epilepsy. The blue line represents the mesial temporal lobe, and the yellow line represents the 50% isodose planned treatment volume.

the confounding effects of tumors or other CNS lesions.[48] Epileptic rats demonstrate no behavioral effects attributable to radiosurgery.[4] In humans, the European prospective trial reports no mean neurocognitive changes through a 2-year follow-up period.[44] Similarly, Srikivilaikul et al reported no group mean changes at 6-months' follow-up, although some individuals showed decline in at least one cognitive domain.[42] McDonald et al reported on 27-month follow-up in three participants who underwent dominant hemisphere low-dose radiosurgery treatment.[43] No long-term consistent changes in neurocognitive parameters were found, although each patient showed a decline in a measure of verbal memory. The authors concluded that neurocognitive changes following radiosurgery appeared similar to those of temporal lobectomy.

Results of a multicenter pilot study sponsored by the National Institutes of Health on the safety of radiosurgery for MTLE have recently become available.[49] In this study, patients who would normally qualify for anterior temporal lobectomy for unilateral MTLE were randomized to either a 20 or 24 Gy dose (**Fig. 16.1**). A total of 30 subjects were enrolled and followed for 3 years. Seizure remission for the purpose of this trial was defined as the absence of complex partial seizures with or without auras (comparable to an Engel's outcome designation of class IB or better[50]) between 24 and 36 months of the 3-year trial.

The first important finding is that in an intent-to-treat, prospective, multicenter trial, the overall rate of patients who experienced seizure remission was 67%, comparable to the European prospective trial[44] and to prospective trials of standard anterior temporal lobectomy (**Fig. 16.2**).[34] Second, higher dose appeared more efficacious than lower dose, although a statistically definitive distinction between the two groups was not possible because of the small numbers of patients within each group. Nevertheless, comparisons

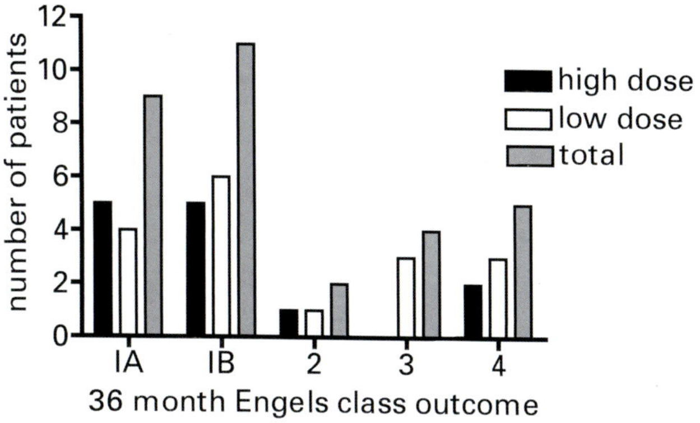

Fig. 16.2 Distribution of seizure outcome as defined by Engel's criteria between months 24 and 36 of the multicenter pilot study sponsored by the National Institutes of Health of radiosurgery for unilateral mesial temporal lobe epilepsy[49] divided by dose. The overall rate of seizure remission (Engel's class IB or better) at 36 months was 76.9% for the high-dose group and 58.8% for the low-dose group (p = .12 by Fisher's exact test).

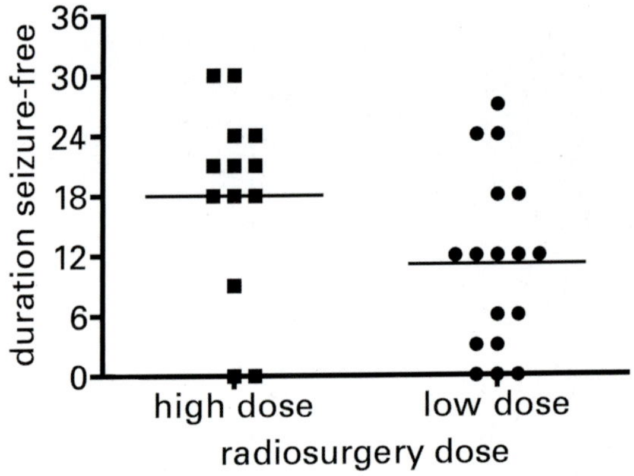

Fig. 16.3 Distribution of continuous duration of seizure remission (defined as Engel's class IB or better) from the final outcome point of 36 months postoperatively in the multicenter pilot study sponsored by the National Institutes of Health.[49] Patients who dropped out early because of "escape" temporal lobectomy or because of loss of follow-up are counted as a duration of zero month. Bar = average, *p* value =.05 from two sample *t*-tests.

between the two dose groups suggest that patients treated with the higher dose experience greater rates of seizure remission, longer durations of and shorter latencies to seizure remission (**Fig. 16.3**), and fewer auras (**Fig. 16.4**) during the development of the radiosurgical lesion. Although higher doses were associated with trends in higher occurrences of new-onset headaches, no particular morbidities occurred disproportionately in higher- versus lower-dose patient groups. Third, neurocognitive outcomes, especially of patients who underwent radiosurgery of the language-dominant hemisphere, were benign. For example, verbal memory impairment was seen in 25% of dominant-surgery patients and in 7% of nondominant patients. Conversely, significant improvement was seen in 16% of dominant and 7% of nondominant patients. In comparison, rates of significant impairment following dominant hemisphere anterior temporal lobectomy range from 10 to 60%.[51–55]

In summary, radiosurgery for MTLE appears to have promise, but optimum dose, patient selection, and relative benefits compared with open surgery have yet to be clearly demarcated.

Other Nonlesional Epilepsies

There are no reports on the use of radiosurgery for non–mass lesion neocortical foci. Because localization of seizure foci in nonlesional neocortical epilepsies usually requires invasive techniques, the noninvasive nature of radiosurgery loses some advantage. One may speculate that if noninvasive localization and brain mapping were rigorous enough to supplant invasive methods, then radiosurgery may have a future role.

Resection of the corpus callosum decreases the severity and number of primary generalized or rapidly propagating secondarily generalized seizures in patients who are not otherwise good surgical candidates. Small case series report that improvement in seizures following radiosurgery resection of the corpus callosum was comparable to that reported after open callosotomy with lack of notable complications.[56,57] The future role of radiosurgery in corpus callosotomy may be more difficult to determine because more epileptologists are currently opting for vagal nerve stimulation in patients who might otherwise qualify for corpus callosotomy.

◆ Summary

Radiosurgery offers an alternative to open surgery in selected patients with epilepsy caused by mass lesions such as tumors and AVMs, with the choice of technique guided by the location and type of the lesion rather than any epilepsy-specific properties of the lesion. Radiosurgery for the seizures arising from CMs appears to have a less than enthusiastic endorsement, given some studies' findings of excessive rebleeding and less efficacy against seizures than open surgery. Radiosurgery for hypothalamic hamartomas, in contrast, appears promising, given the combination of inaccessibility to traditional surgery, severe morbidity of gelastic epilepsy, and good safety profile. Finally, recent trials suggest that certain protocols of radiosurgery for MTLE may offer a noninvasive alternative to open surgery while yielding similar rates of seizure remission. Other possible situations merit consideration of

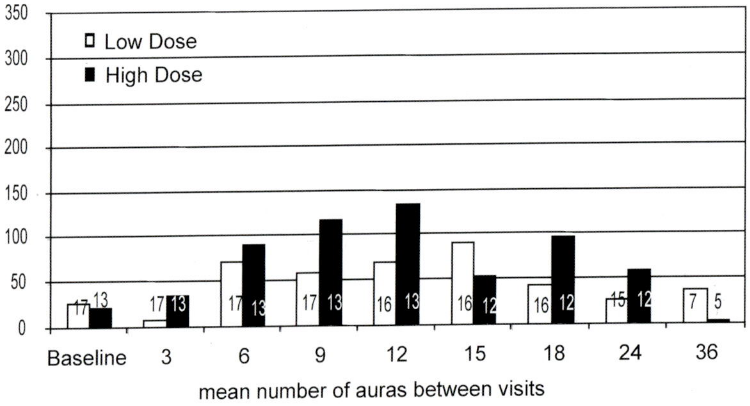

Fig. 16.4 Mean ± standard error of the number of auras per seizure diary interval in patients in the multicenter pilot study sponsored by the National Institutes of Health.[49] As seen in earlier studies, the onset of auras frequently preceded frank magnetic resonance imaging changes and coincided with the diminishment of complex partial seizures.

radiosurgery; one authority proposes that radiosurgery may be useful in cases of (1) epilepsy of temporal lobe origin in those who have medical contraindications to open surgery, (2) temporal lobe epilepsy after failed open resection, and (3) extratemporal epilepsy that can be noninvasively localized, especially following a failed open surgery.[58] Further work is needed to clarify risks and benefits of radiosurgery for these less common but important clinical situations.

References

1. Ferland RJ, Williams JP, Gross RA, Applegate CD. The effects of brain-irradiation-induced decreases in hippocampal mitotic activity on flurothyl-induced epileptogenesis in adult C57BL/6J mice. Exp Neurol 2003;179(1):71–82
2. Sun B, DeSalles AA, Medin PM, et al. Reduction of hippocampal-kindled seizure activity in rats by stereotactic radiosurgery. Exp Neurol 1998;154(2):691–695
3. Chen ZF, Kamiryo T, Henson SL, et al. Anticonvulsant effects of gamma surgery in a model of chronic spontaneous limbic epilepsy in rats. J Neurosurg 2001;94(2):270–280
4. Maesawa S, Kondziolka D, Dixon CE, Balzer J, Fellows W, Lunsford LD. Subnecrotic stereotactic radiosurgery controlling epilepsy produced by kainic acid injection in rats. J Neurosurg 2000;93(6):1033–1040
5. Mori Y, Kondziolka D, Balzer J, et al. Effects of stereotactic radiosurgery on an animal model of hippocampal epilepsy. Neurosurgery 2000; 46(1):157–165
6. Cmelak AJ, Abou-Khalil B, Konrad PE, Duggan D, Maciunas RJ. Low-dose stereotactic radiosurgery is inadequate for medically intractable mesial temporal lobe epilepsy: a case report. Seizure 2001;10(6):442–446
7. Kondziolka D, Lunsford LD, Claassen D, Maitz AH, Flickinger JC. Radiobiology of radiosurgery, I: The normal rat brain model. Neurosurgery 1992;31(2):271–279
8. Tsuchitani S, Drummond J, Kamiryo T, et al. Selective vulnerability of interneurons to low dosage radiosurgery. Paper presented at: Society for Neuroscience Annual Meeting; Nov 8–12, 2003; New Orleans
9. Jenrow KA, Ratkewicz AE, Elisevich KV. Enhanced excitability induced by ionizing radiation in the kindled rat. Exp Neurol 2001;169(1):96–104
10. Schrottner O, Eder HG, Unger F, Feichtinger K, Pendl G. Radiosurgery in lesional epilepsy: brain tumors. Stereotact Funct Neurosurg 1998;70(Suppl 1):50–56
11. Heikkinen ER, Konnov B, Melnikov L, et al. Relief of epilepsy by radiosurgery of cerebral arteriovenous malformations. Stereotact Funct Neurosurg 1989;53(3):157–166
12. Steiner L, Lindquist C, Adler JR, Torner JC, Alves W, Steiner M. Clinical outcome of radiosurgery for cerebral arteriovenous malformations. J Neurosurg 1992;77(1):1–8
13. Gerszten PC, Adelson PD, Kondziolka D, Flickinger JC, Lunsford LD. Seizure outcome in children treated for arteriovenous malformations using Gamma Knife radiosurgery. Pediatr Neurosurg 1996;24(3):139–144
14. Kurita H, Kawamoto S, Suzuki I, et al. Control of epilepsy associated with cerebral arteriovenous malformations after radiosurgery. J Neurol Neurosurg Psychiatry 1998;65(5):648–655
15. Schauble B, Cascino GD, Pollock BE, et al. Seizure outcomes after stereotactic radiosurgery for cerebral arteriovenous malformations. Neurology 2004;63(4):683–687
16. Kim DS, Park YG, Choi JU, Chung SS, Lee KC. An analysis of the natural history of cavernous malformations. Surg Neurol 1997;48(1):9–17, discussion 17–18
17. Del Curling O, Kelly DL, Elster AD, Craven TE. An analysis of the natural history of cavernous angiomas. J Neurosurg 1991;75:702–708
18. Bartolomei F, Régis J, Kida Y, et al. Gamma Knife radiosurgery for epilepsy associated with cavernous hemangiomas: a retrospective study of 49 cases. Stereotact Funct Neurosurg 1999;72(Suppl 1):22–28
19. Kim MS, Pyo SY, Jeong YG, Lee SI, Jung YT, Sim JH. Gamma Knife surgery for intracranial cavernous hemangioma. J Neurosurg 2005; 102(Suppl):102–106
20. Liscak R, Vladyka V, Simonova G, Vymazal J, Novotny J Jr. Gamma Knife surgery of brain cavernous hemangiomas. J Neurosurg 2005; 102(Suppl):207–213
21. Liu KD, Chung WY, Wu HM, et al. Gamma Knife surgery for cavernous hemangiomas: an analysis of 125 patients. J Neurosurg 2005; 102(Suppl):81–86
22. Shih YH, Pan DH. Management of supratentorial cavernous malformations: craniotomy versus Gamma Knife radiosurgery. Clin Neurol Neurosurg 2005;107(2):108–112
23. Baumann CR, Schuknecht B, Lo Russo G, et al. Seizure outcome after resection of cavernous malformations is better when surrounding hemosiderin-stained brain also is removed. Epilepsia 2006;47(3): 563–566
24. Karlsson B, Kihlstrom L, Lindquist C, Ericson K, Steiner L. Radiosurgery for cavernous malformations. J Neurosurg 1998;88(2):293–297
25. Takenaka N, Imanishi T, Sasaki H, et al. Delayed radiation necrosis with extensive brain edema after Gamma Knife radiosurgery for multiple cerebral cavernous malformations—case report. Neurol Med Chir (Tokyo) 2003;43(8):391–395
26. Cappabianca P, Alfieri A, Maiuri F, Mariniello G, Cirillo S, de Divitiis E. Supratentorial cavernous malformations and epilepsy: seizure outcome after lesionectomy on a series of 35 patients. Clin Neurol Neurosurg 1997;99:179–183
27. Cohen DS, Zubay GP, Goodman RR. Seizure outcome after lesionectomy for cavernous malformations. J Neurosurg 1995;83:237–242
28. Régis J, Bartolomei F, de Toffol B, et al. Gamma Knife surgery for epilepsy related to hypothalamic hamartomas. Neurosurgery 2000;47(6):1343–1351
29. Unger F, Schrottner O, Feichtinger M, Bone G, Haselsberger K, Sutter B. Stereotactic radiosurgery for hypothalamic hamartomas. Acta Neurochir Suppl (Wien) 2002;84:57–63
30. Selch MT, Gorgulho A, Mattozo C, Solberg TD, Cabatan-Awang C, DeSalles AA. Linear accelerator stereotactic radiosurgery for the treatment of gelastic seizures due to hypothalamic hamartoma. Minim Invasive Neurosurg 2005;48(5):310–314
31. Barajas MA, Ramirez-Guzman MG, Rodriguez-Vazquez C, Toledo-Buenrostro V, Cuevas-Solorzano A, Rodriguez-Hernandez G. Gamma Knife surgery for hypothalamic hamartomas accompanied by medically intractable epilepsy and precocious puberty: experience in Mexico. J Neurosurg 2005;102(Suppl):53–55
32. Regis J, Scavarda D, Tamura M, et al. Epilepsy related to hypothalamic hamartomas: surgical management with special reference to Gamma Knife surgery. Childs Nerv Syst 2006;22(8):881–895
33. Mathieu D, Kondziolka D, Niranjan A, Flickinger J, Lunsford LD. Gamma Knife radiosurgery for refractory epilepsy caused by hypothalamic hamartomas. Stereotact Funct Neurosurg 2006;84(2–3): 82–87
34. Wiebe S, Blume WT, Girvin JP, Eliasziw M. A randomized, controlled trial of surgery for temporal-lobe epilepsy. N Engl J Med 2001;345:311–318
35. Wellis G, Nagel R, Vollmar C, Steiger HJ. Direct costs of microsurgical management of radiosurgically amenable intracranial pathology in Germany: an analysis of meningiomas, acoustic neuromas, metastases and arteriovenous malformations of less than 3 cm in diameter. Acta Neurochir (Wien) 2003;145(4):249–255
36. Talairach J, Bancaud J, Szikla G, et al. New approaches in epilepsy surgery: stereotactic methods and results. Paper presented at: Neurochirurgie: Congrés Annuel de la Société de Langue Franéaise; 1974; Marseille, France
37. Lindquist C, Kilstrom L, Hellestrand E. Functional neurosurgery—future for the Gamma Knife? Stereotact Funct Neurosurg 1991;57:72–81
38. Barcia JA, Barcia-Salorio JL, Lopez-Gomez L, Hernandez G. Stereotactic radiosurgery may be effective in the treatment of idiopathic epilepsy: report on the methods and results in a series of eleven cases. Stereotact Funct Neurosurg 1994;63(1–4):271–279
39. Régis J, Peragui J, Rey M, et al. First selective amygdalohippocampal radiosurgery for "mesial temporal lobe epilepsy." Stereotact Funct Neurosurg 1995;64(Suppl 1):193–201
40. Régis J, Bartolomei F, Rey M, et al. Gamma Knife surgery for mesial temporal lobe epilepsy. Epilepsia 1999;40(11):1551–1556
41. Kawai K, Suzuki I, Kurita H, Shin M, Arai N, Kirino T. Failure of low-dose radiosurgery to control temporal lobe epilepsy. J Neurosurg 2001;95(5):883–887
42. Srikijvilaikul T, Najm I, Foldvary-Schaefer N, Lineweaver T, Suh JH, Bingaman WE. Failure of Gamma Knife radiosurgery for mesial temporal lobe epilepsy: report of five cases. Neurosurgery 2004;54(6):1395–1402, discussion 1402–1394
43. McDonald CR, Norman MA, Tecoma E, Alksne J, Iragui V. Neuropsychological change following Gamma Knife surgery in patients with left

temporal lobe epilepsy: a review of three cases. Epilepsy Behav 2004;5(6):949–957

44. Régis J, Rey M, Bartolomei F, et al. Gamma Knife surgery in mesial temporal lobe epilepsy: a prospective multicenter study. Epilepsia 2004;45(5):504–515
45. Hoggard N, Wilkinson ID, Griffiths PD, Vaughan P, Kemeny AA, Rowe JG. The clinical course after stereotactic radiosurgical amygdalohippocampectomy with neuroradiological correlates. Neurosurgery 2008;62(2):336–344, discussion 344–336
46. Bartolomei F, Hayashi M, Tamura M, et al. Long-term efficacy of Gamma Knife radiosurgery in mesial temporal lobe epilepsy. Neurology 2008;70(19):1658–1663
47. Régis J, Semah F, Bryan RN, et al. Early and delayed MR and PET changes after selective temporomesial radiosurgery in mesial temporal lobe epilepsy. AJNR Am J Neuroradiol 1999;20(2):213–216
48. Armstrong CL, Gyato K, Awadalla AW, Lustig R, Tochner ZA. A critical review of the clinical effects of therapeutic irradiation damage to the brain: the roots of controversy. Neuropsychol Rev 2004;14(1):65–86
49. Barbaro NM, Quigg M, Broshek DK, et al. A multicenter, prospective pilot study of Gamma Knife radiosurgery for mesial temporal lobe epilepsy: seizure response, adverse events, and verbal memory. Ann Neurol In press
50. Engel JJ, Van Ness P, Rasmussen T. Outcome with respect to epileptic seizures. In: Engel JJ, ed. Surgical Treatment of the Epilepsies. 2nd ed. New York: Raven Press; 1993:609–621
51. Stroup E, Langfitt J, Berg M, McDermott M, Pilcher W, Como P. Predicting verbal memory decline following anterior temporal lobectomy (ATL). Neurology 2003;60(8):1266–1273
52. Hermann BP, Wyler AR, Bush AJ, Tabatabai FR. Differential effects of left and right anterior temporal lobectomy on verbal learning and memory performance. Epilepsia 1992;33(2):289–297
53. Hermann BP, Seidenberg M, Dohan FC Jr, et al. Reports by patients and their families of memory change after left anterior temporal lobectomy: relationship to degree of hippocampal sclerosis. Neurosurgery 1995;36(1):39–44, discussion 44–45
54. Seidenberg M, Hermann B, Wyler AR, Davies K, Dohan FC Jr, Leveroni C. Neuropsychological outcome following anterior temporal lobectomy in patients with and without the syndrome of mesial temporal lobe epilepsy. Neuropsychology 1998;12(2):303–316
55. Chelune GJ, Najm IM. Risk factors associated with postusurgical decrements in memory decline after anterior temporal lobectomy. In: Luders HO, Comair Y, eds. Epilepsy Surgery. 2nd ed. Philadelphia: Raven; 2000:497–504
56. Eder HG, Feichtinger M, Pieper T, Kurschel S, Schroettner O. Gamma Knife radiosurgery for callosotomy in children with drug-resistant epilepsy. Childs Nerv Syst 2006;22(8):1012–1017
57. Pendl G, Eder HG, Schroettner O, Leber KA. Corpus callosotomy with radiosurgery. Neurosurgery 1999;45(2):303–307, discussion 307–308
58. Anschel DJ, Romanelli P. Letter in response to Quigg and Barbaro. Arch Neurol 2008;65:1136–1137

17

Stereotactic Radiosurgery for Ocular Disorders

Roman Liščák and Gabriela Šimonová

Due to its underlying radiobiological principles, radiosurgery is generally used to treat small-volume lesions, and volumes of ocular disorders usually fall within the volume constraints of radiosurgery. The first radiosurgical experience with ophthalmologic indications involved the treatment of patients suffering from uveal melanomas.[1–7,21] However, it would appear that the potential of radiosurgery to provide effective treatment for ophthalmologic indications is broader. In addition to uveal melanomas, the current spectrum of ocular indications includes eye metastases, advanced glaucoma, age-related macular degeneration (ARMD), hemangioblastoma, pseudotumors, and vegetative pain.

Radiosurgery of ocular disorders necessitates a close cooperation with ophthalmologists. This multidisciplinary approach is critical for patient selection, follow-up, and treatment.

◆ Technical Issues Specific to Stereotactic Radiosurgery for Ocular Disorders

The Leksell Gamma Knife (Elekta Instruments AB, Stockholm, Sweden) was originally designed to treat deep brain targets, and stereotactic coordinates are derived from the position of the coordinate head frame, which is rigidly fixed to the skull. Proper eye fixation or an eye motion–monitoring system is required because the eye can move during the treatment procedure. Very eccentric target volume location can also cause some inaccuracies in the treatment-planning calculations, including relative dose distribution and absolute dose calculations. Finally, there may be some technical inconveniences in treating patients due to limitations in the range of the coordinate system in this eccentric target location. Despite these difficulties, radiosurgery is an attractive alternative treatment for ophthalmic lesions mainly because of its accurate and precise delivery of high conformal doses to the treatment target.

Eye Fixation

Several different eye immobilization systems and techniques have been described in the literature.[1,8–15] Tokuuye et al described a mask fixation technique with a plastic mold gently pressed down over the orbit to restrict ocular movements.[14] Zehetmayer et al reported on a suction immobilization technique for radiosurgery of intracranial malignancies using the Gamma Knife.[15] Langmann et al used a fixation method of the globe by means of a retrobulbar anesthetic block for eye treatments using the Gamma Knife.[1] In the Prague center, the treated eye was fixed under a retrobulbar local anesthesia by suturing two rectus eye muscles to the stereotactic frame; this procedure was done by an ophthalmologist. To ensure adequate dose buildup and homogeneous propagation of radiation between the tissues and the air, a partial tarsorrhaphy was performed, and a plastic cover filled with tissue-equivalent gel was used (**Fig. 17.1**). This simultaneously acted as protection for the cornea. This eye fixation technique showed very good stability and rigidity in time. Having the patient in a prone versus supine position had no effect on stereotactic target and eye structure localization.[11,12]

Active eye immobilization techniques, where the patient controls the eye position, for example, by fixating on a light source, have been described for proton/helium ion beam therapy and also for linear accelerator (linac)–based stereotactic radiotherapy of malignant tumors.[8,10] For proton/helium ion beam therapy, a surgical intervention is performed to position tantalum clips at the border of the visible tumor under diaphanoscopical control. These clips are used during treatment planning to define the target volume and to verify the position of the tumor during treatment delivery by using x-rays.[9] Petersch et al described a noninvasive eye fixation system for the application of linac-based stereotactic radiotherapy in the treatment of uveal melanoma.[13] The computer-controlled eye-monitoring system is based on the patient's fixation on a point of light. When the eye position exceeds the preset geometrical limits to that point of light, the system

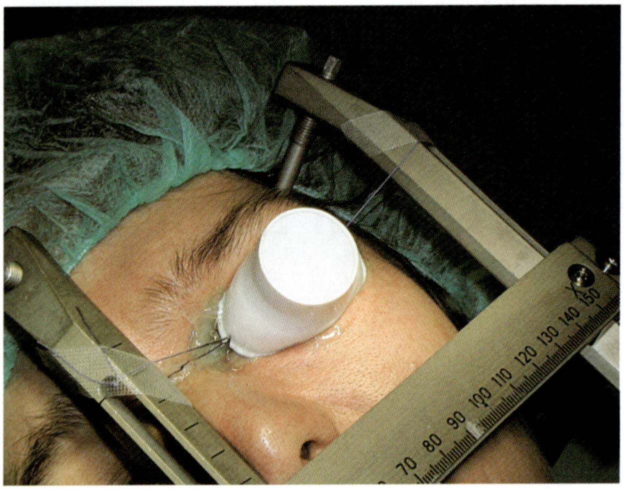

Fig. 17.1 Fixation of the eye.

automatically initiates a cessation of the radiation beam until the eye is repositioned to the proper alignment.

Accuracy of Stereotactic Imaging

Magnetic resonance imaging (MRI) is the preferred imaging modality for radiosurgery. It offers more detailed and artifact-free information than computed tomography (CT). However, whereas CT is supposed to be free of geometric distortions, MRI may produce some geometric image distortions significant for radiosurgery treatment planning. Generally, MRI geometric distortion is mainly a function of the particular MRI scanner employed, MRI sequence used, image slice orientation, position in the imaged object, and material and geometric parameters of the stereotactic frame.[16,17] The issue of image geometric distortion is even more crucial in the case of eye imaging when a target and other structures of interest are in a very frontal location. It is essential to check the extent of geometric distortions for each MRI scanner and sequence employed for ocular imaging.[12]

Dosimetry and Treatment Planning

Due to very eccentric target volume location, some inaccuracies in the treatment-planning calculations, including relative dose distributions and absolute dose calculations (calculation of treatment time or monitor units), can be expected. This issue is even more prominent for surface structures of the eye (e.g., eye lens, eyelid, and cornea) than for target volumes itself.

Petersch et al reported excellent agreement between actual measurements and the treatment-planning system calculations for uveal melanomas at a depth of 15 to 20 mm.[13] However, at small depths (<10 mm), the treatment-planning system cannot model the influence of absorption in the eye motion–monitoring device accurately if the beam passed perpendicularly through it. Consequently, as a means of reducing dosimetric errors, avoidance of frontal beams during radiosurgery to ocular lesions has been suggested.

Detailed dosimetric measurements were also performed at the Prague Na Homolce Hospital. In this case, treatment-planning system calculations of target volume relative dose distributions and absolute dose calculations in different depths were compared with experimental measurements.[12] Various treatment plans for different ophthalmic indications (e.g., uveal melanoma, glaucoma, and retinoblastoma) calculated for the Gamma Knife were evaluated. Absolute doses measured by pinpoint ion chamber at depths of 10 mm and deeper showed relatively good agreement with the treatment-planning system calculated data. Absolute doses delivered during head phantom irradiation were systematically lower than calculated ones, usually within 5% or even within 3%. Absolute doses measured by pinpoint ion chamber at depths < 10 mm showed a relatively large deviation compared with the treatment-planning system's calculated data. In this situation, absolute doses delivered during phantom irradiation were systematically lower by 15 to 20%. To improve on inaccuracies in absolute dose calculations in surface structures, proper tissue-equivalent built-up material attached to the treated eye was recommended (**Fig. 17.1**). Such material should reduce discrepancies between the planned and the delivered radiation dosimetry. Preliminary measurements demonstrated that calculation errors should not exceed more than 10% even at surface structures when built-up material is used. Relative dose distributions measured by polymer gel dosimetry in the region of the target volumes were in good agreement with the Leksell Gamma Plan (Elekta).

Because of the marginal position of the eye, an extreme gamma angle has to be used to avoid collision of the skull with the collimator helmet of the Gamma Knife model B or C. Patients usually do no tolerate backward bending of the head in a supine position. Therefore, the prone position was used in most cases. The treatment could not be performed for this reason on a small number of patients suffering from rigid kyphosis or Bekhterev disease.

Depending on the patient's head shape and volume, it may be difficult to adjust properly the frame position to reach all Leksell stereotactic coordinates. Specifically, the Y (posterior-anterior) coordinate can exceed limits engraved on the commercially available Leksell stereotactic frame. Because of this, a special Y coordinate "extender" was developed at Na Homolce Hospital to be able to treat Y coordinates exceeding standard Gamma Knife limits (**Fig. 17.2**). Fortunately, the problems of collisions and coordinate limits have largely been overcome by the enlarged space of the collimator helmet in the latest model of the Leksell Gamma Knife Perfexion (Elekta).

◆ Specific Disorders

Uveal Melanoma

Natural History and Clinical Presentation

Uveal melanoma represents the most common primary malignant tumor of the eye in adults. There is a peak incidence between 55 and 70 years of age, with a prevalence of 6 or

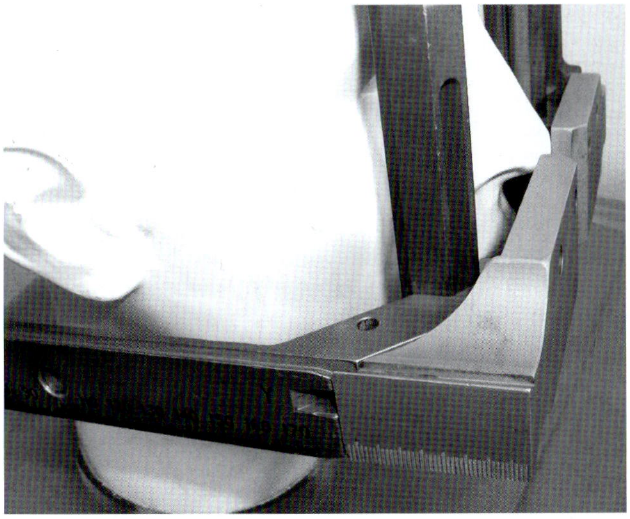

Fig. 17.2 Triangle adapter to expand the stereotactic space Y coordinate.

7 cases per million people per year. The incidence is rare in patients younger than 20 years of age. Approximately 50% of patients with diagnosed melanomas of the choroid or ciliary body will die from this tumor within 15 years.[18,19]

Uveal melanomas are neoplasms arising from the uveal tract that includes the iris, ciliary body, and choroid. The uveal tract is a vascular structure with no lymphatic drainage. Lymphatic node involvement (preauricular, submandibular, and cervical nodes) can be diagnosed on rare occasions when subconjunctival extension of the primary tumor has also been observed. The major routes of extension are local growth and hematogenous spread. The common sites of hematologic dissemination are the liver, lung, and brain. Liver metastases are diagnosed in two thirds of patients with disease dissemination.

Wide variations in the grading of malignancy can be observed, from relatively benign types with several years of survival without dissemination, to other tumors with fast multiorgan dissemination, which can lead to the patient's death within a few months. Tumor growth is also influenced by the potential cell doubling time, which varies widely from 60 to 350 days (median ~70 days).[20] A longer doubling time as compared with a significant proportion of other tumors can explain the relatively long survival of these patients and also the relatively slow tumor response after irradiation.

Iris melanomas (incidence ~10%) are single or multiple elevated lesions with associated changes of iris color. These types of melanomas are much more benign, smaller in size, readily visible, and diagnosed early. It can be difficult to assess the potential of the malignant cells, even in those with documented growth, because iris nevi may also grow. For this reason, local resection is usually effective whenever it is required.

Choroidal melanomas typically (but with some variation) grow in nodular form and in cases of continuing growth cause many tumors to break through the Bruch membrane (a base membrane–connective tissue complex lying between the retina pigment epithelium and the choriocapillaris). When the melanomas break through the Bruch membrane, they extend into the subsensory retinal space, which gives them a mushroom or collar-button shape. These characteristics, as well as including the detachment of the retina, are typical for uveal melanomas. This type of tumor growth is sometimes accompanied by vitreous hemorrhage with symptoms of sudden visual loss.

Melanomas involving the ciliary body are rare, carry a poor prognosis, and are often diagnosed late. Melanomas can also have diffuse, infiltrating growth to the ciliary body and a pattern called ring melanoma. These tumors are difficult to diagnosis because they are accompanied by relatively little visible tumor mass effect, and they occur in the diagnostically "silent" eye area. Any extrascleral extension of the tumor usually confers a poor prognosis. The diffusely growing melanomas are usually more aggressive, with more malignant cell types.

Melanoma of the ciliary body and choroid have typical clinical features, and the correct diagnosis for a majority of patients can be made by taking a history and performing a complete ocular examination. The ophthalmologic examination includes external ocular examination, indirect ophthalmoscopy, fluorescein angiography, and ultrasonography, which plays a basic role at the time of diagnosis. The ophthalmologic examination also plays a role in follow-up and can be used to obtain precise measurement of the tumor base and height. The height of the tumor in particular represents one of the most important factors influencing the treatment decision, and it is used during follow-up to evaluate the tumor's response.

Results of Radiosurgery

The first experiments with radiosurgery for the treatment of uveal melanomas were conducted using the rabbit eye melanoma model. The reported tumor lethal dose in this experiment ranged from 60 to 90 Gy applied in a single session.[4] Several authors reported the results of Gamma Knife radiosurgery in uveal melanomas, and some observed relatively high radiation-related toxicity.[1–3,5,6,21–24] The minimum effective dose for long-lasting local tumor control, as well as the tolerance doses for critical ocular structures, is not yet well defined.

Our own experience represents a group of 126 patients with uveal melanoma treated using the Gamma Knife over a period of 8 years. The LENT SOMA (Late Effects Normal Tissues, subjective, objective, management, and analytic) scoring system[25] was used to measure the radiation side effects (**Table 17.1**). The tumor marginal dose for radiosurgery ranged from 35 to 45 Gy, with a median dose of 41 Gy in our series.

Tumor regression was defined as a decrease in tumor height registered by ultrasonography scans and by control MRI. The tumor regression was achieved in 70% of patients. The maximum local effect has been recorded within 24 months after radiosurgery. Patients with tumor growth progression or without any response 30 months after treatment were candidates for re-treatment by radiosurgery, and patients with a tumor height >10 mm or extrascleral growth were indicated for enucleation (5% in our series).

Table 17.1 Toxicity Scoring System (RTOG/EORTC LENT SOMA)

	Grade 1	Grade 2	Grade 3	Grade 4
Cornea	Increased tearing on exam	Noninfectious keratitis	Infectious keratitis; corneal ulcer	Panophthalmitis; corneal scar; ulceration leading to perforation of globe/loss of globe
Iris	Rubeosis only	Rubeosis; increased intraocular pressure	Neovascular glaucoma; ability to count fingers 1 m	Neovascular glaucoma without ability to count fingers 1 m; complete blindness
Optic nerve	Afferent pupillary defect with normal-appearing nerve	≤ 1/4 pallor with asymptomatic visual field defect	> pallor or central scotoma	Profound sptic atrophy; complete blindness
Lens	Asymmetric lenticular opacities; no visual loss	Moderate lenticular changes with mild–moderate visual loss	Moderate lenticular changes with severe visual loss	Severe lenticular changes
Retina	Microaneurysms, nonfoveal exudates, minor vessel attenuation, and extrafoveal pigment changes	Cotton wool spots	Massive macular exudation; focal retinal detachment	Opaque vitreous hemorrhage; complete retinal detachment; blindness
Sclera	Loss of episcleral vessels	≤ 50% scleral thinning	> 50% scleral thinning	Scleral or periosteal graft required due to perforation

Abbreviations: EORTC, European Organization for Research and Treatment of Cancer; LENT SOMA, Late Effects Normal Tissues, subjective, objective, management, and analytic; RTOG, Radiation Therapy Oncology Group.

Complications from Radiosurgery

The most common late toxicity complications for all types of irradiation are retinopathy, cataract, secondary glaucoma, and optic neuropathy.[6,24,26–30] The most common cause of the toxicity-related enucleation is secondary neovascular glaucoma.[28,31] Secondary glaucoma is typically a late complication, and its incidence increases with longer follow-up. Although the risk of enucleation from this reason is ~6% for a 2-year follow-up period after radiosurgery, it increases to 19% with 8 years of follow-up.[31–35] Secondary glaucoma often accompanies uveal melanoma already before the treatment. The question remains: how much of the treatment itself contributes to its development or accentuation? Differentiation of the natural development of this complication from accentuation of secondary glaucoma caused by radiosurgery is not possible at present.

A study with proton beam treatment identified localization of the tumor in the region of the ciliary body or fovea and a height of the tumor >8 mm as risk factors for subsequent enucleation.[31] Some observations were made on patients after radiosurgery who had their eye secondarily enucleated. Eyes with secondary enucleations presented an initial tumor height >9 mm. The second frequent reason for enucleation was the origin of the tumor in the region of the ciliary body.[24]

An analysis of late toxicity of 126 patients of our series recorded severe grade 3–4 retinopathy in 15% of treated patients, radiation-related late toxicity grade 3–4 in the lens was observed in 26%, optic neuropathy in 9%, and secondary glaucoma in 18% of cases. Eleven percent of patients were enucleated for worsening glaucoma during the first 2 years after radiosurgery. The median time to occurrence of secondary neovascular glaucoma was 18 months, so a higher incidence of enucleation during a longer follow-up cannot be excluded. The worsening of useful vision caused by radiation-related toxicity during 3 years after radiosurgery was observed in 34% of patients and was due to tumor progression in 3%, optic nerve neuropathy in 8%, retinopathy in 9%, and neovascular glaucoma in 14%.

Significantly lower toxicity in the optic nerve was observed when the maximum dose to that structure was < 10 Gy (incidence of late toxicity grade 3–4 in 2.4%), in the cornea when the maximum dose did not exceed 10 Gy (incidence of late toxicity grade 3–4 in 3%), in the lens when the maximum dose did not exceed 7 Gy (incidence of late toxicity grade 3–4 in 7.7%), and in the iris when the maximum dose did not exceed 15 Gy (incidence of late toxicity grade 3–4 in 4.6%).

In a prospective study of helium ion therapy, the incidence of secondary glaucoma was 29% after a mean observation period of 53 months. The incidence of rubeosis iridis in 34% of patients has been observed using proton beam therapy after a median follow-up of 36 months.[33] A major predictive factor for the development of rubeosis iridis and later neovascular glaucoma was a large tumor size unsuitable for brachytherapy. The enucleation rate was 19%—3% for local failure and 16% because of complications.[32]

Prognostic Factors

The prognosis of patients with uveal melanoma is determined by tumor size, cell type, tumor location (poor results for ciliary body tumors), and the extent of the disease.[6,9,32–34,36–49] The most important prognostic factor is the presence or absence of organ dissemination at the time of uveal melanoma diagnosis. Some authors maintain that dissemination from uveal melanomas starts when the tumor is >7 mm in diameter, and growth from a 7 to 10 mm diameter increases the risk of metastatic disease to ~16%. This fact was supported by clinical observations.[20] Five-year survival rates of patients with small tumors (heights < 8 mm) and with no detected metastatic disease outside the eye are >80%. For larger tumors (>10 mm in height) with metastases outside the eye, the 5-year survival period ranged from 10 to 30%. There still exists a knowledge gap regarding growth of melanomas in situ and the documentation of the time intervals between the diagnosis of primary tumor and the appearance of the other organ dissemination.

Tumor growth depends on tumor doubling time; for uveal melanoma, it is estimated to be longer than 69 days. On theoretical grounds, it has been suggested that metastatic death (after the primary tumor has released malignant cells into the systemic circulation) will occur at a time interval derived from the multiplication of the tumor doubling time by 35 to 40.[20] Therefore, the death is unlikely to occur before 6 years after dissemination of the first viable embolus of malignant tumor cells. The minimum latent interval of 6 years implies that metastatic death within 7 to 8 years after local treatment on the uveal melanoma is nearly always due to pretreatment dissemination.

The best prognosis in our group of patients had been for patients with the following: age younger than 50 years, with a preequatorial location of the tumor; tumor height does not exceed 5 mm; gross tumor volume was not larger than 500 mm^3; and no other organ dissemination existed.[6]

Other Treatment Methods

The management of uveal melanomas still remains controversial. Several therapeutic approaches and options for this tumor are available, including expectant observation with periodic ophthalmologic examination only, laser photocoagulation, thermotherapy, resection or enucleation, brachytherapy, charged particle therapy (protons or helium ions), and stereotactic radiotherapy or radiosurgery. It is typically resistant to standard fractionation radiotherapy and chemotherapy. Better results were noticed after application of a higher dose per fraction (hypofractionated scheme) and with immunotherapy. The available data have not yet established whether enucleation or eye preservation treatment including radiosurgery is more effective in prolonging patients' survival, as the treatment results in terms of survival are similar. Comparison of different treatment methods is given in **Table 17.2.**

Small tumors (diameter ≤ 10 mm, height ≤ 3 mm) are sometimes considered for observation only. When risk of dissemination is considered, then resection, transpupillary thermotherapy, laser photocoagulation, charged particle treatment, or brachytherapy could be used. For middle-sized tumors (diameter 10–15 mm, height 3–8 mm), besides brachytherapy, proton therapy and enucleation are used. For bigger tumors, enucleation is preferred, although in some patients brachytherapy and radiotherapy are used.[50]

The most frequently used surgical method is enucleation, which is performed in 35% of patients with uveal melanoma. Five- and 10-year survival rates after enucleation are 63 and 43%, respectively.[51,52] Postoperative external beam radiotherapy has been used in patients with large tumors with extrascleral or extraocular extension.

Charged particle therapy has good results, but the treatment facilities are located in physical research centers with synchrocyclotrons. Operation and treatment are therefore very expensive. The most extensively published charged particle center is the Paul Scherrer Institute in Switzerland.[38] In their group of 2258 patients, 5- and 10-year local tumor control rates were 96 and 95%, respectively. Five- and 10-year survival rates were 82 and 62%, respectively. Seven percent of patients underwent enucleation after proton therapy. Preservation of the eye 5 and 10 years after the treatment was 89 and 85%, respectively.

The most frequently clinically used therapeutic system for delivering radiation is brachytherapy (plaque radiotherapy) with ruthenium 106 and iodine 125. A number of other radionuclides have been used, including cobalt 60, gold 198, iridium 192, and palladium 103, with varying results according to the retrospective studies.[34,37,40,42,44–9,53,54] Brachytherapy leads to long-term local tumor control in 85 to 90% of patients, and secondary enucleation is performed in 6% of patients.

Stereotactic irradiation using linac with applied doses of 45 to 70 Gy delivered usually in three fractions is an effective method, with tumor height reduction achievement in 97% of cases, secondary enucleation performance in 13%, and the incidence of secondary glaucoma in 20%, also including iris or chamber angle neovascularization.[7,8,27]

Treatment Decision

Rationale criteria for selecting a treatment modality in our current practice are the following. Small tumors (<10 mm in height) localized preequatorially can be successfully treated using brachytherapy. Tumors localized equatorially or posterior to the equator and not higher than 10 mm can be irradiated using the Gamma Knife. Tumors >10 mm in height, especially melanomas of the ciliary body, progression of growth after irradiation, tumors combined with neovascular glaucoma, and vitreous hemorrhage are candidates for enucleation.

Table 17.2 Comparison of Different Radiation Treatment Methods

Treatment Method	Median Follow-Up (months)	Minimal Dose (Gy)	Tumor Response (%)	Five-Year Local Tumor Control (%)	Radiation-Related Retinopathy (%)	Neovascular Glaucoma (%)	Enucleation Rate (%)
Brachytherapy[37,42,44,45,47]	39–96	70–250	69–96	82–92	22–63	3–11	10–21
Proton beam therapy[31,38]	40	40–70 F	91–100	87–100	NA	8	9
Helium ion therapy[32,33]	96	50–80 F	87–96	80	NA	35	20
Stereotactic radiotherapy[7,27]	36	45–60 F	94	NA	26	9–20	NA
Radiosurgery[1,2,5,6,24]	36	35–90	70–90	NA	23–70	18–23	18

Abbreviations: F, fractionated treatment; NA, data not available.

Glaucoma

Glaucoma is a chronic, slowly progressive, usually bilateral neuropathy of the optic nerve. Untreated glaucoma eventually leads to complete loss of vision. About 10% of patients with glaucoma become uni- or bilaterally blind.[55,56] We currently understand the pathophysiology of glaucoma to be a progressive loss of ganglion cells resulting in visual field damage related to the intraocular pressure (IOP).[57] Although many clinicians now feel that there are several factors involved in the pathogenesis of glaucoma, the only rigorously proven treatment method is the lowering of IOP.[58] This could be achieved in two ways: by increasing the chamber-liquid drainage or by decreasing its production. The conventional antiglaucomatous treatment—local and systemic pharmacotherapy, laser and cryotherapy, and incisional surgery—takes effect in this way. Surgical treatment is necessary when visual functions deteriorate despite the maximal pharmacological or laser treatment.

Production of intraocular liquid can be decreased by affecting the site of its origin, which is the ciliary body. Irradiation of the ciliary body using the Gamma Knife is one such process. The intention of radiosurgery is not complete destruction of the ciliary body, but reduction of intraocular liquid production through action on its vessels. It thereby achieves a decrease of IOP.

In secondary glaucoma, the goal of the radiosurgical treatment is determined by the stage of the disease. When vision has been totally or partially lost, the main aims are to abolish the elevated IOP and to eliminate severe pain. In the early stages of the disease, when conventional therapy has insufficient effect and visual acuity is still preserved, the treatment has the more difficult task of preventing any further progress of the pathogenic mechanisms.

Because there was no previous experience in the radiosurgical treatment of glaucoma to refer to, we started to evaluate an effective and safe irradiation of the corpus ciliare as the source of intraocular aqueous humor.[59,60] Four isocenters using the 8 mm collimator were displaced in a cruciform manner (**Fig. 17.3**). We delivered 20 Gy at 50% isodose, but for patients with some preserved vision, the dose was lowered to 15 Gy at 50% isodose. The patients are ophthalmologically followed in regular 3-month intervals during the first year after the irradiation, then twice yearly to assess the irradiation influence on pain, IOP, and neovascularization.

In a nonrandomized prospective study, a total of 107 eyes in 103 patients were irradiated in this way. All the patients had a long history of the disease and had exhausted all traditional forms of therapy. Because of advanced painful glaucoma and progressive clinical symptoms, we have focused on following the decrease in pain and the effect on IOP, as well as simplifying pharmacotherapy after the radiosurgery. Positive effect was recorded in all patients in at least one of the following parameters. IOP decreased usually within 12 weeks after the radiosurgery to the painless level in 52% of cases; residual elevation of IOP remains in 45% of cases. Pain, which was present in all patients before the treatment, regressed within 1 to 8 weeks after the treatment. Patients were completely pain free in 66% of cases, and partial relief of pain was recorded in 29% of cases. During the follow-up, which was at least 2 years, there was no further deterioration of the vision (if preserved before the treatment), and there were no significant signs of postirradiation eye-bulb irritation, retinitis, or changes in the anterior segment of the eye. In case of neovascularization, at least partial regression was observed in all affected eyes, usually 4 to 5 months after the radiosurgery. Pharmacotherapy was reduced in 39% of patients within 2 to 3 months after the radiosurgery. Enucleation was performed in eight blind eyes: in five of them the radiosurgery was not sufficiently effective, in two eyes the reason was cosmetic, and in one eye there was a trauma during the follow-up.

Treatment complications were not significant: short-term postoperative lacrimation in 61% of patients caused by mechanical irritation after the eye fixation, postirradiation cataracts in two patients, and noninfectious keratitis in another two patients.

Gamma Knife radiosurgery of the ciliary body leads to a significant alleviation of pain and reduction of IOP in advanced glaucoma. It is effective in secondary glaucoma, especially in terms of neovascularization.[59,60] The latency of the treatment effect is relatively short.

The patients with primary open angle glaucoma suffer less pain, their IOP is less elevated, and their disease is mainly expressed by visual loss as a manifestation of the optic neuropathy. Even in the early stages of glaucoma, this can be detected by confocal laser scanning tomography and nerve fiber layer testing and analysis.[61–65] The treatment effect on optic neuropathy can be evaluated after a longer follow-up by registering visual function and performing other tests for glaucoma neuropathy. We assume that radiosurgery can help to achieve "the target IOP" and thus prevent further progression of optic neuropathy. A long follow-up is needed to evaluate whether progressive optic neuropathy will be stabilized by radiosurgery. Special ophthalmologic examinations have to be performed to make this evaluation. A prospective 5-year clinical study to halt progressive optic neuropathy in the early stages of glaucoma is under way.

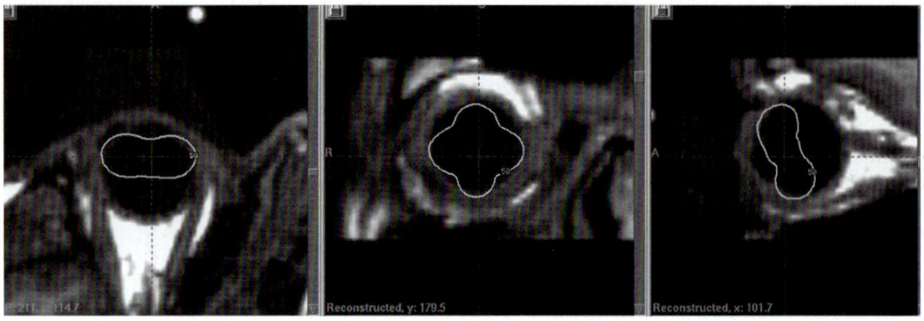

Fig. 17.3 A plan to irradiate the ciliary body using four 8 mm collimators (50% isodose displayed) in the eye bulb with aphakia, therefore, lens is not visible on MRI.

Age-Related Macular Degeneration

ARMD is the most common cause of legal blindness in patients 50 years or older. The two main forms are nonexudative and exudative. ARMD is characterized by the presence of some degree of visual loss in association with drusen and atrophy of the retinal pigment epithelium or changes associated with subretinal neovascularization. Exudative ARMD forms abnormal blood vessels called choroidal neovascular membranes (CNVMs), which develop under the retina, leak fluid and blood, and ultimately cause a blinding disciform scar in and under the retina.

Laser coagulation, photodynamic therapy, transpupillary thermotherapy, and subretinal surgery techniques are successful in small numbers of strictly indicated cases. The effect of those methods—the destruction or reduction of the neovascular complex—is better in well-defined CNVMs. In severe cases of ARMD with "malignant-destroying CNVM," these treatments are ineffective. These advanced forms of CNVM are characterized by the fast growth of subfoveal neovascular tissue with strong exudation, covered with blood and lipid, which can cause damage to the neurosensory retina overlying the CNVM.

ARMD is a degenerative process with a proliferative component, and irradiation can play an antiproliferative role. CNVMs, which are composed of endothelial cells and proliferate more rapidly than the endothelial cells of the retina, may be more sensitive than the retinal vasculature. Consequently, radiation therapy has been suggested as a treatment for subfoveal CNVMs.[66–72] Clinical experience with conventional fractionated irradiation for head and neck malignancies has demonstrated that cumulative doses (multiple fractions) of up to 25 Gy cause minimal to no damage to the retina or optic nerve, and the susceptibility of retinal vasculature endothelial cells has been confirmed in other studies described by Archer et al.[73] Many pilot studies for exudative ARMD show stabilization or regression of CNVMs with different kinds of radiation therapy.[74–76]

Initial results from patients treated with radiosurgery for ARMD show that the Gamma Knife is able to affect tissues beneath the retina without damaging the overlying retinal structures. Haas et al[75] in their pilot study investigated the effect of single-fraction (10 Gy at the 90% isodose) Gamma Knife radiosurgery in patients with subfoveal CNVMs due to ARMD. Ten patients were followed for a period of 12 months. Fluorescein angiography and indocyanine green chorioangiography demonstrated a regression of the neovascular complex in one patient and stabilization in three patients. Enlargement of the CNVM was found in six patients and was associated with a decrease of visual acuity in four patients. Henderson et al[77] followed seven patients with ARMD after Gamma Knife radiosurgery using a marginal dose of 12 Gy. With a median patient follow-up of 2 years, they observed stabilization of disease in five patients; improvement of vision was recorded in one, and impairment also in one patient.

In our study we treated 25 patients with occult forms of CNVM in ARMD with a dose of 15 Gy at a 50% isodose. Both ultrasonography and fluorescein angiography demonstrated a regression of the neovascular complex in 19 patients. An enlargement of the CNVMs was found after 4 to 6 months of a temporary period of stabilization in four patients. As in the study by Haas's group, we did not observe a decrease of vision immediately after treatment, and no severe radiation-related side effects (retinopathy, optic neuropathy, cataract progression, or keratitis) have been detected. One third of the patients reported subjective improvement of vision. Our results show that radiosurgery could play a significant role in advanced forms of CNVMs or large CNVMs, which are not treatable using other procedures. On this basis, we have constructed a new prospective, nonrandomized study, which is now under way.

Ocular Disorders Rarely Treated by Radiosurgery

Retinoblastoma

Retinoblastoma represents the most common primary malignant tumor of the eye in young children (in the first 2 years of life). The treatment strategy depends on clinical staging (disease confined to the retina, disease confined to the globe, extraocular extension, and presentation of distant metastases) and includes tumor resection, enucleation, chemotherapy, and external beam radiotherapy.

Our experience covers treatment of four children who were admitted for stereotactic irradiation using the Gamma Knife and had vitreous seeding of malignant cells. All patients were pretreated by the International Society of Pediatric Oncology protocol and relapsed after standard treatment. The only remaining possibility was enucleation. The whole vitreous body was irradiated using the Gamma Knife in a single session, with a collimator diameter of 14 mm. To avoid growth retardation of the irradiated eye and bony structures, the minimal dose delivered to the eye globe did not exceed 15 Gy in all these patients. For this reason, and also bearing in mind the risk of complications of previous treatment, the applied doses were relatively low. Local progression was observed in three out of four patients, and three patients were enucleated a median 2 months after radiosurgery. The role of radiosurgery in the treatment of retinoblastoma remains unclear.

Orbital and Uveal Metastases of Carcinomas

Metastatic lesions in every location of the eye and the orbit have been described, and autopsy studies estimate the incidence of these metastases to be 4 to 12% in all types of cancer patients.[78]

Brachytherapy is a standard treatment method using the same radionuclides as for uveal melanomas. Candidates for this type of irradiation are patients with a solitary lesion and a mean diameter of the pathologic lesion not exceeding 8 to 10 mm. External beam fractionated radiotherapy represents the local effective treatment with a low rate of late complications. The recommended total dose is 30 to 40 Gy, with a 2 to 3 Gy per fraction per day.[79]

Radiosurgery may extend treatment options for uveal metastases because of its specific advantages: the possibility of applying a high radiation dose and evidence of its sparing effect on the surrounding critical structures. The recommended minimal doses are similar to those for brain metastases, ranging from 20 to 30 Gy and depending on the tumor volume, location, and histology.

Other Ocular Disorders

We have recorded positive experience with treatment of ocular hemangioblastomas. Four patients with von Hippel-Lindau disease suffering from retinal or choroidal hemangioblastomas were treated using Gamma Knife radiosurgery. Radiosurgery had a stable effect, with follow-up exceeding 6 years in all patients even when several lesions in other organs progressed and had to be surgically treated. Regression of the lesion volume by 50% or more was observed.

We irradiated the ciliary ganglion in a 32-year-old woman suffering from severe vegetative orbital pain after a longer history of penetrating bulbar injury, three previous operations for amotio retinae, and a cyclocryocoagulation for secondary glaucoma. The affected eye was blind. The pain disappeared within a week. Two and a half years after treatment, the patient was still pain free after several years of previous continual suffering.

Radiosurgery proved to be effective in the treatment of exophthalmos refractory to conservative treatment. Irradiation of intraorbital muscles or inflammatory intraorbital tissue leads to a regression of exophthalmos within 3 months of the treatment (**Fig. 17.4**).

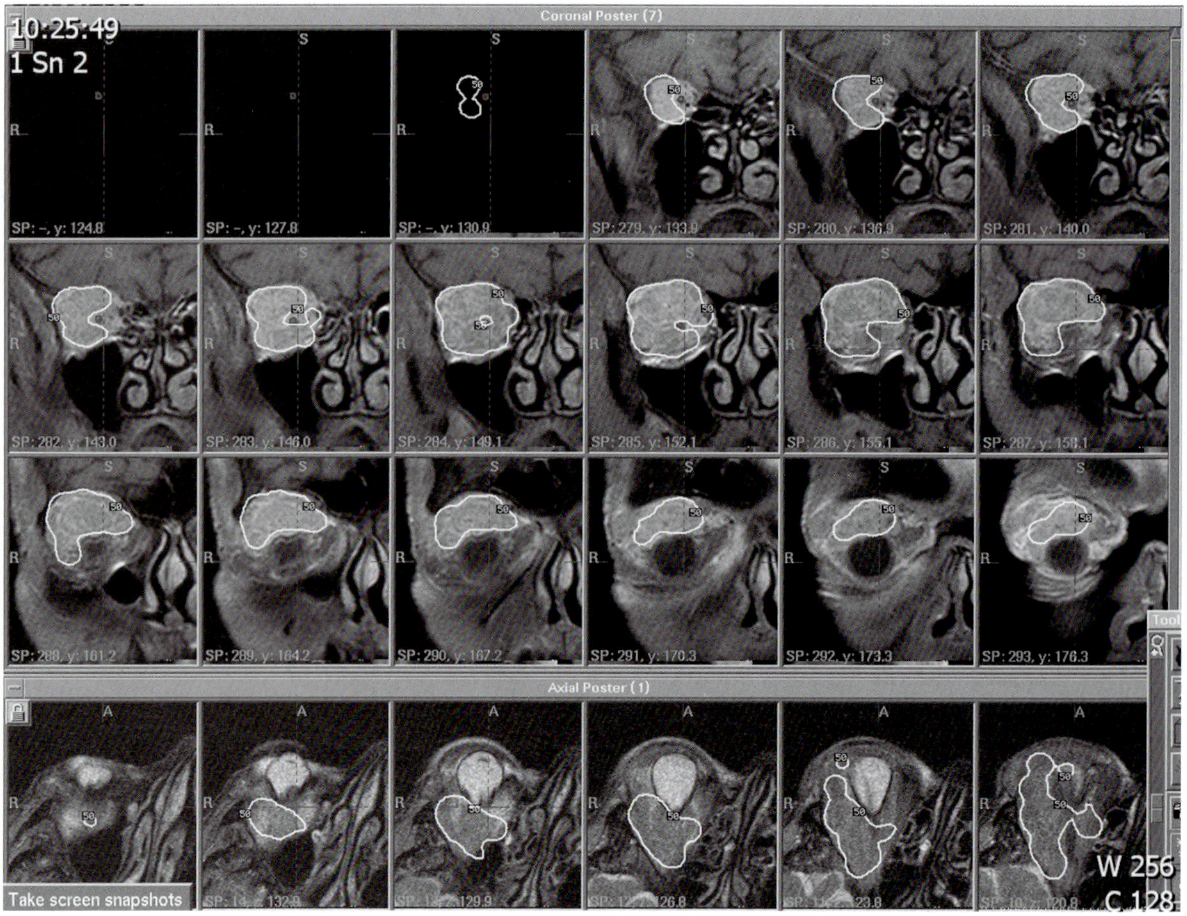

A

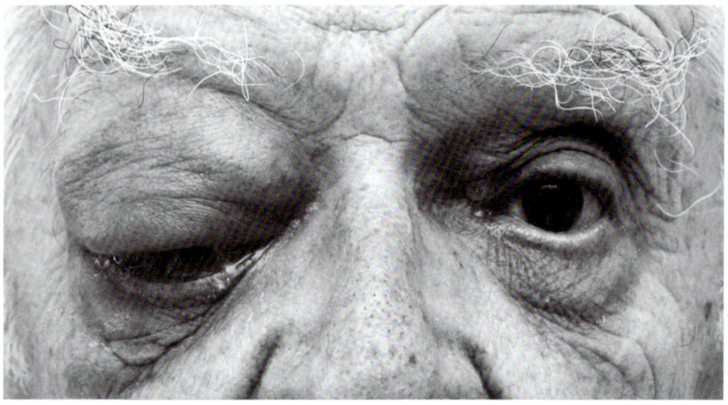

B

Fig. 17.4 **(A,B)** A patient with chronic thyropathy causing exophthalmos of the right eye. The orbit is filled with inflammatory tissue. The 50% isodose represents 8 Gy. The optic nerve receives < 8 Gy.

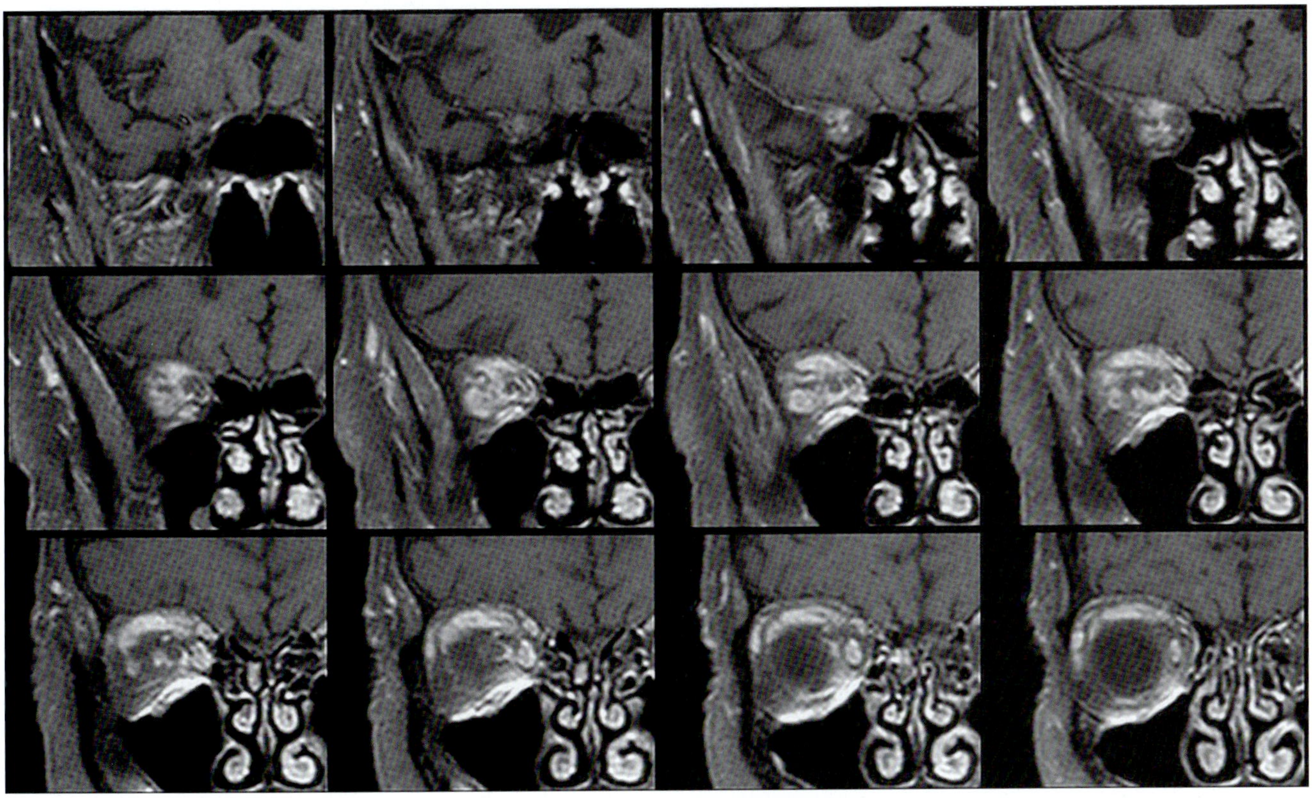

C

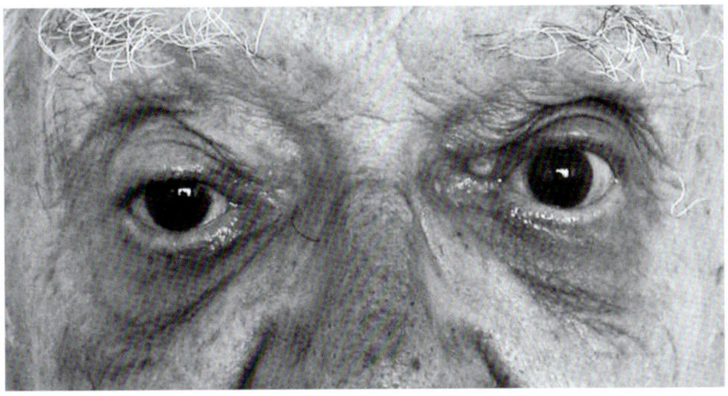

D

Fig. 17.4 *(Continued)* **(C,D)** Six months after radiosurgery, regression of the exophthalmos is observed.

◆ Summary

Radiosurgery of ocular tumors and other eye or orbital lesions represents a reasonable therapeutic option. If successful, it can help to preserve the globe and visual function. Further clinical studies using radiosurgery in ocular disease are necessary to optimize effective doses and to analyze factors influencing the length of survival, with a careful evaluation of the side effects. They are also required to improve local treatment effects while decreasing radiation-related complications.

Acknowledgments We thank our colleagues from the Department of Ophthalmology, first medical faculty, Charles University and the Central Military Hospital, Prague: J. Pašta, MD, PhD; J. Vladyková, MD, DSc; J. Ernest, MD, PhD; P. Němec, MD; and L. Nováček, MD, as well as colleagues from our own department, namely, V. Vladyka, MD, PhD, and J. Novotný Jr., PhD, for their care for our patients and their assistance in the preparation of this chapter.

References

1. Langmann G, Pendl G, Schröttner O. Gamma Knife of uveal melanoma radiosurgery for intraocular melanomas: preliminary report. Spectrum Augenheilkd 1995;9(Suppl 1):16–21
2. Marchini G, Gerosa M, Piovan E, et al. Gamma Knife stereotactic radiosurgery for uveal melanoma: clinical results after 2 years. Stereotact Funct Neurosurg 1996;66(Suppl 1):208–213
3. Pochop P, Pilbauer J, Křepelková J, Vladyka V, Liščák R, Šimonová G. Two years of experience with therapy of uveal melanoma by using the Leksell Gamma Knife [in Czech]. Cesk Slov Oftalmol 1998;54:222–235
4. Rand RW, Khonsary A, Brown WJ, Winter J, Snow HD. Leksell stereotactic radiosurgery in the treatment of eye melanoma. Neurol Res 1987;9:142–146

5. Rennie I, Forster D, Kemeny A, Walton L, Kunkler I. The use of single fraction Leksell stereotactic radiosurgery in the treatment of uveal melanoma. Acta Ophthalmol Scand 1996;74(6):558–562
6. Šimonová G, Novotný J Jr, Liščák R, Pilbauer J. Leksell Gamma Knife treatment of uveal melanoma. J Neurosurg 2002;97(Suppl 5):635–639
7. Zehetmayer M, Kitz K, Menapace R, et al. Local tumor control and morbidity after one to three fractions stereotactic external beam irradiation for uveal melanoma. Radiother Oncol 2000;55(2):135–144
8. Bellmann C, Fuss M, Holz FG. Stereotactic radiation therapy for malignant choroidal tumors, preliminary, short-term results. Ophthalmology 2000;107:358–365
9. Courdi A, Caujolle JP, Grange JD. Results of proton therapy of uveal melanomas treated in Nice. Int J Radiat Oncol Biol Phys 1999;45:5–11
10. Debus J, Fuss M, Engenhart-Cabillic R. Stereotactic conforming irradiation of choroid metastases. Ophthalmologe 1998;95:163–167
11. Liščák R, Vladyka V. Radiosurgery in ocular disorders: clinical applications. Prog Neurol Surg 2007;20:324–339
12. Novotný J Jr, Novotný J, Liščák R, et al. Assessment of the accuracy in opthalmic radiosurgery. In Kondziolka D (ed), Radiosurgery 2006; 6:71–85
13. Petersch B, Bogner J, Dieckmann K, Potter R, Georg D. Automatic real-time surveillance of eye position and gating for stereotactic radiotherapy of uveal melanoma. Med Phys 2004;31(12):3521–3527
14. Tokuuye K, Akine Y, Sumi M, Kagami Y, Ikeda H, Kaneko A. Fractionated stereotactic radiotherapy for choroidal melanoma. Radiother Oncol 1997;43(1):87–91
15. Zehetmayer M, Menapace R, Kitz K, Ertl A. Suction attachment for stereotactic radiosurgery of intraocular malignancies. Ophthalmologica 1994;208(3):119–121
16. Novotny J Jr, Vymazal J, Novotny J, et al. Does new magnetic resonance imaging technology provide better geometrical accuracy during stereotactic imaging? J Neurosurg 2005;102(Suppl):8–13
17. Walton L, Hampshire A, Forster D. Accuracy of stereotactic localization using magnetic resonance imaging: a comparison between two- and three-dimensional studies. Stereotact Funct Neurosurg 1996;66(Suppl): 49–56
18. Egan KM, Seddon JM, Glynn RJ, et al. Epidemiologic aspects of uveal melanoma. Surv Ophthalmol 1988;32(4):239–251
19. Singh AD, Topham A. Incidence of uveal melanoma in the United States:1973–1997. Ophthalmology 2003;110(5):956–961
20. Manschot WA, van Strik R. Uveal melanoma: therapeutic consequences of doubling times and irradiation results. Int Ophthalmol 1992;16:91–99
21. Mueller AJ, Talies S, Schaller UC, Horstmann G, Wowra B, Kampik A. Stereotactic radiosurgery of large uveal melanomas with the Gamma Knife. Ophthalmology 2000;107(7):1381–1387
22. Fakiris AJ, Lo SS, Henderson MA, et al. Gamma Knife based stereotactic radiosurgery for uveal melanoma. Stereotact Funct Neurosurg 2007;85:106–112
23. Woodburn R, Danis R, Timmerman R, et al. Preliminary experience in the treatment of choroidal melanoma with Gamma Knife radiosurgery. J Neurosurg 2000;93(Suppl 3):177–179
24. Zehetmayer M, Menapace R, Kitz K, Ertl A, Strenn K, Rushwurm I. Stereotactic irradiation of uveal melanoma with the Leksell gamma unit. Front Radiat Ther Oncol 1997;30:47–55
25. LENT SOMA tables. Radiother Oncol 1995;35:25–26
26. Collaborative Ocular Melanoma Study Group. Histopathologic characteristics of uveal melanomas in eyes enucleated from Collaborative Ocular Melanoma Study: COMS Report No. 6. Am J Ophthalmol 1998;125:745–766
27. Dieckmann K, Georg D, Zehetmayer M, Bogner J, Georgopoulos M, Potter R. Linac-based stereotactic radiotherapy of uveal melanoma: 4 years clinical experience. Radiother Oncol 2003;67:199–206
28. Kim MK, Char DH, Castro JL, et al. Neovascular glaucoma after helium ion irradiation for uveal melanoma. Ophthalmology 1986;93:189–193
29. Park SS, Walsh SM, Gragoudas ES. Visual field deficits associated with proton beam irradiation for parapapillary chorioidal melanoma. Ophthalmology 1996;103:110–116
30. Saornil MA, Egan KM, Gragoudas ES, Seddon JM, Walsh SM, Albert DM. Histopathology of proton beam-irradiated vs enucleated uveal melanomas. Arch Ophthalmol 1992;110:1112–1118
31. Egan KM, Gragoudas ES, Seddon JM, et al. The risk of enucleation after proton beam irradiation for uveal melanoma. Ophthalmology 1989;96:1377–1383
32. Castro JR, Char D, Petti P, et al. Fifteen years' experience with helium ion radiotherapy for uveal melanoma. Int J Radiat Oncol Biol Phys 1997;39:989–996
33. Char DH, Kroll SM, Castro J. Ten-year follow-up of helium ion therapy for uveal melanoma. Am J Ophthalmol 1998;125:81–89
34. Char DH, Quivey JM, Castro JR, et al. Helium ions versus iodine 125 brachytherapy in the management of uveal melanoma: a prospective, randomized, dynamically balanced trial. Ophthalmology 1993;100: 1547–1554
35. Wilson MW, Hungerford JL. Comparison of episcleral plaque and proton beam radiation therapy for the treatment of choroidal melanoma. Ophthalmology 1999;106:1579–1587
36. Damato BE, Paul J, Foulds WS. Risk factors for residual and recurrent uveal melanoma after trans-scleral local resection. Br J Ophthalmol 1996;80:102–108
37. The Collaborative Ocular Melanoma Study (COMS). Randomized trial of I-125 brachytherapy for medium chorioideal melanoma, III: Initial mortality findings. COMS report. Arch Ophthalmol 2001;119: 969–982
38. Egger E, Zografos L, Giotein G. Proton beam irradiation of choroidal melanoma: techniques and results. In: Sagerman RH, Alberti WE, eds. Radiotherapy of Intraocular and Orbital Tumors. 2nd rev. ed. Berlin: Springer-Verlag; 2003:67–80
39. Fine SL, Straatsma BR, Earle JD, Hawkins BS, McLaughlin JA. Failure of preenucleation radiation to decrease uveal melanoma mortality: the Collaborative Ocular Melanoma Study Steering Committee. Am J Ophthalmol 1989;107(4):440–442
40. Finger PT, Berson A, Syechter A. Palladium-103 plaque radiotherapy for choroidal melanoma: an 11-year study. Int J Radiat Oncol Biol Phys 2002;54(5):1438–1445
41. Finger PT. Radiation therapy for choroidal melanoma (therapeutic review). Surv Ophthalmol 1997;42:215–232
42. Fontanesi J, Meyer D, Xu S, Tai D. Treatment of choroidal melanoma with I-125 plaque. Int J Radiat Oncol Biol Phys 1993;26:619–623
43. Gragoudas ES, Seddon JM, Egan K. A randomized controlled trial of varying radiation doses in the treatment of choroidal melanoma. Arch Ophthalmol 2000;118:773–778
44. Karvat A, Duzenli C, Ma R, Paton K, Pickles T. The treatment of choroidal melanoma with 198 Au plaque brachytherapy. Radiother Oncol 2001;59:153–156
45. Nag S, Quivey JM, Earle JD. The American Brachytherapy Society recommendations for brachytherapy of uveal melanomas. Int J Radiat Oncol Biol Phys 2003;56(2):544–555
46. De Potter P, Shields CL, Shields JA, Cater JR, Brady LW. Plaque radiotherapy for juxtapapillary choroidal melanoma: visual acuity and survival outcome. Arch Ophthalmol 1996;114:1357–1365
47. Potter R, Janssen K, Prott FJ, et al. Ruthenium106 eye plaque brachytherapy in the conservative treatment of uveal melanoma: evaluation of 175 patients treated with 150 Gy from 1981 to 1989. Front Radiat Ther Oncol 1997;30:143–149
48. Straatsma BR, Fine SL, Earley JD, et al. Enucleation versus plaque irradiation for choroidal melanoma. Ophthalmology 1988;95:1000–1004
49. Bergman L, Nilsson B, Lundell G, Lundell M, Seregard S. Ruthenium brachytherapy for uveal melanoma, 1979–2003: survival and functional outcomes in the Swedish population. Ophthalmology 2005;112(5):834–840
50. Shields CL, Shields JA, Gunduz K, Freire JE, Mercado GL. Radiation therapy for uveal malignant melanoma. Ophthalmic Surg Lasers 1998;29:397–409
51. Diener-West M, Hawkins BS, Markowitz JA, Schachat AP. A review of mortality from choroidal melanoma, II: A metaanalysis of 5-year mortality rates following enucleation,1966 through 1988. Arch Ophthalmol (Paris) 1992;110:245–250
52. Shields JA, Shields CL. Current management of posterior uveal melanoma. Mayo Clin Proc 1993;68:1196–1200
53. Blurton AF, De La Garza A, McCoy T, Ekstrand K, Greven C, Greven K. Visual outcomes and eye preservation after iodine-125 brachytherapy for uveal melanoma. Int J Radiat Oncol Biol Phys 2005;63: S159–S167
54. Damato B, Patel I, Campbell IR, Mayles HM, Errington RD. Local tumor control after ^{106}Ru brachytherapy of choroidal melanoma. Int J Radiat Oncol Biol Phys 2005;63(2):385–391
55. Alfonso A. Relationship of structural and functional measurements. In: Weinreb RN, Kitazawa Y, Kriegelstein GK, eds. Glaucoma in the 21st Century. London: Mosby International Ltd; 2000:57–65

56. Fuchs J, Nissen KR, Goldschmidt E. Glaucoma blindness in Denmark. Acta Ophthalmol (Copenh) 1992;70:73–78

57. Harwerth RS, Carter-Dawson L, Shen F, Smith EL, Crawford ML. Ganglion cell losses underlying visual field defects from experimental glaucoma. Invest Ophthalmol Vis Sci 1999;40:2242–2250

58. Langham ME, Farrel R, Krakau T, Silver D. Ocular pulsatile blood flow, hypotensive drugs, and differential light sensitivity in glaucoma. In: Krieglstein GK, ed. Glaucoma Update IV by GK Krieglstein. Berlin: Springer-Verlag; 1991:162–172

59. Vladyka V, Liščák R, Šubrt O, et al. Initial experience with Gamma Knife radiosurgery for advanced glaucoma. J Neurosurg 2000;93:180–183

60. Vladyka V, Liščák R, Šimonová G, Pilbauer J, Hejduková I, Nováček L. Progress in glaucoma treatment research: a nonrandomized prospective study of 102 patients with advanced refractory glaucoma treated by Leksell Gamma Knife irradiation. J Neurosurg 2005;102(Suppl):214–219

61. Brigatti L, Caprioli J. Correlation of visual field with scanning confocal laser optic disc measurements in glaucoma. Arch Ophthal 1995; 113(9):1191–1194

62. Burk RO, Rohrschneider K, Takamoto T, Volcker HE, Schwartz B. Laser scanning tomography and stereophotogrammetry in three-dimensional optic disc analysis. Graefes Arch Clin Exp Ophthalmol 1993;231(4):193–198

63. Chauhan BC, Blanchard JW, Hamilton DC. Technique for detecting serial topographic changes in the optic disc and peripapillary retina using scanning laser tomography. Invest Ophthalmol Vis Sci 2000; 41:775–782

64. Greenfield DS. Optic nerve and retinal nerve fiber layer analyzers in glaucoma. Curr Opin Ophthalmol 2002;13:68–76

65. Mardin CY, Junemann AG. The diagnostic value of optic nerve imaging in early glaucoma. Curr Opin Ophthalmol 2001;12(2):100–104

66. Bergink GJ, Deutman AF, van den Broek JF. Radiation therapy for subfoveal choroidal neovascular membranes in age-related macular degeneration: a pilot study. Graefes Arch Clin Exp Ophthalmol 1994;232(10):591–598

67. Bergink GJ, Deutman AF, van den Broek JE, van Daal WA, van der Maazen RM. Radiation therapy for age-related subfoveal choroidal neovascular membranes: a pilot study. Doc Ophthalmol 1995;90(1):67–74

68. Berkow JW, Flower RW, Orth DH, Kelley JS. Fluorescein and Indocyanine Green Angiography. 2nd ed. San Francisco: American Academy of Ophthalmology; 1997:7

69. Berson AM, Finger PT, Sherr DL, Emery R, Alfieri AA, Bosworth JL. Radiotherapy for age-related macular degeneration: preliminary results of a potentially new treatment. Int J Radiat Oncol Biol Phys 1996; 36(4):861–865

70. Valmaggia C, Ries G, Ballinari P. Radiotherapy for subfoveal choroidal neovascularization in age-related macular degeneration: a randomized clinical trial. Am J Ophthalmol 2002;133(4):521–529

71. Finger PT, Berson A, Ng T, Szechter A. Ophthalmic plaque radiotherapy for age-related macular degeneration associated with subretinal neovascularization. Am J Ophthalmol 1999;127(2):170–177

72. Weinberger AW, Wolf S, Kube T. Radiation therapy of occult choroidal neovascularisation (CNV) in age-related macular degeneration (AMD). Klin Monatsbl Augenheilkd 1999;214(2):96–99

73. Archer DB, Amoaku WM, Gardiner TA. Radiation retinopathy—clinical, histopathological, ultrastructural and experimental correlations. Eye 1991;5(2):239–251

74. Chakravarthy U, Houston RF, Archer DB. Treatment of age-related subfoveal neovascular membranes by teletherapy: a pilot study. Br J Ophthalmol 1993;77(5):265–273

75. Haas A, Papaefthymiou G, Langmann G, et al. Gamma Knife treatment of subfoveal, classic neovascularization in age-related macular degeneration: a pilot study. J Neurosurg 2000;93(Suppl 3):172–176

76. Spaide RF, Guyer DR, McCormick B, et al. External beam radiation therapy for choroidal neovascularization. Ophthalmology 1998; 105(1):24–30

77. Henderson MA, Valluri S, Lo SS, et al. Gamma Knife radiosurgery in the treatment of choroidal neovascularizattion (wet-type macular degeneration). Stereotact Funct Neurosurg 2007;85:11–17

78. Bloch RS, Gartner S. The incidence of ocular metastatic carcinoma. Arch Ophthalmol 1971;85:673–675

79. Rudoler SB, Corn BW, Shields CL, et al. External beam irradiation for chorioid metastases: identification of factors predisposing to long-term sequelae. Int J Radiat Oncol Biol Phys 1997;38(2):251–256

18

Stereotactic Radiosurgery for Gliomas

Gregory J. A. Murad and William A. Friedman

The management of patients diagnosed with gliomas is wide ranging. Depending on the primary pathology of the tumor, a combination of surgical resection, therapeutic radiation, and chemotherapy can be used for treatment.[1–6] With the advent of radiosurgery, neuro-oncologists have another tool to accurately and safely treat intracranial pathology. Unlike conventional radiotherapy, stereotactic radiosurgery allows for very high doses of radiation to be delivered to a small volume of tissue with very little dose to surrounding tissue. This feature makes it ideal for any lesion that is readily discernible from normal structures on imaging; thus, the majority of experience has been with extra-axial lesions, such as meningiomas,[7] acoustic neuromas,[8] and pituitary tumors,[9] or with intra-axial lesions that have readily discernible structures, such as arteriovenous malformations.[10] The only intra-axial tumors that have been extensively treated with stereotactic radiosurgery are brain metastases. Metastases are different from gliomas in that they are usually distinct, contrast-enhancing lesions that are much less likely to infiltrate surrounding brain tissue.[11] Stereotactic radiosurgery also allows for doses of radiation that make radiosensitivity of tumors much less of an issue. Gliomas are by nature more infiltrative and are more difficult to target as separate from normal brain; thus, stereotactic radiosurgery for these lesions would not seem optimal. However, in the case of malignant gliomas, not only is radiation therapy the most effective management tool, but overall survival appears to be correlated with the total dose delivered, up to a total dose of 60 Gy.[12,13] Also, the majority of tumor recurrences occur within 2 cm of the enhancing margin of the original tumor, leading to the theory that increasing dose to this area may allow for higher local dose of radiation, and improve survival and progression-free survival.[14,15] This realization led to the initial interest in and use of interstitial brachytherapy for the treatment of malignant gliomas.[16] In this technique, radioisotopes, usually iodine 125, are implanted directly into the tumor cavity after resection to provide maximum radiation dose to the surrounding tissue. Early evidence in the 1990s appeared to show that brachytherapy increased survival rates in patients with brain tumors.[16] However, since that time, three separate clinical trials, most recently in 2007, have shown no evidence of a survival benefit but an increased risk of radiation necrosis, toxicity, and reoperations,[17–19] and it became clear that selection bias led to the erroneous conclusion that brachytherapy had a positive treatment effect. Despite the hazards of selection bias, several reports describe the use of radiosurgery in the treatment of glial neoplasms. In this chapter we review this experience, by pathologic category.

◆ Anaplastic Astrocytomas and Glioblastomas

Most of the reported experience with stereotactic radiosurgery to treat gliomas has been for patients with these tumors. In the 1990s, some reports appeared to show good efficacy and increased survival benefit with the use of stereotactic radiosurgery at the time of surgical resection in conjunction with conventional radiotherapy and chemotherapy[20–49] (**Table 18.1**). Similar to the experience with brachytherapy, selection bias is likely to have been the driving force behind the apparent efficacy of stereotactic radiosurgery in these early reviews.[50] In an attempt to address the problem of selection bias, the Radiation Therapy Oncology Group (RTOG) 93–05 protocol was established for a randomized comparison of stereotactic radiosurgery followed by conventional radiotherapy and carmustine (BCNU) chemotherapy versus conventional radiotherapy and BCNU chemotherapy alone.[43] A total of 203 patients with supratentorial glioblastoma multiforme (GBM) < 40 mm were randomized to receive stereotactic radiosurgery plus radiotherapy (60 Gy) and BCNU or radiotherapy and BCNU alone (**Fig. 18.1**). Stereotactic radiosurgery dose ranged from 15 to 24 Gy depending on the tumor size. At a median

Table 18.1 Radiosurgery for Malignant Glioma

Study	Form of Radiosurgery	Timing of SRS	No. of Cases Analyzed (GBM/AA)	Prescription Dose (Gy)	Median Survival (GBM/AA) (months)
Loeffler et al[20]	Linac	Initial	23/14	12–15	26/not reached
Chamberlain et al[22]	Linac	Recurrent	5/14	12–15	8 (not broken down)
Masciopinto et al[25]	Linac	Initial	31/0	12.0–18.75	9.5
Hall et al[27]	Linac	Recurrent	26/9	20	18/24
Sarkaria et al[28]	Linac	Initial	96/19	6–20	21.8/not reached
Larson et al[30]	GK	Initial and recurrent	97/43	5.0–37.5	13/21
Kondziolka et al[32]	GK	Initial and recurrent	64/43	15.5	26/32
Shrieve at al[34]	Linac	Initial	78/0	6–24	19.9
Sanghavi et al[35]	Linac	Recurrent	20/10	10–20	7/11
Nwokedi et al[36]	GK	Initial	31/0	17.1	25
Wang et al[38]	Linac	Initial	30/28	19.4	13/22.5
Cho et al[41]	Linac	Initial	14/0	15–24	16
Souhami et al[43]	Linac and GK	Initial	89/0	15–24	13.5
Mahajan et al[45]	Linac	Recurrent	41/0	Not reported	26
Ulm et al[46]	Linac	Initial and recurrent	74/26	15	16.2 (not broken down)
Hsieh at al[47]	GK	Initial and recurrent	51/0	12	14.3
Combs et al[48]	GK	Recurrent	32/0	15	22
Yoshikawa et al[49]	Linac	Initial	18/7	20.3	20.7/not reached

Abbreviations: AA, anaplastic astrocytoma; GBM, glioblastoma multiforme; GK, Gamma Knife; linac, linear accelerator; SRS, stereotactic radiosurgery.

follow-up of 61 months, patients in the stereotactic radiosurgery group had a median survival time of 13.5 months versus 13.6 months in the conventional treatment group. The data were also analyzed to see if there was a tail effect, leading to more long-term survivors, but 2- and 3-year survival rates were not significantly different. Recurrence patterns, cognitive decline, quality of life, and type of stereotactic radiosurgery used (Gamma Knife [Elekta Instruments AB, Stockholm, Sweden] versus linear accelerator [linac]) were also analyzed, but the groups did not have significant differences in these areas. The results of this trial proved that upfront stereotactic radiosurgery is not of benefit for patient survival or quality of life, and prior reports of efficacy were likely due to selection bias.

Subsequently, in 2005, the American Society for Therapeutic Radiology and Oncology (ASTRO) published an evidence-based review of the role of stereotactic radiosurgery for malignant glioma.[44] In this review, the previously mentioned randomized trial was reviewed, along with five prospective[20,21,23,29,31] and seven retrospective studies.[26,28,30,33,34,36,37] These studies did not have significant improvement in survival, quality of life, or tumor progression. Toxicity did not appear to be increased as a result of the therapy. Overall, there was no evidence that stereotactic radiosurgery was of benefit as an upfront treatment. A second portion of the review concentrated on stereotactic radiosurgery as salvage therapy for recurrent or progressive malignant gliomas. There have been no randomized trials to address this issue.

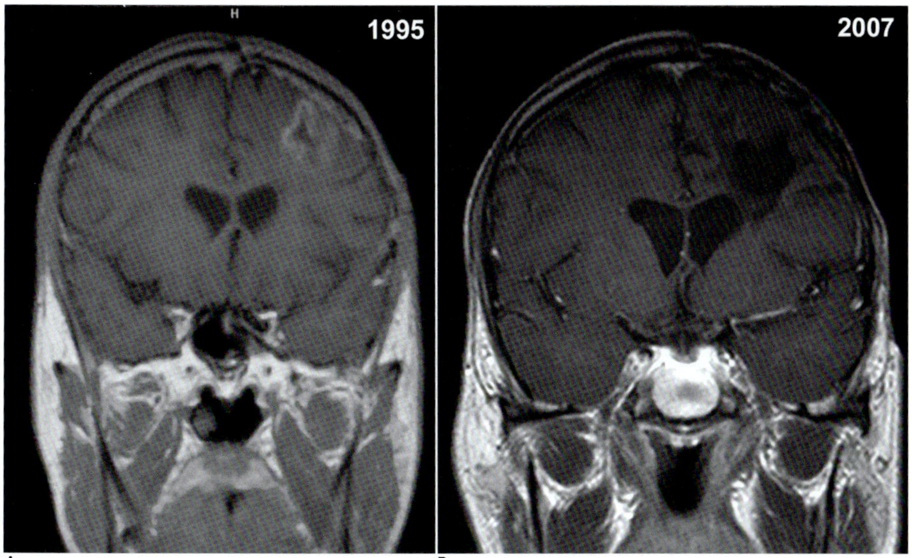

Fig. 18.1 **(A)** A 39-year-old man following resection of a left frontal glioblastoma multiforme in April 1994, followed by external radiation, hydrea, and procarbazine, lomustine, and vincristine (PCV) chemotherapy. He underwent radiosurgical boost of 1000 Gy to the tumor bed in March 1995. **(B)** Magnetic resonance imaging from September 2007 shows complete resolution of the enhancing tumor and moderate encephalomalacic defect.

There were three prospective[22,27,39] and four retrospective[24,30,35,40] studies that tried to assess it. These studies did not demonstrate a survival benefit for stereotactic radiosurgery, and none of them addressed quality of life issues. Recurrence patterns on these patients also did not change. As a result, stereotactic radiosurgery was not recommended as a salvage treatment.

Multiple other retrospective studies have been published on the subject of stereotactic radiosurgery for malignant gliomas. The University of Florida experience[46] with linac stereotactic radiosurgery for malignant gliomas, which was updated in 2005, reviewed a total of 100 patients. These patients were then compared with historical controls from the RTOG's recursive portioning categories, in an attempt to eliminate selection bias. Sixty-seven of these patients received upfront stereotactic radiosurgery. The remainder had stereotactic radiosurgery as a treatment boost at the time of recurrence or progression. Overall, survival rates were similar to historical controls except in those patients in recursive partitioning analysis (RPA) class V, where the median survival time was 15.6 months for the stereotactic radiosurgery group versus 8.9 months for the historical control. Of course, this study was limited by selection bias, as it was a retrospective review. Hsieh et al[47] published results of 51 patients treated with Gamma Knife stereotactic radiosurgery either upfront (25 patients) or at the time of progression (26 patients). They found that those patients treated at the time of progression had increased survival time (16.7 months vs 10 months), but this did not reach statistical significance ($p = .09$). The authors concluded, however, that there was likely a benefit to stereotactic radiosurgery for patients treated at the time of recurrence. Combs et al[48] published their results for linac salvage treatment without adjuvant chemotherapy in 32 patients with GBM. The median interval from primary treatment to stereotactic radiosurgery was 10 months, and the median overall survival time after stereotactic radiosurgery was 10 months. Progression-free survival time was 7 months. This review compared these results to those of chemotherapy alone, with a mean survival time of 5 months. Again, this study was likely limited by selection bias of those patients who had already survived with continued good neurologic function.

Overall, stereotactic radiosurgery appears to be another treatment option for malignant gliomas, but further randomized, controlled studies of stereotactic radiosurgery at the time of recurrence of these tumors are indicated to answer the question of whether or not there is benefit to stereotactic radiosurgery. As is clear from RTOG 93–05, upfront stereotactic radiosurgery is not of benefit and cannot be recommended as a treatment option at this time. The safety of stereotactic radiosurgery has also not been proven. Lesion enlargement after stereotactic radiosurgery can be due to tumor recurrence, radiation necrosis, or both. Without tissue diagnosis, it is impossible to determine the true incidence of symptomatic radiation necrosis. It is likely that radionecrosis is underreported.

◆ Low-Grade Gliomas

Low-grade gliomas include pilocytic astrocytomas, grade II astrocytomas, oligoastrocytomas, oligodendrogliomas, and, less commonly, glial neoplasms, such as pleomorphic xanthoastrocytoma, ganglioglioma, and subependymoma. Of these tumors, pilocytic astrocytoma and grade II astrocytoma have been most frequently treated with stereotactic radiosurgery. These two tumor types are somewhat distinct in terms of their clinical course. Pilocytic astrocytomas are most common in pediatric patients, are often surgically curable with total resection, and behave in a slow-growing, nonaggressive fashion. Ten-year survival rates for pilocytic astrocytomas are up to 94%. The location of these tumors in unresectable areas such as the hypothalamus, thalamus, optic tract, pons, and cerebellar peduncle can, however, make other treatment options more attractive (**Fig. 18.2**).[4] Grade II astrocytomas are more likely to occur in young adults and

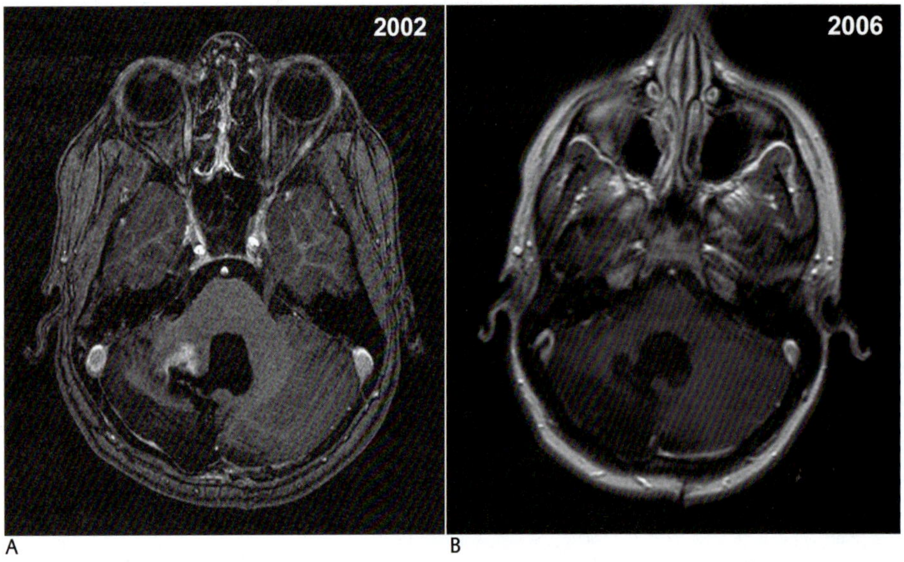

Fig. 18.2 **(A)** A 13-year-old female patient status postresection of pilocytic astrocytoma in January 2002, with recurrence on imaging that enlarged over 6 months postoperatively. **(B)** The patient was treated with 1500 Gy to the 70% isodose line in December 2002 and has no residual effect evident on follow-up in August 2006.

Table 18.2 Radiosurgery for Low-Grade Gliomas

Study	Form of Radiosurgery	Timing of SRS	No. of Cases Analyzed (Pilocytic/Grade II)	Prescription Dose	Median Survival
Grabb et al[51]	GK	Initial and recurrent	8/5	15.2	Not reached (all alive at 6–48 months)
Somaza et al[52]	GK	Recurrent	9/0	15	Not reached (all alive at 13–41 months)
Kida et al[53]	GK	Recurrent	12/39	12.5/15.7	27.6 months, 91% tumor control
Hadjipanayis et al[54]	GK	Initial and recurrent	37/0	15	Not reached, 59 months f-up
Boëthius et al[55]	GK	Initial and recurrent	19/0	9–20	18/19 progression free at 5.9 years
Hadjipanayis et al[56]	GK	Initial and recurrent	0/12	16	8/12 no growth at 52 months
Giller at al[58]	Linac	Recurrent	3	18.8	No growth at 17 months
Heppner at al[59]	GK	Initial and recurrent	21/28	15	44-month PFS, no growth in 37/49
Szeifert et al[60]	GK	Initial and recurrent	15/17	12.6/13.4	All grade 1 alive at 28.8 months, 16/17 grade 2 at 33.4 months

Abbreviations: f-up, follow-up; GK, Gamma Knife; linac, linear accelerator; PFS, progression-free survival; SRS, stereotactic radiosurgery.

have a more aggressive course, with recurrence and malignant transformation leading to a median survival time of 7 to 10 years. These lesions can also have focal areas that are difficult to access with open surgery.[2,3] Treatment of these tumor types with stereotactic radiosurgery has largely been for residual lesions after resection or biopsy or for focal areas of nodular recurrence.

There are no randomized trials of stereotactic radiosurgery for low-grade gliomas, but there are some retrospective reviews of patients who were treated with stereotactic radiosurgery as part of a multimodality approach (**Table 18.2**).[40,51–61] Kida et al[53] reported on 51 patients treated over an 8-year period. Twelve patients had pilocytic astrocytomas, and 39 had grade II astrocytomas. Of those with pilocytic tumors, after a mean follow-up of 25 months, one patient had complete radiographic resolution of tumor, five had partial reduction in volume, one was slightly reduced in volume, four were unchanged, and one increased in size, for a control rate of 91.7%. For grade II lesions, at a mean of 28.5 months, 5 had complete resolution, 13 had partial reduction, 6 had slight reduction, 10 were unchanged, and 5 increased in size, for a control rate of 87.2%. Forty-one percent of these patients developed radiation edema, and half of these required 2 to 3 months of steroid medication for symptom management. There did not appear to be any long-term complications.

Hadjipanayis et al[57] reported on 49 patients treated with Gamma Knife stereotactic radiosurgery over a 13-year period. Thirty-seven patients had pilocytic astrocytomas, and 12 had grade II astrocytomas. All diagnoses were confirmed with tissue sampling. Of those treated, 11 had complete tumor resolution, 12 had reduced tumor volume, 10 had stable tumor volume, and 16 had progression. At a median of 32 months after stereotactic radiosurgery and 63 months after diagnosis, 45 of 49 patients were alive, with 3 deaths due to tumor progression. Heppner at al[59] reported on Gamma Knife stereotactic radiosurgery for low-grade gliomas in 49 patients over a 13-year period. Pathology included 21 pilocytic tumors, 2 subependymal giant cell astrocytomas (grade II), and 26 grade II astrocytomas. Mean clinical follow-up was 63 months, and mean imaging follow-up was 59 months. Mean clinical progression-free survival period was 44 months, with radiologic progression-free survival period of 37 months. At final follow-up, 37 of 49 patients had either stable or decreased tumor volume, and 7 patients died due to tumor progression. Four patients developed radiation-associated complications, one of which was permanent and required urgent reoperation due to mass effect.

Overall, these studies appear to provide some early evidence for tumor control in low-grade gliomas. The incidence of complications for these reviews is subject to some skepticism, as it is often difficult to assess tumor regrowth versus radiation effects. Also, the indolent nature of many of these tumors makes evidence of local control hard to assess, as most of these reviews have limited follow-up. Making generalizable conclusions about treating these tumors is difficult, as these studies are limited by selection bias, small patient numbers, combining different pathologies, and relatively short patient follow-up times.

◆ Ependymomas

Ependymomas represent a small percentage of intracranial glial tumors. These tumors are more common in the pediatric population and often occur in the posterior fossa. Currently, therapeutic options for ependymoma include surgical resection followed by external beam radiation therapy (EBRT) for localized disease. Residual tumor remaining after surgery and distant central nervous system (CNS) spread of disease have been shown to be poor prognostic factors.[5] For these lesions, there are no randomized trials of the use of stereotactic radiosurgery. However, there do exist some small case series of patients treated with stereotactic radiosurgery boost at the time of initial radiotherapy or for recurrent disease (**Fig. 18.3**)[62–70] (**Table 18.3**). Jawahar et al[63] reported on 22 patients with progressive anaplastic ependymomas treated with Gamma Knife stereotactic radiosurgery. At a median follow-up of 21 months, 16 of the patients had stable or decreased disease volume. The median survival time after

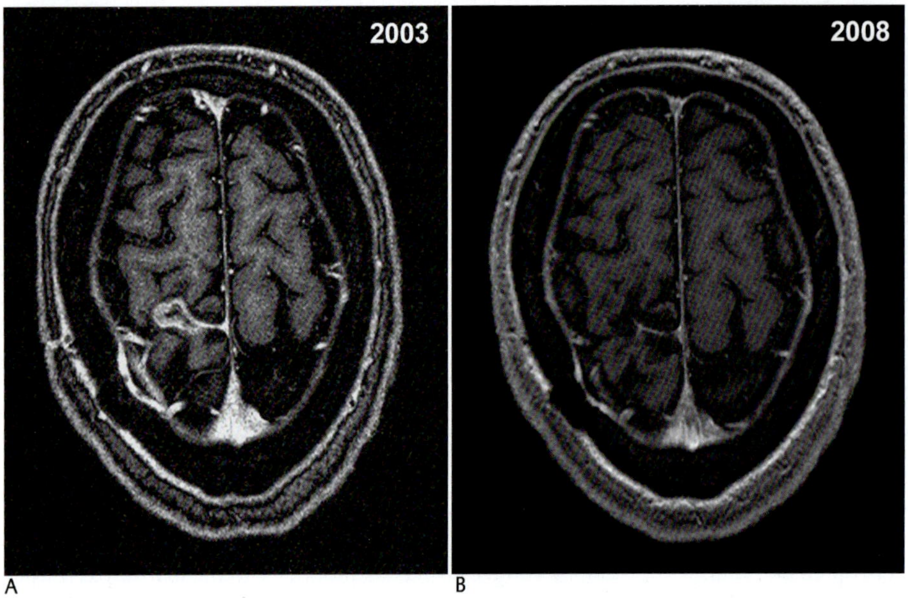

Fig. 18.3 **(A)** A 60-year-old man following resection of an ependymoma in June 2003, followed by stereotactic radiosurgery of 1500 Gy to the 70% isodose line to the above residual in September 2003. **(B)** The patient received no other treatment except for stereotactic radiosurgery and had complete resolution of the enhancing tumor at the time of the last follow-up examination in May 2008.

stereotactic radiosurgery was 2.2 years, and the median overall survival time from diagnosis was 10.1 years. There were no complications. Stafford et al[64] reported on 12 patients with a total of 17 recurrent ependymomas. Eleven of the patients had undergone surgery followed by EBRT, and one had undergone surgery alone. After a median imaging follow-up of 22.5 months, in-field local control was maintained in 14 of 17 patients, and the median survival time was 3.4 years. One patient developed radiation-induced complications. Hodgson et al[65] reported on 90 patients treated with stereotactic radiosurgery for multiple different tumors, of which 28 were ependymomas. Median follow-up for all patients was 24 months. Progression-free survival for the ependymoma group was 8.5 months, and the 3-year actuarial control rate was 29%. There were 19 complications, but these were not broken down by histology. Mansur et al[66] reported on nine ependymomas treated with Gamma Knife and linac stereotactic radiosurgery. Two patients had grade III lesions, and seven patients had grade II lesions. Eight of the patients received prior radiotherapy. Median follow-up was 28 months, and median age at treatment was 35 years. Four patients (44%) developed progressive disease, and two died due to progressive disease. Four patients had stereotactic radiosurgery as an initial treatment. All of these patients were progression free. Of the five remaining patients, four were treated at recurrence and subsequently had radiographic disease progression. Lo et al[70] reported on eight patients with a total of 13 lesions. Of these, five were treated for recurrence, two were treated for gross residual disease after surgery and EBRT, and one (age 1.3 years) was treated with stereotactic radiosurgery alone. Of the lesions, the 1-year actuarial in-field control rate was 76.2%, with a 3-year control rate of 61%. Overall survival was 75% at a median of 30 months, with a 50% progression-free survival rate. The two patients treated with radiosurgical boost were both alive without disease progression at 39 and 65 months.

These case series show that stereotactic radiosurgery can be used as an adjunct to radiotherapy, both in the initial treatment of ependymoma and at recurrence. Efficacy and safety are still debatable without any randomized trials. Complication rates in these series are hard to assess in the setting of possible recurrent tumor. Similar to the previous tumor types, the retrospective nature of the data available, the small numbers of patients, and selection bias make

Table 18.3 Radiosurgery for Ependymoma

Study	Form of Radiosurgery	Timing of SRS	No. of Cases Analyzed	Prescription Dose (Gy)	Outcomes
Aggarwal et al[62]	Linac	Initial and recurrent	5	10	15- to 40-month f-up with 1 patient w/progressive disease
Jawahar et al[63]	GK	Progressive	22	16.1	Survival 2.2 years post-SRS, 10.1 years overall
Stafford et al[64]	GK	Recurrent	12	18	3.4-year survival, 68% local control at 3 years
Hodgson et al[65]	Linac	Initial and recurrent	28	12.5	PFS 8.5 months, 29% 3-year actuarial survival
Mansur et al[66]	GK/linac	Initial and recurrent	9	16.1	3-year survival 71% (100% initial, 20% recurrent)
Lo et al[69]	GK	Initial and recurrent	8	14	3-year survival 75% (100% for 2 patients treated as boost therapy)

Abbreviations: GK, Gamma Knife; linac, linear accelerator; PFS, progression-free survival; SRS, stereotactic radiosurgery.

drawing real conclusions from these reports difficult. Still, because of some specific reports of tumor control in those patients treated upfront with stereotactic radiosurgery, further investigation of this technique as a boost treatment at the time of initial radiotherapy to provide better long-term tumor control may be warranted.

Brainstem Gliomas

Brainstem gliomas are a heterogeneous population of tumors. These lesions range from highly aggressive and infiltrative to focal and indolent. Their location by definition makes them difficult to access surgically in a safe manner. Focal lesions are often treated with a combination of open surgical resection (although most often subtotal), biopsy, or imaging follow-up with possible radiotherapy.[6] Stereotactic radiosurgery has been investigated as an alternative for primary treatment as well as an adjunct for residual disease after surgery. There have been no controlled trials of this technology for these lesions, but multiple small case series do appear to show that stereotactic radiosurgery is safe and at least fairly effective for brainstem lesions[71–75] (**Table 18.4**). Unfortunately, some of these series are contaminated by the fact that pathologic tissue is not available for all of the tumors, making generalization of their treatment outcomes impossible.

Kihlström et al[71] reported on seven patients treated with Gamma Knife stereotactic radiosurgery for tectal tumors. These tumors were all proven by biopsy to be low-grade astrocytomas. After a median follow-up of 6.9 years, four tumors disappeared, two remained the same, and one progressed. Clinically, four patients improved, and one worsened. Fuchs et al[73] reported on 21 patients with tumors of the midbrain, pons, and medulla who were treated with stereotactic radiosurgery. All tumors were histologically verified, with 12 low-grade gliomas and 9 high-grade tumors. After a mean follow-up of 41 months for the low-grade tumors, six tumors had decreased in size, five were unchanged, and one was larger. Clinically, four patients improved, two worsened, and three died during the follow-up period. In the high-grade group, eight patients had follow-up. Three patients with glioblastomas died after a median of 5.5 months, three with anaplastic astrocytomas died after a median of 28 months, and the remaining three with anaplastic pathology were alive after a median of 74 months. Yen et al[75] reported on 20 patients with tumors of the midbrain, pons, and medulla. Ten of these patients had histologic diagnosis, five of pilocytic tumor and five of low-grade astrocytoma. After a median follow-up of 78 months, these patients had 4 tumors disappear, 12 regress, and 4 increase in size. Clinically, eight patients improved, three worsened, and one died over the follow-up period. One patient had transient radiation-induced complications.

These results appear to be in keeping with those of the prior reviews of stereotactic radiosurgery for glial tumors. Stereotactic radiosurgery is a safe technology that appears to have a low risk of acute complications and evidence of some benefit in a retrospective review. Again, the limiting factors for these studies are their retrospective nature, patient selection, and limited numbers of patients, as well as the mixed pathologies for which stereotactic radiosurgery was applied.

Medulloblastomas

Medulloblastomas are the most common form of pediatric brain tumor and are highly malignant. Most are located in the posterior fossa, and there is a 2:1 male predominance. Survival for these lesions is as low as 50%, but newer treatment methods with radiotherapy, high-dose chemotherapy, and stem cell rescue have led to 5-year survival rates as high as 80%.[76] Adult medulloblastoma appears to be a somewhat different pathologic entity, although most treatment is in keeping with pediatric tumor protocols. Newer data with results of pediatric treatments for adult patients show 5-year survival rates of up to 80%, although 10-year survival rates drop to 40 to 50%.[77,78] Medulloblastomas have a higher propensity to metastasize throughout the CNS than do other glial tumors. Focal recurrences outside the radiation treatment field are common. Stereotactic radiosurgery was originally suggested as a treatment option in 1993[79] in the hopes of lowering total radiation dose and subsequent radiation-induced complications, and has since been reported as an adjunct for nodular residual, recurrent, or metastatic disease[80–85] (**Table 18.5**). Patrice et al[81] reported on 14 pediatric patients with medulloblastomas treated with stereotactic radiosurgery. Three patients underwent treatment with boost stereotactic radiosurgery for residual tumor after initial treatment, and all were alive at a median of 27 months after treatment. Eleven patients had treatment of recurrent disease. Six of these patients died, and overall survival from the time of treatment was a median of 10 months. Progressive disease occurred outside the treatment volume in all six of the patients who died, and there were two marginal recurrences. One patient developed acute complications, two developed transient complications, and

Table 18.4 Radiosurgery for Brainstem Gliomas

Study	Form of Radiosurgery	No. of Cases Analyzed	Prescription Dose (Gy)	F-up Period	Tumor Outcome
Kihlström et al[71]	GK	7	14–30	6.9 years	1/7 progressed
Fuchs et al[73]	GK	12	12	41 months	1/12 progressed
Yen et al[75]	GK	20	12.8	78 months	4/20 progressed

Abbreviations: f-up, follow-up; GK, Gamma Knife.

Table 18.5 Radiosurgery for Medulloblastomas

Study	Form of Radiosurgery	No. of Cases Analyzed	Prescription Dose (Gy)	F-up Period	Tumor Outcome
Patrice et al[81]	Linac	14	6–16	21 months	3 initial participants alive, 5/11 w/recurrence alive
Woo et al[82]	Linac	4	4.5–10.0	30 months	All alive w/o evidence of disease
Hodgson et al[65]	Linac	16	6–25	24 months	57% 3-year control
Milker-Zabel et al[84]	Linac	8	10–18	No reported	4 stable, 4 smaller after 3 months
Germanwala et al[83]	GK	12	11–25	72.4 months (from Dx)	5 w/o disease, 3 with stable disease, 4 progression (all died)

Abbreviations: Dx, diagnosis; f-up, follow-up; GK, Gamma Knife; linac, linear accelerator.

one had a cerebellar hemorrhage in the treatment field. Hodgson et al[65] reported on 16 pediatric patients treated with stereotactic radiosurgery. Median progression-free survival in these patients was 11 months, with a 57% 3-year local control rate. Six patients were treated with upfront stereotactic radiosurgery; of these, three were alive without progression at a mean of 47 months. More detailed information about all 16 patients was not reported, nor were specific complication rates. Woo et al[82] reported on four patients (two pediatric, two adult) treated with boost stereotactic radiosurgery after initial resection and radiotherapy. These patients were alive without progression of disease at 12 to 48 months. There were no complications aside from one episode of nausea and vomiting. One patient developed panhypopituitarism, although this was likely related to his prior conventional radiotherapy. Germanwala et al[83] reported on 12 adult patients treated with stereotactic radiosurgery. Six of the patients had posttreatment residual tumors, and six had recurrent disease, including distant metastases. Three patients had two stereotactic radiosurgery treatments, and three had three treatments. At a mean follow-up period of 72.4 months, five patients are alive without disease, three are alive with stable disease, and four had progressive disease, all of whom died. There were no acute radiation complications or delayed radionecrosis.

Stereotactic radiosurgery for medulloblastoma appears to have similar evidence for usage as in other glial tumors. All of the available data are of small numbers of patients and are retrospective in nature. There do not appear to be significant stereotactic radiosurgery–related complications, and some patients have regression of disease. Again, a randomized, controlled trial of stereotactic radiosurgery to decide optimal timing, dose, and treatment volume would likely shed much more light on the true safety and effectiveness of this treatment modality for these tumors.

◆ Summary

In conclusion, stereotactic radiosurgery for gliomas has not been rigorously proven to be effective. The only randomized, controlled trial of this technology in the treatment of glial tumors, as upfront treatment for glioblastomas, showed no benefit. Stereotactic radiosurgery as a treatment for recurrent malignant gliomas is of uncertain benefit, although a similar randomized, controlled trial is warranted to address this issue. The use of stereotactic radiosurgery for other glial tumors, including low-grade astrocytomas, ependymomas, brainstem gliomas, and medulloblastomas, has been shown in many retrospective reports to be of possible value. These reports, however, are very much limited by small numbers, selection bias, and short periods of follow-up. Finally, it is likely that complications from stereotactic radiosurgery are underreported due to the difficulty of differentiating progressive disease from radiation necrosis.

References

1. Stupp R, Hegi ME, Gilbert MR, Chakravarti A. Chemoradiotherapy in malignant glioma: standard of care and future directions. J Clin Oncol 2007;25(26):4127–4136
2. Grier JT, Batchelor T. Low-grade gliomas in adults. Oncologist 2006; 11(6):681–693
3. Norden AD, Wen PY. Glioma therapy in adults. Neurologist 2006; 12(6):279–292
4. Koeller KK, Rushing EJ. From the archives of the AFIP: pilocytic astrocytoma—radiologic-pathologic correlation. Radiographics 2004; 24(6):1693–1708
5. Jaing TH, Wang HS, Tsay PK, et al. Multivariate analysis of clinical prognostic factors in children with intracranial ependymomas. J Neurooncol 2004;68(3):255–261
6. Mauffrey C. Paediatric brainstem gliomas: prognostic factors and management. J Clin Neurosci 2006;13(4):431–437
7. Friedman WA, Murad GJ, Bradshaw P, et al. Linear accelerator surgery for meningiomas. J Neurosurg 2005;103(2):206–209
8. Chopra R, Kondziolka D, Niranjan A, Lunsford LD, Flickinger JC. Long-term follow-up of acoustic schwannoma radiosurgery with marginal tumor doses of 12 to 13 Gy. Int J Radiat Oncol Biol Phys 2007;68(3): 845–851
9. Zipfel GJ, Bradshaw P, Bova FJ, Friedman WA. Do the morphological characteristics of arteriovenous malformations affect the results of radiosurgery? J Neurosurg 2004;101(3):393–401
10. Sheehan JP, Niranjan A, Sheehan JM, et al. Stereotactic radiosurgery for pituitary adenomas: an intermediate review of its safety, efficacy, and role in the neurosurgical treatment armamentarium. J Neurosurg 2005;102(4):678–691
11. McDermott MW, Sneed PK. Radiosurgery in metastatic brain cancer. Neurosurgery 2005; 57(5, Suppl):S45–S53, discussion S1–S4
12. Walker MD, Strike TA, Sheline GE. Analysis of dose–effect relationship in the radiotherapy of malignant gliomas. Int J Radiat Oncol Biol Phys 1979;5(10):1725–1731
13. Bleehen NM, Stennings SP. A Medical Research Council trial of two radiotherapy doses in grades 3 and 4 astrocytoma: the Medical Research Council Brain Tumour Working Party. Br J Cancer 1991; 64(4):769–774
14. Hochberg FH, Pruitt A. Assumptions in the radiotherapy of glioblastoma. Neurology 1980;30(9):907–911
15. Wallner KE, Galicich JH, Krol G, Arbit E, Malkin MG. Patterns of failure following treatment for glioblastoma multiforme and anaplastic astrocytoma. Int J Radiat Oncol Biol Phys 1989;16(6):1405–1409

16. Vitaz TW, Warnke PC, Tabar V, Gutin PH. Brachytherapy for brain tumors. J Neurooncol 2005;73(1):71–86
17. Laperriere NJ, Leung PM, McKenzie S, et al. Randomized study of brachytherapy in the initial management of patients with malignant astrocytoma. Int J Radiat Oncol Biol Phys 1998;41(5):1005–1011
18. Selker RG, Shapiro WR, Burger P, et al. The Brain Tumor Cooperative Group NIH Trial 87-01: a randomized comparison of surgery, external radiotherapy, and carmustine versus surgery, interstitial radiotherapy boost, external radiation therapy, and carmustine. Neurosurgery 2002;51(2):343–355, discussion 355–357
19. Chen AM, Chang S, Pouliot J, et al. Phase I trial of gross total resection, permanent iodine-125 brachytherapy, and hyperfractionated radiotherapy for newly diagnosed glioblastoma multiforme. Int J Radiat Oncol Biol Phys 2007;69(3):825–830
20. Loeffler JS, Alexander E III, Shea WM, et al. Radiosurgery as part of the initial management of patients with malignant gliomas. J Clin Oncol 1992;10(9):1379–1385
21. Stea B, Rossman K, Kittelson J, et al. A comparison of survival between radiosurgery and stereotactic implants for malignant astrocytomas. Acta Neurochir Suppl (Wien) 1994;62:47–54
22. Chamberlain MC, Barba D, Kormanik P, Shea WM. Stereotactic radiosurgery for recurrent gliomas. Cancer 1994;74(4):1342–1347
23. Mehta MP, Masciopinto J, Rozental J, et al. Stereotactic radiosurgery for glioblastoma multiforme: report of a prospective study for evaluating prognostic factors and analyzing long-term survival advantage. Int J Radiat Oncol Biol Phys 1994;30(3):541–549
24. Shrieve DC, Alexander E III, Wen PY, et al. Comparison of stereotactic radiosurgery and brachytherapy in the treatment of recurrent glioblastoma multiforme. Neurosurgery 1995;36(2):275–282
25. Masciopinto JE, Levin AB, Mehta MP, Rhode BS. Stereotactic radiosurgery for glioblastoma: a final report of 31 patients. J Neurosurg 1995;82:530–535
26. Buatti JM, Friedman WA, Bova FJ, Mendenhall WM. Linac radiosurgery for high grade gliomas: the University of Florida experience. Int J Radiat Oncol Biol Phys 1995;32(1):205–210
27. Hall WA, Djalilian HR, Sperduto PW, et al. Stereotactic radiosurgery for recurrent malignant gliomas. J Clin Oncol 1995;13(7):1642–1648
28. Sarkaria JN, Mehta MP, Loeffler JS, et al. Radiosurgery in the initial management of malignant gliomas: survival comparison with the RTOG recursive partitioning analysis. Int J Radiat Oncol Biol Phys 1995;32(4):931–941
29. Gannett D, Stea B, Lulu B, Adair T, Verdi C, Hamilton A. Stereotactic radiosurgery as an adjunct to surgery and external beam radiotherapy in the treatment of patients with malignant gliomas. Int J Radiat Oncol Biol Phys 1995;33(2):461–468
30. Larson DA, Gutin PH, McDermott M, et al. Gamma Knife for glioma: selection factors and survival. Int J Radiat Oncol Biol Phys 1996;36(5): 1045–1053
31. Shenouda G, Souhami L, Podgorsak EB, et al. Radiosurgery and accelerated radiotherapy for patients with glioblastoma. Can J Neurol Sci 1997;24(2):110–115
32. Kondziolka D, Flickinger JC, Bissonette DJ, Bozik M, Lunsford LD. Survival benefit of stereotactic radiosurgery for patients with malignant glial neoplasms. Neurosurgery 1997;41(4):776–785
33. Selch MT, DeSalles AF, Goetsch SJ, et al. Single-fraction radiosurgery for primary and recurrent malignant gliomas. J Radiosurg. 1998;1(3): 155–168
34. Shrieve DC, Alexander E, Black P, et al. Treatment of patients with primary glioblastoma multiforme with standard postoperative radiotherapy and radiosurgical boost: prognostic factors and long-term outcome. J Neurosurg 1999;90:72–77
35. Sanghavi S, Skrupky R, Badie B, Robbins I, Tome W, Mehta MP. Recurrent malignant gliomas treated with radiosurgery. J Radiosurg. 1999;2(3):119–125
36. Nwokedi EC, Dibiase SJ, Jabbour S, Herman J, Amin P, Chin LS. Gamma Knife stereotactic radiosurgery for patients with glioblastoma multiforme. Neurosurgery 2002;50(1):41–46
37. Prisco FE, Weltman E, de Hanriot RM, Brandt RA. Radiosurgical boost for primary high-grade gliomas. J Neurooncol 2002;57(2):151–160
38. Wang YY, Bao XF, Li SY, Wu CY. Prognostic factors for deep situated malignant gliomas treated with linac radiosurgery. Ai Zheng 2002; 21(10):1149–1153
39. Larson DA, Prados M, Lamborn KR, et al. Phase II study of high central dose Gamma Knife radiosurgery and Marimistat in patients with recurrent malignant glioma. Int J Radiat Oncol Biol Phys 2002;54(5):1397–1404
40. Sarkar A, Pollock BE, Brown PD, Gorman DA. Evaluation of Gamma Knife radiosurgery in the treatment of oligodendrogliomas and mixed oligoastrocytomas. J Neurosurg 2002;97(5, Suppl):653–656
41. Cho KH, Hall WA, Lo SS, Dusenbery KE. Stereotactic radiosurgery versus fractionated stereotactic radiotherapy boost for patients with glioblastoma multiforme. Technol Cancer Res Treat 2004;3(1):41–49
42. Crowley RW, Pouratian N, Sheehan JP. Gamma Knife radiosurgery for glioblastoma multiforme. Neurosurg Focus 2006;20(4):E17:1–5
43. Souhami L, Seiferheld W, Brachman D, et al. Randomized comparison of stereotactic radiosurgery followed by conventional radiotherapy with carmustine to conventional radiotherapy with carmustine for patients with glioblastoma multiforme: report of Radiation Therapy Oncology Group 93-05 protocol. Int J Radiat Oncol Biol Phys 2004; 60(3):853–860
44. Tsao MN, Mehta MP, Whelan TJ, et al. The American Society for Therapeutic Radiology and Oncology (ASTRO) evidence-based review of the role of radiosurgery for malignant glioma. Int J Radiat Oncol Biol Phys 2005;63(1):47–55
45. Mahajan A, McCutcheon IE, Suki D, et al. Case-control study of stereotactic radiosurgery for glioblastoma multiforme. J Neurosurg 2005; 103(2):210–217
46. Ulm AJ III, Friedman WA, Bradshaw P, Foote KD, Bova FJ. Radiosurgery in the treatment of malignant gliomas: the University of Florida experience. Neurosurgery 2005;57(3):512–517
47. Hsieh PC, Chandler JP, Bhangoo S, et al. Adjuvant Gamma Knife stereotactic radiosurgery at the time of tumor progression potentially improves survival for patients with glioblastoma multiforme. Neurosurgery 2005;57(4):684–692
48. Combs SE, Widmer V, Thilmann C, Hof H, Debus J, Schulz-Ertner D. Stereotactic radiosurgery (SRS): treatment option for recurrent glioblastoma multiforme (GBM). Cancer 2005;104(10):2168–2173
49. Yoshikawa K, Saito K, Kajiwara K, Nomura S, Ishihara H, Suzuki M. CyberKnife stereotactic radiotherapy for patients with malignant glioma. Minim Invasive Neurosurg 2006;49(2):110–115
50. Irish WD, Macdonald DR, Cairncross JG. Measuring bias in uncontrolled brain tumor trials—to randomize or not to randomize? Can J Neurol Sci 1997;24(4):307–312
51. Grabb PA, Lunsford LD, Albright AL, Kondziolka D, Flickinger JC. Stereotactic radiosurgery for glial neoplasms of childhood. Neurosurgery 1996;38(4):696–702
52. Somaza SC, Kondziolka D, Lunsford LD, Flickinger JC, Bissonette DJ, Albright AL. Early outcomes after stereotactic radiosurgery for growing pilocytic astrocytomas in children. Pediatr Neurosurg 1996;25(3): 109–115
53. Kida Y, Kobayashi T, Mori Y. Gamma Knife radiosurgery for low-grade astrocytomas: results of long-term follow-up. J Neurosurg 2000; 93(Suppl 3):42–46
54. Hadjipanayis CG, Kondziolka D, Gardner P, et al. Stereotactic radiosurgery for pilocytic astrocytomas when multimodal therapy is necessary. J Neurosurg 2002;97:56–64
55. Boëthius J, Ulfarsson E, Rähn T, Lippittz B. Gamma Knife radiosurgery for pilocytic astrocytomas. J Neurosurg 2002;97(5, Suppl):677–680
56. Hadjipanayis CG, Niranjan A, Tyler-Kabara E, Kondziolka D, Flickinger JC, Lunsford LD. Stereotactic radiosurgery for well-circumscribed fibrillary grade II astrocytomas: an initial experience. Stereotact Funct Neurosurg 2002;79(1):13–24
57. Hadjipanayis CG, Kondziolka D, Flickinger JC, Lunsford LD. The role of sterotactic radiosurgery for low-grade astrocytomas. Neurosurg Focus 2003;14(5):E15:1–7
58. Giller CA, Berger BD, Pistenmaa DA, et al. Robotically guided radiosurgery for children. Pediatr Blood Cancer 2005;45(3):304–310
59. Heppner PA, Sheehan JP, Steiner LE. Gamma Knife surgery for low-grade gliomas. Neurosurgery 2005;57(6):1132–1139
60. Szeifert GT, Prasad D, Kamyrio T, Steiner M, Steiner LE. The role of Gamma Knife in the management of cerebral astrocytomas. Prog Neurol Surg 2007;20:150–163
61. Han SR, Yoon SW, Yee GT, et al. Novalis radiosurgery of optic gliomas in children: preliminary report. Pediatr Neurosurg 2007;43:251–257
62. Aggarwal R, Yeung D, Kumar P, Muhlbauer M, Kun LE. Efficacy and feasibility of stereotactic radiosurgery in the primary management of unfavorable pediatric ependymoma. Radiother Oncol 1997;43(3): 269–273
63. Jawahar A, Kondziolka D, Flickinger JC, Lunsford LD. Adjuvant stereotactic radiosurgery for anaplastic ependymoma. Stereotact Funct Neurosurg 1999;73(1–4):23–30

64. Stafford SL, Pollock BE, Foote RL, Gorman DA, Nelson DF, Schomberg PJ. Stereotactic radiosurgery for recurrent ependymoma. Cancer 2000;88(4):870–875
65. Hodgson DC, Goumnerova LC, Loeffler JS, et al. Radiosurgery in the management of pediatric brain tumors. Int J Radiat Oncol Biol Phys 2001;50(4):929–935
66. Mansur DB, Drzymala RE, Rich KM, Klein EE, Simpson JR. The efficacy of stereotactic radiosurgery in the management of intracranial ependymoma. J Neurooncol 2004;66(1–2):187–190
67. Endo H, Kumabe T, Jokura H, Shirane R, Tominaga T. Stereotactic radiosurgery for nodular dissemination of anaplastic ependymoma. Acta Neurochir (Wien) 2004;146(3):291–298, discussion 298
68. Kinoshita M, Izumoto S, Kagawa N, Hashimoto N, Maruno M, Yoshimine T. Long-term control of recurrent anaplastic ependymoma with extracranial metastasis: importance of multiple surgery and stereotactic radiosurgery procedures—case report. Neurol Med Chir (Tokyo) 2004;44(12):669–673
69. Lo SS, Chang EL, Sloan AE. Role of stereotactic radiosurgery and fractionated stereotactic radiotherapy in the management of intracranial ependymoma. Expert Rev Neurother 2006;6(4):501–507
70. Lo SS, Abdulrahman R, Desrosiers PM, et al. The role of Gamma Knife radiosurgery in the management of unresectable gross disease or gross residual disease after surgery in ependymoma. J Neurooncol 2006;79(1):51–56
71. Kihlström L, Lindquist C, Lindquist M, Karlsson B. Stereotactic radiosurgery for tectal low-grade gliomas. Acta Neurochir Suppl (Wien) 1994;62:55–57
72. Hirato M, Nakamura M, Inoue HK, et al. Gamma Knife radiosurgery for the treatment of brainstem tumors. Stereotact Funct Neurosurg 1995;64(Suppl 1):32–41
73. Fuchs I, Kreil W, Sutter B, Papaethymiou G, Pendl G. Gamma Knife radiosurgery of brainstem gliomas. Acta Neurochir Suppl (Wien) 2002;84:71–76
74. Pollock BE. Gamma Knife surgery for focal brainstem gliomas. J Neurosurg 2007;106:6–7
75. Yen CP, Sheehan J, Steiner M, Patterson G, Steiner L. Gamma Knife surgery for focal brainstem gliomas. J Neurosurg 2007;106:8–17
76. Gajjar A, Chintagumpala M, Ashley D, et al. Risk-adapted craniospinal radiotherapy followed by high-dose chemotherapy and stem-cell rescue in children with newly diagnosed medulloblastoma (St. Jude Medulloblastoma-96): long-term results from a prospective, multicentre trial. Lancet Oncol 2006;7(10):813–820
77. Spreafico F, Massimino M, Gandola L, et al. Survival of adults treated for medulloblastoma using paediatric protocols. Eur J Cancer 2005;41:1304–1310
78. Brandes AA, Ermani M, Amista P, et al. The treatment of adults with medulloblastoma: a prospective study. Int J Radiat Oncol Biol Phys 2003;57(4):755–761
79. Inoue HK, Nakamura M, Ono N, Kawashima Y, Hirato M, Ohye C. Long-term clinical effects of radiation therapy for primitive gliomas and medulloblastomas: a role for radiosurgery. Stereotact Funct Neurosurg 1993;61(Suppl 1):51–58
80. Suh JH, Barnett GH. Stereotactic radiosurgery for brain tumors in pediatric patients. Technol Cancer Res Treat 2003;2(2):141–146
81. Patrice SJ, Tarbell NJ, Goumenerova LC, Shrieve DC. Black PM, Loeffler JS. Results of radiosurgery in the management of recurrent and residual medulloblastoma. Pediatr Neurosurg 1995;22:197–203
82. Woo C, Stea B, Lulu B, Hamilton A, Cassady JR. The use of stereotactic radiosurgical boost in the treatment of medulloblastomas. Int J Radiat Oncol Biol Phys 1997;37(4):761–764
83. Germanwala AV, Mai JC, Tomycz N, et al. Boost Gamma Knife surgery during multimodality management of adult medulloblastoma. J Neurosurg 2008;108(2):204–209
84. Milker-Zabel S, Zabel A, Thilmann C, et al. Results of three-dimensional stereotactically-guided radiotherapy in recurrent medulloblastoma. J Neurooncol 2002;60(3):227–233
85. Abe M, Tokumaru S, Tabuchi K, Kida Y, Takagi M, Imamura J. Stereotactic radiation therapy with chemotherapy in the management of recurrent medulloblastomas. Pediatr Neurosurg 2006;42(2):81–88

19

Stereotactic Radiosurgery for Brain Metastases

Mayur Jayarao, Lawrence S. Chin, and William F. Regine

Brain metastases are a significant cause of mortality and morbidity, with an annual incidence of ~170,000.[1] Most commonly, these lesions originate from primary tumors of the lung, breast, kidney, skin (especially melanomas), and colon. An estimated 20 to 30% of patients with cancer are at risk of developing metastases to the brain,[2] with ~40% of patients presenting with a single lesion.[3]

The prognosis for these patients remains poor despite advances in surgical technique, chemotherapy, and radiation therapy, with those receiving no form of therapy having a median survival of ~1 month. Based on historical studies, it has been determined that medical treatment with steroids alone yields a median survival of 1 to 2 months, whereas the addition of whole brain radiation therapy (WBRT) affords a median survival of 4 to 7 months.[4–8] Undoubtedly, brain metastasis is one of the most feared developments for a cancer patient, and hence represents a serious and often difficult therapeutic challenge for both neurosurgeons and oncologists.

The treatment of brain metastases historically has included WBRT, a therapeutic modality first reported in the early 1950s.[9,10] The Radiation Therapy Oncology Group (RTOG) conducted numerous trials from 1971 to 1993 to investigate various doses of WBRT and their modalities of delivery.[11–19] Additionally, the RTOG investigated the use of radiation sensitizers, such as bromodeoxyuridine (a synthetic nucleoside that is the analogue of thymidine) and hyperfractionation, and found no overall improvement in survival. From the outcome of these studies, it was determined that the use of 3000 Gy in 10 fractions was an acceptable regimen. However, although neurologic symptoms improved in the majority of patients, local control rates were low, and neurologic death still occurred in 25 to 54% of patients.[11] To offset the poor prognosis in patients with brain metastases, alternative techniques to WBRT were simultaneously sought. Described by Lars Leksell in 1951, stereotactic radiosurgery (SRS) employs the use of a single high dose of radiation directed by stereotaxis to the target with the use of narrow radiation beams to spare the normal surrounding brain tissue.[20] Since the initial report of 12 patients treated by a modified linear accelerator (LINAC) in 1987,[21] numerous studies have supported the benefit of SRS therapy in newly diagnosed as well as recurrent brain metastases. Today, brain metastases represent the most common indication for SRS. **Table 19.1** shows a comparison of studies for surgery versus WBRT versus SRS in categories of study design, average dose, and rates of local control, local recurrence, and median overall survival.

◆ Patient Selection and Prognostic Factors

The prognostic scale most commonly used for patients with brain metastases is the RTOG recursive partitioning analysis (RPA), as described by Gaspar et al in 1997.[22] Based on data obtained from 1200 consecutive patients enrolled in three RTOG trials from 1979 to 1993, the RPA scale identified three major variables predictive of outcome: patient age ≥ 65 years, functional independence as defined by a Karnofsky Performance Scale (KPS) score ≥ 70, and uncontrolled compared with controlled extracranial disease. Patients were then stratified into class 1, 2, or 3 according to these variables. **Table 19.2** lists the various classes, their components, and their mean survival time. The single most important predictor of outcome was functional status; patients with KPS scores < 70 had the worst prognosis, whereas young, functionally independent patients with controlled extracranial disease had the best prognosis. Corroborating this, a study by Lagerwaard et al reviewed 1292 patients with brain metastases and found the most important factors to be KPS, treatment modality, extracranial disease, and response to steroid treatment.[23]

Table 19.1 Comparison of Studies for Surgery versus Whole Brain Radiation Therapy versus Stereotactic Radiosurgery

Study	Design	No. of Patients	Dose (Gy)	Local Control	Recurrence Rate	Median Survival (months)
Bindal et al[39]	SRS Surgery	13 62	20 N/A	N/A N/A	21% 8%	7.5 16.4
Noordijk et al[24]	WBRT Surgery + WBRT	N/A N/A	40 Gy/wk 40 Gy/wk	N/A N/A	N/A N/A	6 10
Patchell et al[25]	WBRT Surgery + WBRT	23 25	N/A N/A	48% 80%	N/A N/A	3.75 10.0
Auchter et al[38]	SRS + WBRT	122	10–27/25–40	86%	N/A	14
Sanghavi et al[46]	WBRT WBRT + SRS	502 (t)	12–58 12–58 + N/A	N/A N/A	N/A N/A	16.1 (RPA1) 7.1 (RPA1)
Andrews et al[48]	WBRT WBRT + SRS	164 167	37.5/3 weeks 37.5/3 weeks + 15–24	71% 82%	43% greater N/A	6.5 4.9
Shehata et al[35]	SRS SRS + WBRT	228 240	7–30 7–30/6.75–50.4	87% 97%	N/A N/A	N/A N/A
Aoyama et al[53]	SRS SRS + WBRT	67 65	18–25 18–25 + 30	72.5% 88.7%	76.4% 46.8%	8 7.5
Sneed et al[67]	SRS SRS + WBRT	268 301	N/A 30–50.4 in fx	N/A N/A	N/A N/A	8.2 14 (RPA1) 8.6 15.2 (RPA1)
Hasegawa et al[68]	SRS	172	11–22	87%	N/A	8
Lutterbach et al[69]	SRS	101	18	91%	N/A	7.6
Regine et al[71]	SRS	36	8–25	N/A	80%	9

Abbreviations: fx, fractions; N/A, not applicable/not available; RPA1, recursive partitioning analysis class 1; RTOG, Radiation Therapy Oncology Group; SRS, stereotactic radiosurgery; t, total; WBRT, whole brain radiation therapy.

◆ Results of Surgical Resection

Although RPA class is the most significant predictor of survival, aggressive local resection for metastatic foci in addition to WBRT improves survival in selected patients.[24–26] Additionally, surgery can establish or confirm the diagnosis while offering immediate and effective palliation of symptomatic mass effect as well as the perceived premise of improved survival (**Fig. 19.1**).

In Europe, Noordijk et al's study included 63 patients with computed tomography (CT)–confirmed single metastases who were randomized to surgery with WBRT versus WBRT alone.[24] Surgery with WBRT improved survival (10 vs 6 months; $p = .04$) and functional independence (7.5 vs 3.5 months; $p = .06$) more than WBRT alone. There was no surgical benefit for patients with active extracranial disease. Similarly, Patchell et al's study at a single center in the United States randomly assigned 48 patients with single brain metastases to two treatment groups and demonstrated that surgery with WBRT improved survival (40 vs 15 weeks; $p < .01$), local control (80% vs 48%; $p < .02$), and functional independence (38 vs 8 weeks; $p < .005$) compared with that of biopsy and WBRT alone.[25] A third trial by Mintz et al included 83 patients but did not demonstrate a survival benefit for

Table 19.2 Determination of Recursive Partitioning Analysis Classes Based on Karnofsky Performance Scale Score, Age, and Extracranial Status

RPA Class	KPS Score	Age (years)	Primary Disease Control	Mean Survival (months)
1	70–100	< 65	Good	7.1
2	70–100	> 65	Bad	4.2
3	< 70	N/A	N/A	2.3

Abbreviations: KPS, Karnofsky Performance Scale. N/A, not applicable (irrelevant); RPA, recursive partitioning analysis; RTOG, Radiation Therapy Oncology Group.

Source: Data from Gaspar L, Scott C, Rotman M, et al. Recursive partitioning analysis (RPA) of prognostic factors in three Radiation Therapy Oncology Group (RTOG) brain metastases trials. Int J Radiat Oncol Biol Phys 1997; 37:745–751.

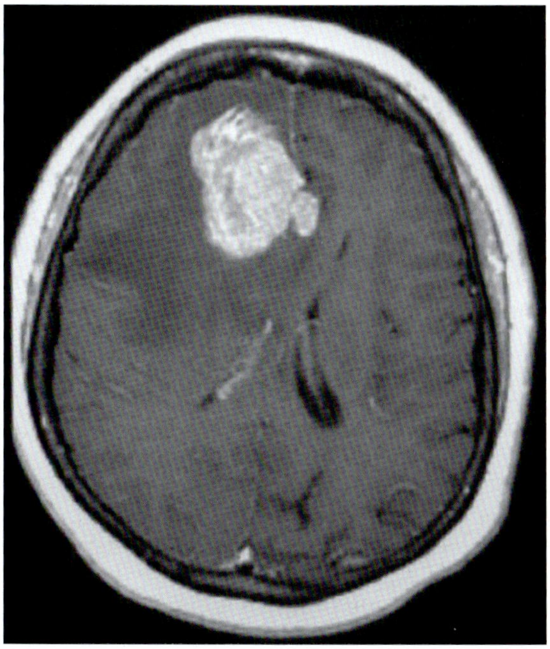

Fig. 19.1 A large right frontal metastatic tumor with mass effect and edema is seen on contrast-enhanced magnetic resonance imaging. This tumor required surgical resection.

surgical patients (6.3 vs 5.6 months; $p = .24$).[26] The lack of benefit in this study has been attributed to the influence of RPA class on survival where patients with lower KPS scores were included and the fact that the study consisted of a large percentage of patients with active extracranial disease.

We recommend surgical resection of brain metastases > 3.5 cm when in a surgically accessible location. Smaller tumors that cause significant mass effect or edema may also benefit from surgery over radiation therapy, particularly when the patient has neurologic deficit. The use of multiple craniotomies for multiple metastases remains controversial, but they may be indicated in good performance patients with large, symptomatic tumors. In general, WBRT follows every surgical resection.

Stereotactic Radiosurgery of Brain Metastases

The success of aggressive resection for control of a single metastasis has allowed neurosurgeons to use a complementary approach with SRS for control of single and multiple brain metastases. Indeed, in a relatively short time, SRS has emerged as one of the most important noninvasive options in the armamentarium against brain metastases.

Brain metastases are generally discrete, pseudo- or semispherical in shape, located in the gray-white junction, have a maximum diameter < 4 cm, and, unlike primary gliomas, are noninfiltrative. These features lend them the characteristics that allow for accurate target localization, planning, and treatment delivery. Importantly, a single large fraction of radiation appears to have a similar effect irrespective of the tumor type.[27–31] Nieder et al reviewed the images of 332 patients with brain metastases to evaluate local control and time to local progression based on dose.[32] Total doses of 25 to 60 Gy were administered (single doses 1.8–5.0 Gy). Biologically effective doses were derived for each patient, from which it was determined that higher doses were needed to improve local control. Brain metastases are considered "category IV" targets, which are targets with early-responding tissue (tumor) surrounded by late-responding normal tissue (brain).[33] Because the biologically effective dose in early-responding tissue is smaller than an equivalent dose in late-responding tissue, a higher single dose is needed in brain metastases than in benign tumors. SRS allows a high central dose to be given, yet has a rapid drop-off in dose that protects the surrounding brain tissue.

As determined from the Noordijk et al[24] and Patchell et al[25] studies comparing surgery with WBRT versus WBRT alone, local tumor control led to improved survival. These results combined with the potential advantages of SRS led to an increased interest in the use of SRS as an alternative to surgery for local tumor control.

Dose Characteristics and Tumor Size

An SRS radiation dose is described as energy per mass and is expressed in units of gray delivered to the prescribed isodose line. The prescription isodose line reflects the minimum amount of radiation delivered to every tumor cell within its area and in most cases is the isodose line that most closely approximates the outline of the tumor. This line is most conveniently described as a percentage of the maximum or central dose delivered to the tumor (**Fig. 19.2**). For example, if 20 Gy is given to the 50% isodose,

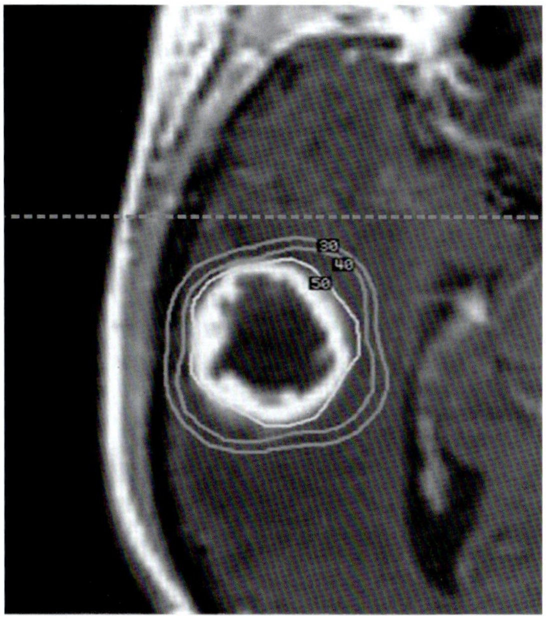

Fig. 19.2 A right temporal metastasis is seen with superimposed isodose curves from a stereotactic radiosurgery treatment plan. The 30, 40, and 50% lines are seen. In this case, the 50% line encompasses the prescription isodose volume.

then the center of the tumor receives 40 Gy. Obviously, the goal of SRS is to include the entire gross tumor volume (GTV) within the prescription isodose volume (PIV) with as little overlap to the normal brain as possible. The ratio PIV/GTV is one description of the treatment plan's conformality. Ideally, the PIV/GTV ratio is < 2, which implies that there is less normal tissue than tumor tissue irradiated in the prescription volume. In addition to being conformal, the treatment plan should ensure that at least 95% of the GTV is covered by the PIV. These relationships can be determined from an examination of the dose–volume histograms (DVHs) that should be generated with each treatment plan. Modern radiosurgery systems can accurately contour the isodose line for small tumors, but if larger tumors are to be treated, this presents a difficulty, as the amount of radiation delivered needs to be increased to allow for equivalent local control. Consequently, the radiation exposure of normal tissue is increased, and therefore treatment of large tumors is performed using the process of hypofractionation, where a lower radiation dosage is delivered over multiple fractions (generally three to five fractions) to prevent radiation toxicity.[34]

To determine the maximum tolerated doses of single-fraction radiosurgery, the RTOG conducted dose escalation studies that were reported from the RTOG 9005 trial.[34] Although the study included patients with primary gliomas and brain metastases, the primary stratification variable was size. From this study it was determined that the maximum tolerated doses were 24, 18, and 15 Gy for tumors ≤ 20 mm, 21 to 30 mm, and 31 to 40 mm in maximum diameter, respectively. However, for tumors < 20 mm, the investigators' reluctance to escalate to 27 Gy, rather than excessive toxicity, determined the maximum tolerated dose. This study provided the guideline and framework for dosing, although it failed to account for other variables, such as location. For example, the cranial nerves and brainstem are more sensitive to radiation than are other regions of the brain parenchyma; consequently, dose prescription must be reduced as necessary to protect these structures.

On the basis of institutional experience at the University of Kentucky and guided by the results from the RTOG 9005 trial, Shehata et al[35] conducted a study to determine the optimal SRS dose and influence of WBRT on local tumor control among metastases ≤ 2 cm in size. Between 1992 and 2001, 160 patients (468 metastases) were treated with SRS (dose range 7–30 Gy; median 20). A total of 240 metastases received planned WBRT (range 6.75–50.4 Gy; median 40.5) versus 228 metastases that did not. The variables tested included histological type, site of metastasis, primary diagnosis, tumor volume, SRS dose, newly diagnosed versus recurrent metastasis, and planned WBRT versus no planned WBRT, with the addition of WBRT alone being the most significant predictor of local tumor control. Overall, patients who received WBRT had superior local tumor control rates (97% vs 87% in those who did not receive WBRT; $p = .0001$). Additionally, patients receiving WBRT and SRS ≥ 20 Gy achieved local control rates of 99% compared with 91% control rates when treated with WBRT and SRS < 20 Gy ($p = .0029$), allowing the investigators to conclude that optimal control of brain metastasis ≤ 2 cm was seen with 20 Gy SRS combined with planned WBRT. Finally, increasing the SRS dose to > 20 Gy resulted in no improvement in local tumor control, but rather a higher rate of neurotoxicity.

Stereotactic Radiosurgery versus Surgery

The potential advantages of SRS include elimination of general anesthesia, outpatient delivery, minimal risk for bleeding or infection, lower risk of complications, short convalescence time, and, frequently, lower cost.[35–37] Additionally, SRS is not limited by the number or location of lesions, coagulopathic state, or other concomitant comorbidities. For these reasons, SRS has become a viable alternative to surgery, although there have been conflicting results from various studies.[38–41]

In a multi-institutional retrospective outcome and prognostic analysis from the University of Wisconsin at Madison for resectable single brain metastasis, 122 patients with newly diagnosed and potentially resectable single brain metastases were treated by SRS and WBRT.[38] In this study, the local control rate was 86%, with a median survival of 56 weeks and 25% of the deaths being related to tumor progression. Based on these results, the investigators concluded that SRS could be used as an alternative to surgery. Another study from the M D Anderson Cancer Center in 1996 compared retrospectively matched patients treated by SRS ($n = 13$) with those treated by surgery alone ($n = 62$).[39] The median survival was 7.5 months for the SRS group compared with 16.4 months for the surgery group; the local recurrence rate was 21% for the SRS group versus 8% for the surgery group. Based on these results, it was concluded that surgery should be the preferred modality of therapy for patients with surgically accessible lesions.

In contrast to the previously described studies, a retrospective Mayo Clinic review comparing SRS with surgical resection in the treatment of solitary brain metastasis found no difference in 1-year survival rates for either group.[40] Further, in a retrospective study by Muacevic et al, the outcome of patients who underwent surgery with radiotherapy were compared with those who underwent Gamma Knife (Elekta Instruments AB, Stockholm, Sweden) SRS alone.[41] Only patients with a single lesion of ≤ 3.5 cm were included. For the surgical and radiotherapy group versus SRS group, 1-year survival rates, 1-year local control rates, and 1-year neurologic death rates were found not to be statistically significant.

It is plausible that patient selection bias was the primary contributor to the previously described results, as they were retrospectively conducted studies. Indeed, when the Joint Center for Radiation Therapy (JCRT) attempted to enroll patients in a phase III trial comparing surgery with SRS in the 1990s, only six patients were enrolled because of patient or physician preference.[42] Currently, it is generally agreed that for lesions > 3.5 cm or for those without histological diagnosis, surgical resection should be considered as the primary modality of therapy rather than SRS. Additionally, surgical resection affords a quicker improvement in neurologic function, minimizes chronic steroid use, and alleviates symptoms secondary to mass effect.

Stereotactic Radiosurgery and Whole Brain Radiation Therapy

Fueled by the encouraging results of studies using SRS for recurrent brain metastases,[43–45] the use of SRS with WBRT was investigated for newly diagnosed patients under the hypothesis that the combination would be superior for local and regional control of brain metastases.

A multi-institutional retrospective study reported by Sanghavi et al from 10 institutions analyzed the outcome for 502 patients with brain metastases treated by SRS with WBRT.[46] The patients were stratified using the RTOG RPA method. The overall median survival period was 10.7 months, with a higher KPS and lower RPA class predicting improved survival. The addition of SRS boosted results in median survival (16.1, 10.3, and 8.7 months for classes 1, 2, and 3, respectively) compared with the median survival (7.1, 4.2, and 2.3 months for classes 1, 2, and 3, respectively; $p < .05$) of patients treated with WBRT alone.

To assess the effectiveness of SRS alone or in combination with WBRT compared with surgery and/or WBRT in prolonging survival and improving the quality of life and functional status of patients with brain metastases, a meta-analysis of randomized, controlled trials and concurrent cohort studies was performed in 2006.[47] The review identified three randomized, controlled trials and one cohort study. Among patients with multiple metastases, no difference in survival between those treated with SRS plus WBRT versus those treated with WBRT alone was found. However, in patients with one metastasis, a statistically significant difference, favoring those treated with SRS plus WBRT, was observed. Regarding local tumor control at 24 months, rates were significantly higher in the SRS plus WBRT treatment arm, regardless of the number of metastases. The investigators concluded that adding SRS to WBRT not only improved survival in patients with one brain metastasis, but also improved local tumor control and functional independence.

The largest and most influential study conducted to date in patients with brain metastasis treated with SRS plus WBRT (3750 Gy, 15 fractions) versus WBRT alone comes from the RTOG 9508 trial.[48] Reported by Andrews et al in 2004, this multi-institutional randomized clinical trial comprised 333 patients from 55 participating RTOG institutions with one to three newly diagnosed brain metastases on magnetic resonance imaging (MRI), each ≤ 4 cm in diameter. One hundred sixty-seven patients were assigned WBRT and stereotactic radiosurgery, and 164 were allocated WBRT alone. Univariate analysis showed that there was a survival advantage in the WBRT and SRS group for patients with a single brain metastasis (median survival time 6.5 vs 4.9 months; $p = .0393$) despite the fact that 19% of the patients failed to receive the intended treatment (31 of 164 patients assigned to the SRS group did not actually undergo SRS, and 28 of 167 patients in the WBRT arm received salvage SRS). Patients in the SRS group were also more likely to have a stable or improved KPS score at 6 months follow-up than were patients allocated to WBRT alone (43% vs 27%, respectively; $p = .03$). By multivariate analysis, survival improved in patients with an RPA class 1 ($p < .0001$) or a favorable histological status ($p = .0121$). Steroid use was also lower in the SRS and WBRT arm, as was local control at 1 year (82% vs 71%; $p = .01$). The risk of developing a local recurrence was 43% greater with WBRT alone ($p = .0021$). Based on these results, the investigators concluded that WBRT and SRS boost treatment improved functional autonomy (KPS) for all patients and survival for patients with a single unresectable brain metastatic lesion. Further, they recommended that SRS with WBRT be considered as the standard treatment for patients with a single unresectable brain metastasis, but at the same time also be considered for patients with two or three brain metastatic lesions.

To follow up the results of RTOG 9508, a phase III trial comparing WBRT and SRS alone versus WBRT and SRS with temozolomide or erlotinib in patients with non–small cell lung cancer (NSCLC) and one to three brain metastases is currently under way.

◆ Stereotactic Radiosurgery as Sole Treatment

The use of SRS with WBRT for treatment of a single brain metastasis has been well proven.[27,28,35,46–53] Nevertheless, the use of SRS alone has gained popularity in part because of concerns over deleterious effects of WBRT, which may affect the quality of life and neurologic function of long-term survivors.[54–57] From a tumor control standpoint, the rationale against the use of WBRT with SRS is that the benefit of WBRT on nonvisualized brain metastases is mitigated by the fact that once WBRT ends, any new metastases are now untreated. Therefore, recurrent brain metastases are best treated expectantly by delayed WBRT or repeat SRS. Several institutional studies have attempted to demonstrate the validity of the use of SRS alone, with local control rates ranging from 63 to 97% for SRS with WBRT versus 42 to 87% with SRS alone.[44,58–68] In the report by DeAngelis et al, the delayed effects of WBRT were reported in 12 patients who underwent surgery with WBRT ($n = 8$) or WBRT alone ($n = 4$).[56] Within 5 to 36 months (median 14 months) all patients developed progressive dementia, ataxia, and urinary incontinence, causing severe disability in all and leading to death in seven. The total dose of WBRT was 2500 to 3900 Gy, but daily fractions of 300 to 600 Gy were also employed. The investigators concluded that these fractionation schedules predisposed patients to delayed neurologic toxicity, and that more protracted schedules should have been used instead.

Interestingly, although the use of prophylactic cranial irradiation routinely demonstrated a decrease in the development of brain metastases, it has only recently offered a noteworthy overall survival advantage demonstrated among patients with extensive stage disease.[63–66,68,69] In the meantime, the RTOG is currently conducting a phase II/III randomized trial (RTOG 0212) of two doses (phase III: standard [25 Gy] vs high [36 Gy]) and two high dose schedules (phase II: once vs twice daily) for delivering prophylactic cranial irradiation for patients with limited disease small cell lung cancer.

In an attempt to determine if SRS alone was effective versus SRS plus WBRT, data were collected from 10 institutions and reviewed to compare the survival of patients with newly diagnosed brain metastases.[67] Of 569 patients, 268 had SRS alone initially (24% of whom ultimately had salvage WBRT), and 301 had SRS plus upfront WBRT. For all RPA classes, the median survival times for patients were comparable between the two treatment groups (RPA class 1: 14 months vs 15 months; RPA class 2: 8 months vs 7 months; RPA class 3: 5 months vs 6 months). Despite adjustment by RPA class, there was no survival difference, which suggested that upfront WBRT did not improve survival better than SRS alone.

A retrospective review of 172 patients with brain metastases $\leq$ 3.5 cm in diameter managed by SRS alone was performed by Hasegawa et al.[68] The mean marginal tumor dose and volume were 18.5 Gy and 4.4 mL, respectively, with 80% of the patients having solitary tumors. The overall median survival time was 8 months, with the median survival time in patients with no evidence of primary tumor disease or stable disease being 13 and 11 months, respectively. At 2 years, the rates of local control, remote brain control, and total intracranial control were 75, 41, and 27%, respectively. Tumor volume alone was significant for local control (p = .02), with tumor volumes of at least 4 mL having a local control rate of ~49% at 1 and 2 years. Based on these results, the authors advocated that WBRT be avoided in selected patients with one or two lesions (with good control of their primary cancer), KPS $\geq$ 90, and age < 60 years. Similar results were also obtained in a study by Lutterbach et al.[70] In this study, median survival was 13.4 months, 9.3 months, and 1.5 months for patients in RPA classes 1, 2, and 3, respectively ($p < .0001$). At 1 year, local control, distant brain freedom from progression (FFP), and overall brain FFP were 91, 53, and 51%, respectively, thereby allowing the investigators to conclude that, although the RPA system successfully predicted survival, SRS alone also yielded high local control. Additionally, an interval > 2 years between diagnosis of the primary tumor and diagnosis of brain metastases and the presence of a single brain metastasis were associated with significantly higher overall brain FFP.

In a retrospective report by Rades et al,[71] the efficacy of SRS alone versus surgical resection plus WBRT was evaluated. Two hundred six patients in RPA classes 1 and 2 who had one or two brain metastases were enrolled to assess overall survival, brain tumor control, and local control. Ninety-four patients received between 18 and 25 Gy of SRS alone, and 112 patients underwent surgical resection of their metastases and received 10 $\times$ 3 Gy/20 $\times$ 2 Gy of WBRT. A comparison of the two treatment groups as well RPA subgroup analyses did not reveal significant overall survival, brain tumor control, or local control. On multivariate analysis, improved overall survival was associated with age $\leq$ 60 years (p = .002), better performance status (p = .015), no extracranial metastases ($p < .001$), interval from tumor diagnosis to treatment > 12 months (p = .003), and RPA class 1 (p = .016). Improved brain tumor control was associated with a single metastasis (p = .034) and an interval from tumor diagnosis to treatment > 12 months (p = .019), whereas improved local control was associated with an interval from tumor diagnosis to treatment > 12 months (p = .047). Based on these results, the investigators concluded that SRS alone appeared to be as effective as surgical resection plus WBRT in the treatment of one or two brain metastases for patients in RPA classes 1 and 2.

The randomized controlled trial by Aoyama et al attempted to determine if WBRT combined with SRS resulted in improvement in survival, brain tumor control, functional preservation rate, and frequency of neurologic death versus patients undergoing SRS alone.[53] One hundred thirty-two patients with one to four brain metastases, each < 3 cm in diameter, were enrolled between 1999 and 2003 and randomized to SRS alone (n = 67) versus SRS plus WBRT (n = 65). The primary end point was overall survival, with secondary end points being brain tumor recurrence, salvage brain treatment, functional preservation, toxic effects of radiation, and cause of death. The 12-month brain tumor recurrence rate was 46.8% in the SRS plus WBRT group versus 76.4% for the SRS alone group ($p < .001$). Salvage brain treatment was also less frequently required in the SRS plus WBRT group (n = 10) versus that of SRS alone (n = 29) ($p < .001$). No significant difference in survival, cause of death, toxic effects of radiation, or preservation of neurologic or systemic function was noted. Aoyama et al concluded that WBRT was likely not necessary and could be safely omitted primarily to avoid the long-term neurotoxic effects. An alternative conclusion is that WBRT decreases tumor recurrence without significant increase in neurotoxicity.[52] The Aoyama et al study to date reinforces this view. In a subsequent publication from this study in which neurocognitive function was prospectively evaluated by Mini-Mental State Examination, the most important factor found to influence stabilization of neurocognitive function was brain tumor control. The average duration until neurocognitive deterioration was 16.5 months in the SRS plus WBRT group versus 7.6 months in the SRS alone group (p = .05).[71]

Although the results previously described are encouraging regarding the use of SRS alone, it is important to consider that patients who undergo SRS alone may in fact be at a higher risk for morbidity due to recurrence of brain metastases. A retrospective study of 36 patients focusing on the risk of symptomatic brain tumor recurrence and neurologic deficit after radiosurgery alone in patients with newly diagnosed brain metastases was conducted by Regine et al.[73] In this study, the SRS dose ranged from 8 to 25 Gy (median 20 Gy). Factors evaluated in analysis of treatment outcome included the number of metastases, site of metastasis, primary tumor site, histology, extent of intracranial and extracranial disease, and interval to diagnosis of brain metastasis. Median survival time and 1-year survival rate for the entire group were 9 months and 36%, respectively. Brain tumor recurrence (BTR) occurred in 47% (17/36) of patients. Of these, 71% (12/17) of the patients were symptomatic at the time of recurrence, and 59% (10/17) had an associated neurologic deficit. Multivariate analysis found that only the extent of disease was a predictor of BTR. Patients who had disease limited to the brain only had a BTR rate of 80% (8/10) versus 35% (9/26) who had disease involving the

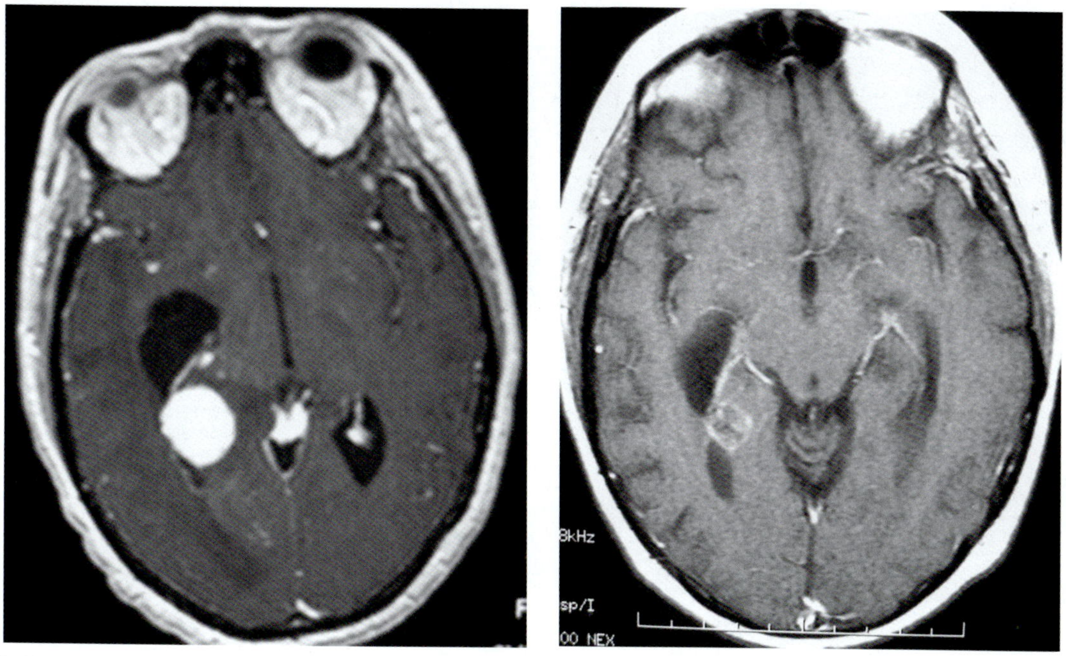

A B

Fig. 19.3 Magnetic resonance imaging scans of a renal cell carcinoma metastasis **(A)** before and **(B)** after stereotactic radiosurgery.

brain, primary site, and/or other extracranial metastatic sites ($p = .03$). The investigators concluded that use of SRS alone in this study was associated with an increasingly significant risk of BTR with increasing survival time. Additionally, the majority of recurrences were symptomatic and associated with a neurologic deficit.

Most retrospective SRS reports for the treatment of radioresistant cancers have found no survival advantage when compared with WBRT. To address the feasibility of using SRS alone, the Eastern Cooperative Oncology Group conducted a prospective, phase II trial evaluating the use of SRS alone in the treatment of primary radioresistant cancers.[73] Thirty-one patients with renal cell carcinoma, melanoma, or sarcoma; one to three brain metastases; and performance status of 0 to 2 were enrolled. Exclusion criteria were leptomeningeal disease; metastases in the medulla, pons, or midbrain; and liver metastases. On the basis of tumor size, patients received 24, 18, or 15 Gy. The median survival time was 8.3 months, with 3- and 6-month intracranial failure rates of 25.8 and 48.3%, respectively, allowing the investigators to conclude that omitting WBRT from the management of intracranial metastases, especially those that are radioresistant, should be approached judiciously and therefore be reserved for select patients only.

At this time, there is no clear consensus regarding the use of SRS alone to manage metastatic brain tumors. Overall, the data indicate that both local and distant tumor controls are improved with the addition of WBRT, but survival is not affected. It is not known whether the lack of survival benefit is a true finding or if the studies to date lack sufficient power to distinguish a difference. Certain patients would be expected to be better candidates for upfront SRS alone therapy: younger patients with a small, single metastasis from a radioresistant tumor, such as melanoma or renal cell carcinoma (**Fig. 19.3**). Obviously, these patients need close follow-up every 3 months with MRI scans following initial treatment.

Impact of Location on Treatment

Lesions in areas such as the brainstem, skull base, and pituitary are often difficult to treat due to nearby critical structures (**Fig. 19.4**). Multiple studies have attempted to examine the efficacy of SRS for the treatment of brainstem,[75–78] skull base,[79,80] and sellar metastases.[81–82]

In the study by Yen et al, 53 patients with metastatic brainstem lesions underwent Gamma Knife SRS, with metastatic deposits located in the midbrain in 8 patients, the pons in 42, and the medulla oblongata in 3.[76] Lung cancer was the most common primary malignancy, followed by breast cancer, melanoma, and renal cell carcinoma. The mean volume of the metastatic deposits at the time of treatment was 2.8 cm^3. The prescription doses varied from 9 to 25 Gy (mean 17.6 Gy). Of 37 patients who underwent an imaging follow-up evaluation at a mean of 9.8 months (range 1–25 months), the tumors disappeared in 7, shrank in 22, remained unchanged in 3, and grew in 5. All but 1 of 18 patients with asymptomatic brainstem deposits remained free of symptoms. In 35 patients with symptomatic brainstem deposits, neurologic symptoms improved in 21, remained stable in 11, and worsened in 3. The overall median survival period was 11 months after Gamma Knife SRS. In terms of survival, the absence of active extracranial

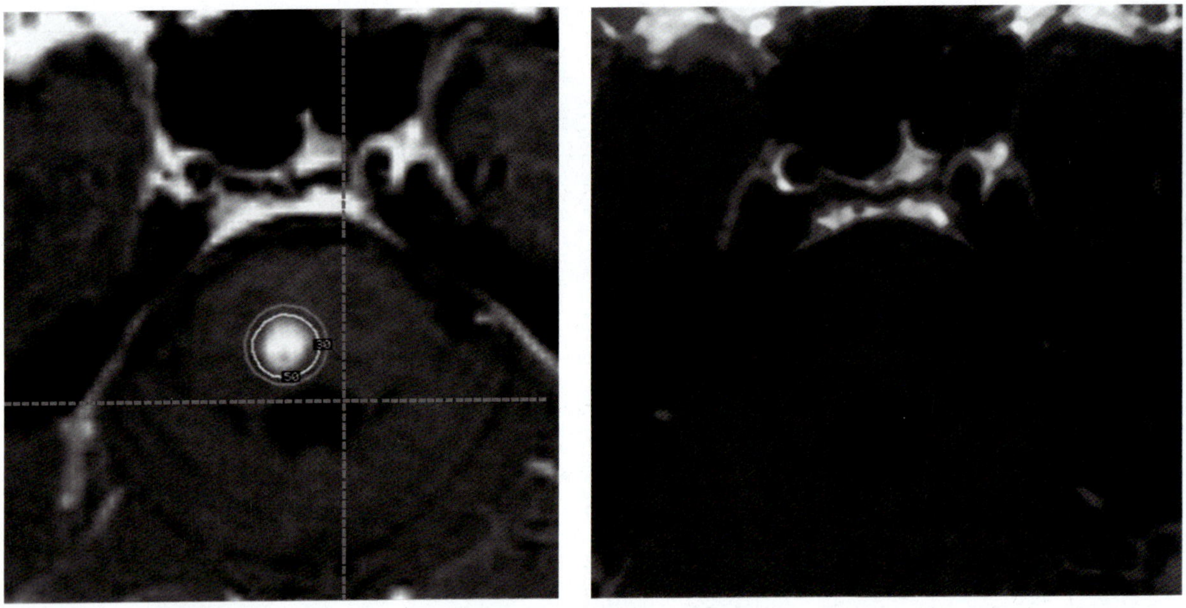

Fig. 19.4 Magnetic resonance imaging scans showing a brainstem metastasis **(A)** before and **(B)** after stereotactic radiosurgery. The 30 and 50% isodose are seen in **(A)**. The patient was treated to a dose of 15 Gy at the 50% line.

disease was the only favorable prognostic factor, thereby allowing the investigators to conclude that compared with allowing a metastatic brainstem lesion to take its natural course, SRS prolonged survival.

In regard to local control, Cmelak et al investigated 37 patients (48 lesions) with skull base metastases or local recurrences from primary head and neck cancers that were treated with linac SRS.[80] Radiation doses of 7 to 35 Gy (median 20 Gy) were delivered to recurrent lesions, usually as a single fraction. Thirty-three of the 48 (69%) recurrent/metastatic lesions were locally controlled. Follow-up for these patients with recurrent lesions ranged from 1 to 60 months (median 9 months). Local control did not correlate with lesion size (p = .80), histology (p = .78), or radiosurgical dose (p = .44), allowing the investigators to conclude that SRS afforded better local control and was a viable treatment modality for skull base metastases or local recurrences from primary head and neck cancers.

Obviously, the treatment of brainstem lesions is restricted by the location of the lesion and the critical surrounding structures. Generally, the safe dose for the brainstem is around 15 Gy, with the safe dose for the optic chiasm being 8 Gy, although some prefer to use 10 Gy.

Recurrent Brain Metastases and Stereotactic Radiosurgery

One of the first reports of SRS use for brain metastases was of patients with recurrent brain metastases following surgery and/or WBRT. In this seminal study, Loeffler et al reported the retrospective results of 18 patients (21 lesions) who underwent SRS using a modified linac.[43] All but one patient had received prior radiotherapy. Local control was achieved in all patients (median follow-up of 9 months), with a majority of them improving neurologically and being able to be withdrawn from steroid therapy. A follow-up report from Alexander et al retrospectively analyzed 248 consecutive patients (421 lesions) treated by SRS between 1986 and 1993.[44] Median overall survival was found to be 9.4 months, with local control rates of 85 and 65% at 1 year and 2 years, respectively. Further, in a study by Noël et al of 54 consecutive patients (97 metastases) relapsing after WBRT who received SRS, the 1- and 2-year local control rates were 91.3 and 84%, respectively.[45] The 1- and 2-year brain control rates were 65 and 57%, respectively, with 1- and 2-year overall survival rates of 31 and 28%, respectively.

Typically, WBRT has been used in the salvage therapy of patients who have undergone previous craniotomy or radiosurgery. In a study by Chen et al,[84] 190 patients with brain metastases were treated primarily with gamma unit radiosurgery. A subset of 45 patients, who underwent radiosurgical salvage for new tumors in a region remote from an initially treated tumor, formed the population base for this study. In this subgroup of patients, a total of 176 tumors were treated. The median time from the first radiosurgical procedure to the first salvage was 17.4 weeks, and the median survival from the second radiosurgical intervention was 28 weeks. Of the 45 study patients, 34 underwent a single salvage procedure, 10 underwent two salvage procedures, and 1 had three salvage procedures. The actuarial FFP for treated tumors at 52 weeks was 92.4%, with patients undergoing upfront whole brain irradiation being less likely to require salvage therapy (p = .008). There were 33 deaths after salvage radiosurgery during the reporting period. Central nervous system causes accounted for 13 deaths, whereas 19 deaths resulted from systemic disease. No statistically significant advantage in overall survival could be demonstrated in patients treated with whole brain irradiation, allowing the investigators to conclude that SRS could be used for salvage therapy with equivalent overall survival to patients receiving salvage WBRT.

Based on the results from the previously described studies, it is evident that SRS is effective in the local control of recurrent brain metastases. The treatment of brain metastases that fail initial SRS either with or without WBRT is more problematic. Repeat SRS can be effective but increases the risk of radiation necrosis (see the next section). Frequently, the best treatment for these tumors is surgical resection.

Complications

Although the immediate risk of mortality due to SRS is zero, there are several early, intermediate, and delayed complications that can cause significant morbidity for patients undergoing SRS. Serious complications include radiation-induced necrosis, peritumoral edema, tumoral hemorrhage, and radiation-induced neoplasia.

Most early complications of SRS include headache (secondary to frame placement), nausea and/or vomiting, infection of pin sites, transient worsening of baseline neurologic function, and fatigue. The risk of seizures ranges from 2 to 6%,[44,48,85] with the risk being higher for patients with cortical lesions and those with a prior history of seizures.

Intermediate complications generally occur within the first 6 months after SRS, with alopecia being reported in 5.6% of patients.[44] It has since been understood that these patients had superficial tumors that resulted in radiation being delivered to the scalp. Seizures may also occur, but these are generally related to tumor location, size, and associated mass effect. Neurologic deterioration can occur in some patients, but this can usually be managed successfully with steroids. In a review of 189 patients with 264 brain metastases secondary to renal cell carcinoma, melanomas, and sarcomas, Chang et al reported a hemorrhage rate of 6.4% (17 lesions) within 2.5 months of SRS therapy and a peritumoral edema rate of 3.8% (10 lesions).[86] Eight of the 17 hemorrhagic metastases and 5 of the 10 peritumoral edema lesions required resection at a median of 2.9 months after treatment (range 1.6–22.0 months).

Of the delayed complications, radiation-induced necrosis is the most serious, with the risk increasing with the use of higher doses, prior stereotactic radiation, and larger tumor volume. Radiation-induced necrosis can be difficult to diagnose, as standard imaging cannot adequately distinguish between necrosis and residual or recurrent tumor (**Fig. 19.5**). More intensive imaging techniques such as positron emission tomography (PET), magnetic resonance spectroscopy, and, on occasion, surgery may be required to adequately diagnose this complication. Data collected from the RTOG 9005 trial[34] demonstrated the rate of radiation necrosis after SRS to be 5, 8, 9, and 11% at 6, 12, 18, and 24 months, respectively. In a study by Chin et al to determine risk factors for radiation necrosis, patients (17/243) who developed radiation necrosis following Gamma Knife surgery were identified.[87] Integral DVHs were calculated and dose–volume treatment parameters determined, and a comparison was made with both the established Kjellberg and Flickinger isonecrosis risk lines. Clinical outcome was assessed according to time to resolution of symptoms and

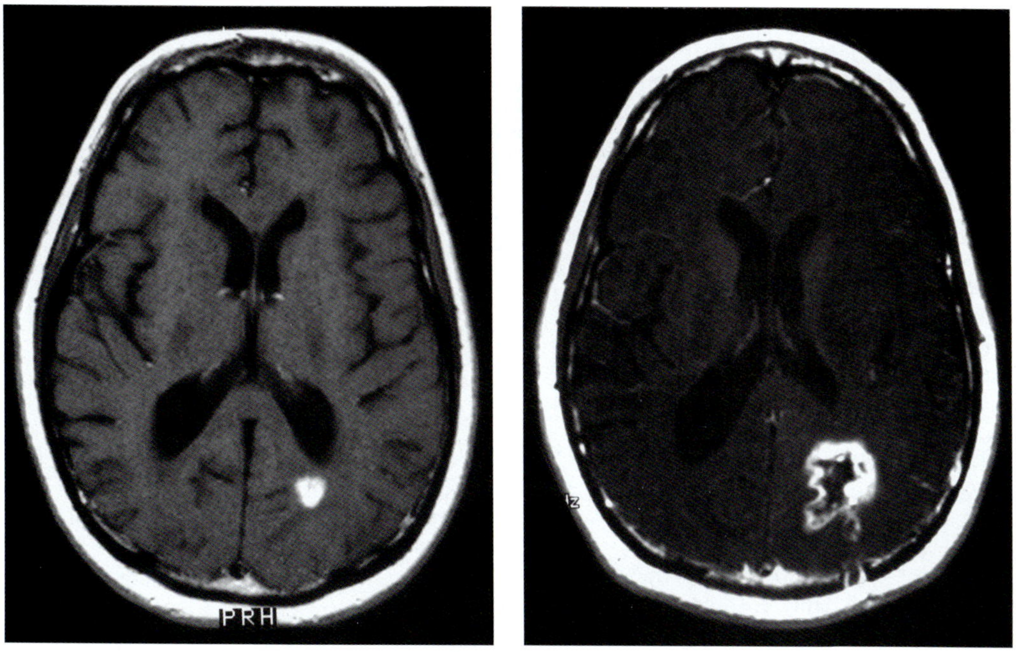

A B

Fig. 19.5 Magnetic resonance imaging scans showing the development of radiation necrosis following stereotactic radiosurgery treatment. **(A)** A small left occipital metastasis was treated, and **(B)** 9 months later developed radiation necrosis, which was confirmed by biopsy.

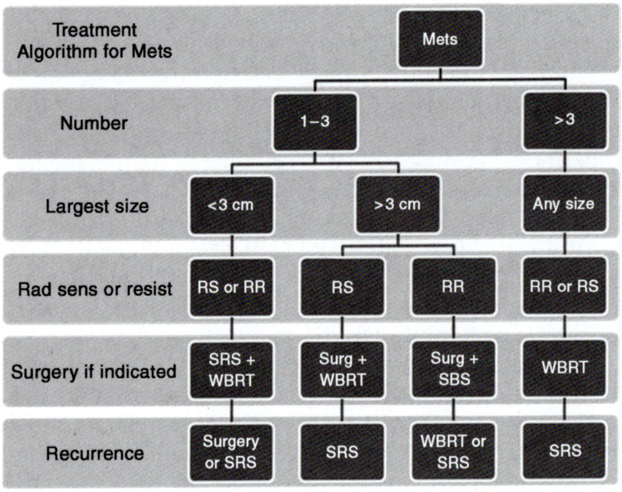

Fig. 19.6 Flowchart showing a proposed treatment algorithm for patients with brain metastases. Mets, metastases; cm, centimeter; RS/Rad Sens, radiosensitive; RR/Resist, radiosistant; SRS, stereotactic radiosurgery; WBRT, whole brain radiation therapy; Surg, surgery.

return to normal radiographic appearance. Based on these, it was determined that the treatment plan variables associated with the risk of necrosis were increased tumor volume integral dose, increased tumor volume, and increased 10 Gy volume. Other risk factors were repeated radiosurgery to the same lesion and histologically identified gliomas. The Kjellberg 1% risk line predicted a 5% risk of radiation necrosis, and the Flickinger 3% risk line predicted a 3% risk. The median time to development of necrosis was 4 months, and symptomatic and radiographic recovery times were 7.5 and 10.5 months, respectively. Avoidance of radiation necrosis is best accomplished by using the lowest effective dose with a highly conformal plan to reduce normal brain exposure. If possible, the same tumor should not undergo a repeat radiosurgery treatment. When symptomatic edema from radiation necrosis occurs, it is best treated with high-dose steroids, but when the diagnosis is in doubt, or when significant mass effect exists, and/or the patient is intolerant of steroids, patients may need a craniotomy for diagnosis and resection of the mass.

The use of hyperbaric oxygen (HBO) has been explored for the treatment and prevention of radiation-induced brain injury.[88] In this study of 78 patients with brain metastases who underwent SRS, prophylactic HBO was used in 32 patients. Radiation-induced brain injuries were divided into two categories, white matter injury (WMI) and radiation necrosis (RN), on the basis of imaging findings. Radiation-induced brain injury occurred in 5 lesions (11%) in the HBO group (2 WMIs and 3 RNs) and in 11 (20%) in the non-HBO group (9 WMIs and 2 RNs). The 1-year actuarial probability of WMI was significantly better for the HBO group (2%) than for the non-HBO group (36%) ($p < .05$), allowing the investigators to conclude that prophylactic HBO could possibly prevent the development of radiation-induced WMI.

◆ Summary

Stereotactic radiosurgery has emerged as an effective, noninvasive therapeutic modality for local tumor control, as well as a means of improving patient survival. A proposed algorithm for treating patients is seen in **Fig. 19.6.** Multiple studies have consistently demonstrated the benefit of SRS either alone, in concert with WBRT, or as a salvage after WBRT, as have studies that demonstrate similar outcomes between surgery and SRS. RTOG 9508 provides level 1 evidence for the use of SRS with WBRT versus that of WBRT alone for patients with a single lesion. Further, the use of SRS without WBRT is now being explored, although the exclusion of WBRT is not without risk, as some studies have demonstrated an increased risk of tumor recurrence and an increased need for salvage treatment.

References

1. Greenberg H, Chandler WF, Sandler HM. Brain metastases. In: Greenberg H, Chandler WF, Sandler HM, eds, Brain Tumors. Oxford: Oxford University Press; 1999:299–317
2. Wen PY, Loeffler JS. Management of brain metastasis. Oncology 1999;13(7):941–954
3. Lohr F, Pirzkall A, Hof H, et al. Adjuvant treatment of brain metastases. Semin Surg Oncol 2001;20:50–56
4. Zimm S, Wampler GL, Stablein D, et al. Intracerebral metastases in solid-tumor patients: natural history and results of treatment. Cancer 1981;48(2):384–394
5. Posner JB. Intracranial metastases. In: Posner JB (ed.), Neurologic Complications of Cancer. Vol 45. Philadelphia: FA Davis; 1995:77–110
6. Nussbaum ES, Djalilian HR, Cho KH, et al. Brain metastasis: histology, multiplicity, surgery and survival. Cancer 1996;78:1781–1788
7. Hazra T, Mullins GM, Lott S. Management of cerebral metastases from bronchogenic carcinoma. Johns Hopkins Med J 1972;130: 377–383
8. Markesbery WR, Brooks WH, Gupta GD, Young AB. Treatment for patients with cerebral metastases. Arch Neurol 1978;35:754–756
9. Chao JH, Phillips R, Nickson JJ. Roentgen-ray therapy of cerebral metastases. Cancer 1954;7:682–689
10. Chu FC, Hilaris BB. Value of radiation therapy on the management of intracranial metastases. Cancer 1961;4:577–581
11. Borgelt B, Gelber R, Kramer S, et al. The palliation of brain metastasis: final results of the first two studies by the Radiation Therapy Oncology Group. Int J Radiat Oncol Biol Phys 1980;6:1–9
12. Gelber RD, Larson M, Borgelt BB, et al. Equivalence of radiation schedules for the palliative treatment of brain metastases in patients with favorable prognosis. Cancer 1981;48:1749–1753
13. Borgelt B, Gelber R, Larson M, et al. Ultra-rapid high-dose irradiation schedules for the palliation of brain metastasis: final result of the first two studies by the Radiation Therapy Oncology Group. Int J Radiat Oncol Biol Phys 1981;7:1633–1638
14. Kurtz JM, Gelber R, Brady LW, et al. The palliation of brain metastasis in a favorable patient population: a randomized clinical trial by the Radiation Therapy Oncology Group. Int J Radiat Oncol Biol Phys 1981; 7:891–895
15. Sause WT, Scott C, Krisch R, et al. Phase I/I1 trial of accelerated fractionation in brain metastasis RTOG 85–28. Int J Radiat Oncol Biol Phys 1993;26:653–657
16. Murray KJ, Scott C, Greenberg HM, et al. A randomized phase III study of accelerated hyperfractionated versus standard in patients with unresected brain metastasis: a report of the Radiation Therapy Oncology Group (RTOG) 9104. Int J Radiat Oncol Biol Phys 1997;39: 571–574
17. Komarnicky LT, Philips TL, Martz K, et al. A randomized phase III protocol for the evaluation of misonidazole combined with radiation in the treatment of patients with brain metastases (RTOG 7916). Int J Radiat Oncol Biol Phys 1991;20:53–58

18. Phillips TL, Scott CB, Leibel S, et al. Results of a randomized comparison of radiotherapy and bromodeoxyuridine with radiotherapy alone for brain metastasis: a report of RTOG trial 89-05. Int J Radiat Oncol Biol Phys 1995;33:339–348
19. Sneed PK, Larson DA, Wara WM. Radiotherapy for cerebral metastases. Neurosurg Clin N Am 1996;7:505–515
20. Leksell L. The stereotactic method and radiosurgery of the brain. Acta Chir Scand 1951;102:316–319
21. Sturm V, Kober B, Hover KH, et al. Stereotactic percutaneous single dose irradiation of brain metastases with a linear accelerator. Int J Radiat Oncol Biol Phys 1987;13:279–282
22. Gaspar L, Scott C, Rotman M, et al. Recursive partitioning analysis (RPA) of prognostic factors in three Radiation Therapy Oncology Group (RTOG) brain metastases trials. Int J Radiat Oncol Biol Phys 1997;37:745–751
23. Lagerwaard FJ, Levendag PC, Novak PJ, et al. Identification of prognostic factors in patients with brain metastases: a review of 1292 patients. Int J Radiat Oncol Biol Phys 1999;43:795–801
24. Noordijk EM, Vecht CJ, Haaxma-Reiche H, et al. The choice of treatment of single brain metastasis should be based on extracranial tumor activity and age. Int J Radiat Oncol Biol Phys 1994;29:711–717
25. Patchell RA, Tibbs PA, Walsh JW, et al. A randomized trial of surgery in the treatment of single metastases to the brain. N Engl J Med 1990; 322:494–500
26. Mintz AH, Kestle J, Rathbone MP, et al. A randomized trial to assess the efficacy of surgery in addition to radiotherapy in patients with a single cerebral metastasis. Cancer 1996;78:1470–1476
27. Chin LS, Regine WF. Principles and Practice of Stereotactic Radiosurgery. New York: Springer-Verlag; 2008
28. Flickinger JC, Kondziolka D, Lunsford LD, et al. A multi-institutional experience with stereotactic radiosurgery for solitary brain metastasis. Int J Radiat Oncol Biol Phys 1994;28:797–802
29. Yu C, Chen JCT, Apuzzo MLJ, et al. Metastatic melanoma to the brain: prognostic factors after Gamma Knife radiosurgery. Int J Radiat Oncol Biol Phys 2002;52:1277–1287
30. Goyal LK, Suh JH, Reddy CA, et al. The role of whole brain radiotherapy and stereotactic radiosurgery on brain metastasis from renal cell carcinoma. Int J Radiat Oncol Biol Phys 2000;47:1007–1012
31. Leibel SA, Sheline GE. Radiation therapy for neoplasms of the brain. J Neurosurg 1987;66:1–22
32. Nieder C, Nestle U, Walter K, et al. Dose/effect relationships for brain metastases. J Cancer Res Clin Oncol 1998;124:346–350
33. Larson DA, Flickinger JC, Loeffler JS, et al. The radiobiology of radiosurgery. Int J Radiat Oncol Biol Phys 1993;25:557–561
34. Shaw E, Scott C, Souhami L, et al. Single dose radiosurgical treatment of recurrent previously irradiated primary brain tumors and brain metastases: final report of RTOG protocol 90-05. Int J Radiat Oncol Biol Phys 2000;47:291–298
35. Shehata MK, Young B, Reid B, et al. Stereotactic radiosurgery of 468 brain metastases ≤ 2 cm: implications for SRS dose and whole brain radiation therapy. Int J Radiat Oncol Biol Phys 2004;59:87–93
36. Mehta M, Noyes W, Craig B, et al. A cost-effectiveness and cost-utility analysis of radiosurgery vs. resection for single brain metastases. Int J Radiat Oncol Biol Phys 1997;39:445–454
37. Sperduto PW, Hall WA. Radiosurgery, cost-effectiveness, gold standards, the scientific method, cavalier cowboys, and the cost of hope. Int J Radiat Oncol Biol Phys 1996;36:511–513
38. Auchter RM, Lamond JP, Alexander E, et al. A multi-institutional outcome and prognostic factor analysis of radiosurgery for resectable single brain metastasis. Int J Radiat Oncol Biol Phys 1996;35:27–35
39. Bindal AK, Bindal RK, Hess KR, et al. Surgery versus radiosurgery in the treatment of brain metastases. J Neurosurg 1996;84:748–754
40. O'Neill BP, Iturria NJ, Link MJ, et al. A comparison of surgical resection and stereotactic radiosurgery in the treatment of solitary brain metastases. Int J Radiat Oncol Biol Phys 2003;55:1169–1176
41. Muacevic A, Kreth FW, Horstmann GA, et al. Surgery and radiotherapy compared with Gamma Knife radiosurgery in the treatment of solitary cerebral metastases of small diameter. J Neurosurg 1999;91: 35–43
42. Loeffler JS, Shrieve DC. What is appropriate therapy for a patient with a single brain metastasis? Int J Radiat Oncol Biol Phys 1994;29: 915–917
43. Loeffler JS, Kooy HM, Wen PW, et al. The treatment of recurrent brain metastasis with stereotactic radiosurgery. J Clin Oncol 1990;8:576–582
44. Alexander E III, Moriarty TM, Davis RB, et al. Stereotactic radiosurgery for the definitive, noninvasive treatment of brain metastasis. J Natl Cancer Inst 1995;87:34–40
45. Noël G, Proudhom MA, Valery CA, et al. Radiosurgery for re-irradiation of brain metastases: results in 54 patients. Radiother Oncol 2001;60: 61–67
46. Sanghavi SN, Miranpuri SS, Chappell R, et al. Radiosurgery for patients with brain metastases: a multi-institutional analysis, stratified by the RTOG recursive partitioning analysis method. Int J Radiat Oncol Biol Phys 2001;51:426–434
47. Stafinski T, Jhangri GS, Yan E, Menon D. Effectiveness of stereotactic radiosurgery alone or in combination with whole brain radiotherapy compared to conventional surgery and/or whole brain radiotherapy for the treatment of one or more brain metastases: a systematic review and meta-analysis. Cancer Treat Rev 2006;32(3): 203–213
48. Andrews DW, Scott CB, Sperduto PW, et al. Whole brain radiation therapy with or without stereotactic radiosurgery boost for patients with one to three brain metastases: phase III results of the RTOG 9508 randomised trial. Lancet 2004;363:1665–1672
49. Chidel MA, Suh JH, Reddy CA, et al. Application of recursive partitioning analysis and evaluation of the use of whole brain radiation among patients treated with stereotactic radiosurgery for newly diagnosed brain metastases. Int J Radiat Oncol Biol Phys 2000;47:993–999
50. Pirzkall A, Debus J, Lohr F, et al. Radiosurgery alone or in combination with whole-brain radiotherapy for brain metastases. J Clin Oncol 1998;16:3563–3569
51. Sneed PK, Lamborn KR, Forstner JM, et al. Radiosurgery for brain metastases: is whole brain radiotherapy necessary? Int J Radiat Oncol Biol Phys 1999;43:549–558
52. Patchell RA, Regine WF, Loeffler JS, et al. Radiosurgery plus whole-brain radiation therapy for brain metastases. JAMA 2006;296(17):2089–2090, author reply 2090–2091
53. Aoyama H, Shirato H, Tago M, et al. Stereotactic radiosurgery plus whole-brain radiation therapy vs stereotactic radiosurgery alone for treatment of brain metastases: a randomized controlled trial. JAMA 2006;295(21):2483–2491
54. Kihlstrom L, Karlsson B, Lindquist C. Gamma Knife surgery for cerebral metastases: implications for survival based on 16 years' experience. Stereotact Funct Neurosurg 1993;61:45–50
55. Valentino V. The results of radiosurgical management of 139 single cerebral metastases. Acta Neurochir Suppl (Wien) 1995;63:95–100
56. DeAngelis LM, Posner LB. Radiation-induced dementia in patients cured brain metastases. Neurology 1989;39:789–796
57. So NK, O'Neill BP, Frytak S, et al. Delayed leukoencephalopathy in survivors with small cell lung cancer. Neurology 1987;37:1198–1201
58. Shiau CY, Sneed PK, Shu HK, et al. Radiosurgery for brain metastases: relationship of dose and pattern of enhancement to local control. Int J Radiat Oncol Biol Phys 1997;37:375–383
59. Matsuo T, Shibata S, Yasunaga A, et al. Dose optimization and indication of linac radiosurgery for brain metastases. Int J Radiat Oncol Biol Phys 1999;45:931–939
60. Schoeggl A, Kitz K, Ertl A, et al. Prognostic factor analysis for multiple brain metastases after Gamma Knife radiosurgery: results in 97 patients. J Neurooncol 1999;42:169–175
61. Simonova G, Liscak R, Novotny J. Solitary brain metastases treated with the Leksell Gamma Knife: prognostic factors for patients. Radiother Oncol 2000;57:207–213
62. Joseph J, Adler JR, Cox RS, et al. Linear accelerator-based stereotaxic radiosurgery for brain metastases: the influence of number of lesions on survival. J Clin Oncol 1996;14:1085–1092
63. Cox JD, Stanley K, Petrovich Z, et al. Cranial irradiation in cancer of the lung of all cell types. JAMA 1981;245:469–472
64. Russell AH, Pajak TE, Selim HM, et al. Prophylactic cranial irradiation for lung cancer patients at high risk for development of cerebral metastasis: results of a prospective randomized trial conducted by the Radiation Therapy Oncology Group. Int J Radiat Oncol Biol Phys 1991;21:637–643
65. Umsawasdi T, Valdivieso M, Chen TT, et al. Role of elective brain irradiation during combined chemoradiotherapy for limited disease non-small cell lung cancer. J Neurooncol 1984;2:253–259
66. Mamon HJ, Yeap BY, Reblando J, et al. High risk of brain metastases in surgically staged IIIA non-small cell lung cancer patients treated with surgery, chemotherapy, and radiation. J Clin Oncol 2005;23: 1530–1537

67. Sneed PK, Suh JH, Goesch SJ, et al. A multi-institutional review of radiosurgery alone vs. radiosurgery with whole brain radiotherapy as the initial management of brain metastases. Int J Radiat Oncol Biol Phys 2002;53:519–526
68. Hasegawa T, Kondziolka D, Flickinger JC, et al. Brain metastases treated with radiosurgery alone: an alternative to whole brain radiotherapy? Neurosurgery 2003;52:1318–1326
69. Slotman B, Faivre-Finn C, Kramer G, et al. Prophylactic cranial irradiation in extensive small-cell lung cancer. N Engl J Med 2007; 357(7): 664–672
70. Lutterbach J, Cyron D, Henne K, et al. Radiosurgery followed by planned observation in patients with one to three brain metastases. Neurosurgery 2003;52:1066–1074
71. Rades D, Bohlen G, Pluemer A, et al. Stereotactic radiosurgery alone versus resection plus whole-brain radiotherapy for 1 or 2 brain metastases in recursive partitioning analysis class 1 and 2 patients. Cancer 2007;109(12):2515–2521
72. Aoyama H, Tago M, Kato N, et al. Neurocognitive function of patients with brain metastasis who received either whole brain radiotherapy plus stereotactic radiosurgery or radiosurgery alone. Int J Radiat Oncol Biol Phys 2007;68(5):1388–1395
73. Regine WF, Huhn JL, Patchell RA, et al. Risk of symptomatic brain tumor recurrence and neurologic deficit after radiosurgery alone in patients with newly diagnosed brain metastases: results and implications. Int J Radiat Oncol Biol Phys 2002;52:333–338
74. Manon R, O'Neill A, Knisely J, et al. Phase II trial of radiosurgery for one to three newly diagnosed brain metastases from renal cell carcinoma, melanoma, and sarcoma: an Eastern Cooperative Oncology Group study (E 6397). J Clin Oncol 2005;23(34):8870–8876
75. Huang CF, Kondziolka D, Flickinger JC, Lunsford LD. Stereotactic radiosurgery for brainstem metastases. J Neurosurg 1999;91(4):563–568
76. Yen CP, Sheehan J, Patterson G, Steiner L. Gamma Knife surgery for metastatic brainstem tumors. J Neurosurg 2006;105(2):213–219
77. Hussain A, Brown PD, Stafford SL, Pollock BE. Stereotactic radiosurgery for brainstem metastases: survival, tumor control, and patient outcomes. Int J Radiat Oncol Biol Phys 2007;67(2):521–524
78. Kased N, Huang K, Nakamura JL, et al. Gamma Knife radiosurgery for brainstem metastases: the UCSF experience. J Neurooncol 2008;86(2): 195–205
79. Iwai Y, Yamanaka K, Yoshimura M. Gamma Knife radiosurgery for cavernous sinus metastases and invasion. Surg Neurol 2005;64(5):406–410, discussion 410
80. Cmelak AJ, Cox RS, Adler JR, et al. Radiosurgery for skull base malignancies and nasopharyngeal carcinoma. Int J Radiat Oncol Biol Phys 1997;37(5):997–1003
81. Iwai Y, Yamanaka K, Honda Y, Matsusaka Y. Radiosurgery for pituitary metastases. Neurol Med Chir (Tokyo) 2004;44(3):112–116, discussion 117
82. Piedra MP, Brown PD, Carpenter PC, Link MJ. Resolution of diabetes insipidus following Gamma Knife surgery for a solitary metastasis to the pituitary stalk: case report. J Neurosurg 2004;101(6):1053–1056
83. Elias B, Uhl E. Intra- and parasellar manifestation of an Ewing's sarcoma before detection of the primary tumour. Acta Neurochir (Wien) 2002;144(7):747–748
84. Chen JC, Petrovich Z, Giannotta SL, Yu C, Apuzzo ML. Radiosurgical salvage therapy for patients presenting with recurrence of metastatic disease to the brain. Neurosurgery 2000;46(4):860–866, discussion 866–867
85. Breneman JC, Warnick RE, Albright RE Jr, et al. Stereotactic radiosurgery for the treatment of brain metastases: results of a single institution series. Cancer 1997;79:551–557
86. Chang EL, Selek U, Hassenbusch SJ III, et al. Outcome variation among "radioresistant" brain metastases treated with stereotactic radiosurgery. Neurosurgery 2005;56(5):936–945
87. Chin LS, Ma L, DiBiase S. Radiation necrosis following Gamma Knife surgery: a case-controlled comparison of treatment parameters and long-term clinical follow-up. J Neurosurg 2001;94(6):899–904
88. Ohguri T, Imada H, Kohshi K, et al. Effect of prophylactic hyperbaric oxygen treatment for radiation-induced brain injury after stereotactic radiosurgery of brain metastases. Int J Radiat Oncol Biol Phys 2007; 67(1):248–255

20

Stereotactic Radiosurgery for Pediatric Brain Tumors

Simon S. Lo, Gene H. Barnett, and John H. Suh

Brain tumors constitute 20% of all pediatric cancers and are the most common solid tumors in childhood.[1,2] Surgical resection is usually the mainstay of treatment, and maximal safe resection is the goal in most cases. Conventional fractionated radiation therapy is indicated for high-grade or incompletely resected or unresectable tumors.

Stereotactic radiosurgery (SRS) refers to a strategically delivered high dose of radiation to a target volume using megavoltage photons generated by a linear accelerator (linac), gamma rays from a Gamma Knife (Elekta Instruments AB, Stockholm, Sweden) unit, or protons generated by a cyclotron or synchrotron unit,[1,2] typically performed in one, but up to five, session(s). SRS has been used extensively to treat brain tumors in adults and has become one of the standard treatments for certain tumors. There is a moderate amount of literature on the use of SRS in the treatment of pediatric brain tumors. Unlike adult patients, there are substantial concerns of radiation-induced damage to the brain, leading to subsequent neurocognitive, neurologic, and neuroendocrine dysfunction. As a result of its favorable dosimetric characteristics, SRS represents a very attractive treatment modality for some pediatric patients with brain tumors. The physics and radiobiology of SRS are covered in other chapters of this textbook. This chapter will focus on the clinical applications and results of SRS in the treatment of pediatric brain tumors.

◆ Technical Issues Specific to Stereotactic Radiosurgery in Pediatric Patients

Unless a frameless radiosurgical system is used, rigid fixation is typically required in SRS because little or no margin around the target volume is given in treatment planning. As opposed to adults, where rigid fixation of the skull is readily achievable, younger children have thin skulls, which may not be completely fused. An alternative to insertion of pins into the outer skull table is the fabrication of a cast or aquaplast with piers where the pins can be inserted[2] (**Fig. 20.1**). A body cast for neck support is necessary because these patients are under general anesthesia, and their body sizes are small.

General anesthesia is generally required for younger children and older children who are psychologically too immature to withstand the whole radiosurgical procedure, because the patient needs to remain still during head frame placement, acquisition of computed tomography (CT) or magnetic resonance (MR) images, and treatment

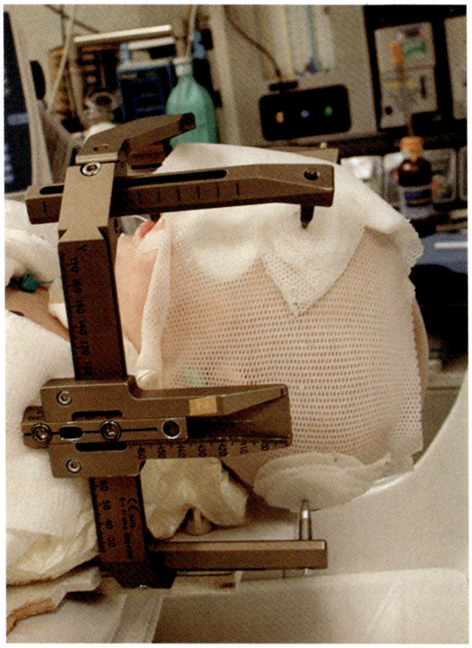

Fig. 20.1 An aquaplast was fabricated with piers where the pins can be inserted for fixation. (From Witt TC, Lo SS, Timmerman RD. Successful treatment of a skull base malignant rhabdoid tumor with surgery, chemotherapy and Gamma Knife-based stereotactic radiosurgery in a young child. Stereotact Funct Neurosurg 2007;85:310–313, with permission from Karger AG, Basel.)

delivery.[1,2] SRS is typically a 1-day procedure that entails lengthy processes mentioned above, complex treatment planning, and transportation of the patient to different parts of the hospital and sometimes a different hospital. Depending on the complexity of the planning and the treatment-planning system used, the time required can vary significantly. The treatment time can be prolonged, especially in circumstances where a Gamma Knife unit with old sources is used to deliver the radiation using trunnions and multiple small shots (isocenters). Prolonged anesthesia of those children undergoing SRS can be expected. To avoid unnecessary radiation exposure to support staff in the treatment area, patients are usually monitored by the anesthesiologist in the control area. When treatment planning is performed, the neurosurgeon and radiation oncologist involved in SRS should strike a balance between the time required in treatment planning and delivery and the extra conformality achieved with more complex planning. A new model of Gamma Knife, the Perfexion (Elekta), allows for shortened treatment and planning times. Radiation dose sculpting is also facilitated. These features may be beneficial for pediatric patients receiving SRS.

A frameless robotically controlled radiosurgical system such as CyberKnife (Accuray, Inc., Sunnyvale, CA) can potentially solve some of the problems associated with frame-based radiosurgical systems. The feasibility, safety, and efficacy of the use of this system in the treatment of brain tumors in pediatric patients, including very young children, have been demonstrated.[3]

◆ Specific Tumors

Ependymomas

Ependymomas account for 5 to 10% of all pediatric brain tumors.[4] Histologically, ependymomas are well-delineated, moderately cellular gliomas that have a sharp demarcation from the surrounding brain parenchyma.[5] Because of this characteristic, they are very well suited for SRS, where the prescribed isodose conforms highly to the target volume, and there is a rapid fall-off of the radiation dose beyond the target volume. Although not specifically categorized by Larson et al, based on their characteristics, ependymomas can be regarded as class IV targets (tumor composed of early-responding tissue with no intermingling normal brain tissue).[6]

The most important factor that determines survival for patients with ependymomas is the extent of surgical resection.[4,7–11] The presence of gross disease predicts a poor prognosis. SRS is used in this disease in children mainly in three settings, namely, as a boost after external beam radiation therapy, as a salvage treatment of recurrent disease, and, less commonly, as the sole treatment.

Boost Therapy

In pediatric patients with ependymomas treated in the primary setting, a radiation dose response has been demonstrated.[12–14] This is particularly relevant in patients with high-risk disease (incompletely resected tumor). In a Pediatric Oncology Group (POG) 9132 study, in which radiation dose escalation to 69.6 Gy was achieved by hyperfractionation, the 19 patients who underwent subtotal resection had superior survival outcomes compared with historic controls from an earlier POG 8532 trial.[4] SRS can deliver a single focused high dose of radiation to a target volume and has been used as a boost therapy after external beam radiation therapy for high-risk patients.

Investigators from St. Jude Children's Research Hospital reported their early experience with this approach. Five pediatric patients with residual enhancing ependymoma measuring ≤ 3 cm received a boost with linac-based SRS after external beam radiation therapy to doses of 50.4 to 55.8 Gy.[15] The SRS dose was 10 Gy (range 9–15 Gy) prescribed to the 80% isodose line. With a median follow-up time of 24 months (range 15–40 months), 80% (four of five patients) survived with no evidence of tumor progression.[15] Complete response was achieved in three (60%) of the five patients. Radionecrosis occurred in one (20%) of the five patients. In a pediatric SRS series from Harvard University, 3 of the 28 patients with ependymoma treated with SRS received it as a boost therapy after external beam radiation therapy. Two (67%) of the three patients survived without evidence of disease progression at 30 and 62 months, respectively.[16] In a series of nine patients treated with SRS for ependymoma from Washington University, three were treated with SRS as a boost therapy after external beam radiation therapy to doses of 45.0 to 53.6 Gy.[17] With follow-up times ranging from 56 to 91 months, the relapse-free survival rate was 100%.[17] Two (67%) of the three patients developed complications (seizures in one patient and facial nerve palsy in the other) after SRS. In the series from Indiana University, two pediatric patients were treated with SRS as boost therapy after external beam radiation therapy to doses of 54.0 to 55.8 Gy. Both patients remained progression free at 40 and 65 months, respectively.[18] One of the two patients developed radionecrosis, which was controlled with hyperbaric oxygen and steroid therapy.

In summary, the combination of external beam radiation therapy and boost with SRS is associated with excellent local control of gross residual disease in ependymoma, although some patients developed late radiation complications. Out of the 13 patients treated with this approach in the literature, 11 (85%) achieved long-term progression-free survival. However, prospective data supporting this approach are lacking. A prior POG phase II trial involving the use of SRS as a boost therapy for pediatric patients with high-risk ependymoma was closed, secondary to poor accrual. Future trials testing this approach may be worthwhile.

Salvage Therapy for Recurrent Disease

The recommended treatment for patients with recurrent ependymoma after prior surgery and postoperative external beam radiation therapy is salvage surgical resection. However, a complete resection may not be safely achievable in some cases. The response to chemotherapy is usually suboptimal in ependymoma. SRS provides a salvage option for patients where a complete resection is not possible and has been used for the treatment of recurrent ependymoma in pediatric patients.

In an early series from the University of Pittsburgh, seven pediatric patients with recurrent ependymoma (grade not specified) were treated with Gamma Knife radiosurgery. The reported recurrence rate was 100%, and the time to progression was 6 months.[19] In a subsequent study from the same institution, 22 patients (including adults and children) with progressive or recurrent anaplastic ependymoma were treated with Gamma Knife radiosurgery. The median dose was 16.1 Gy (range 10–20 Gy). With a median follow-up of 21 months, the 3-year local and cranial control rates were 62.3 and 32.4%, respectively.[20] Hodgson et al from Harvard University reported that among the 28 pediatric patients treated with SRS for ependymoma (3 treated with SRS as boost therapy after external beam radiation therapy and the remaining treated for recurrent disease), the median progression-free survival time was 8.5 months, and the 3-year local control was only 29%.[16] Out of the 25 patients treated for recurrent disease, only 3 remained disease free. In a series from the Mayo Clinic, 12 adult and pediatric patients with 16 recurrent ependymomas were treated with Gamma Knife radiosurgery. Eleven of them had prior external beam radiation therapy. The median prescribed dose was 18 Gy (range 12–24 Gy). With a median follow-up of 22.5 months, the 3-year local control was 68%, and 2 (17%) of the 12 patients developed distant neuraxis failure.[21] Two (17%) patients developed complications. In the Indiana University series, five patients (two children) with 10 recurrent ependymomas were treated with Gamma Knife radiosurgery. Out of the five patients who received SRS as salvage treatment, three (60%) were alive, two (40%) were alive without recurrence, two (40%) developed distant failure, and three (60%) had in-field control.[18] The 3-year in-field control for the 10 recurrent tumors was 62.5%.[18]

Most children with recurrent ependymomas have a prior history of external beam radiation therapy. If a complete surgical resection of the gross tumor is not achievable, they are left without other effective options. Chemotherapy has been used in ependymomas in various settings but with limited success. Local tumor progression is uniformly fatal. SRS provides a minimally invasive treatment modality, and dramatic responses to SRS have been observed. However, distant failure remains a significant issue. To address this problem, more effective chemotherapy treatments need to be developed.

Stereotactic Radiosurgery as the Sole Treatment

SRS is seldom used as the sole treatment for gross disease in ependymoma because most patients usually undergo external beam radiation therapy. There are scarce data in the literature on this approach. In a series from Indiana University, a 16-month-old child who had partial response to a subtotally resected cerebellopontine angle ependymoma received SRS as the sole treatment to delay external beam radiation therapy. The ependymoma progressed after 13 months, and salvage treatment with further chemotherapy and conformal radiation therapy was given.[18]

Although this approach appears to be sound, given the lack of adequate data from the literature documenting its efficacy and safety in this setting, SRS should typically not be offered as the sole treatment outside of a clinical trial setting. **Table 20.1** summarizes the treatment outcomes of selected series.

Low-Grade Astrocytomas

World Health Organization (WHO) grade I and II astrocytomas are collectively known as low-grade astrocytomas, which can occur in both adult and pediatric patients. Pilocytic astrocytomas (WHO grade I) represent the most indolent subtype of low-grade astrocytomas, with 10-year survival rates of over 90% in the pediatric population.[22] Diffuse astrocytomas (WHO grade II) carry a slightly worse prognosis in the pediatric population, with 10-year survival rates of ~80%.[22] The mainstay of treatment is maximal safe surgical resection, if achievable. If a complete resection is

Table 20.1 Summary of Treatment Outcomes of Stereotactic Radiosurgery for Ependymoma in Children

Study	No. of Patients	Histology	Marginal Dose (Gy)	Setting of Treatment	Local Control (%)
Aggarwal et al[15]	5	Ependymoma	10	Boost	80
Grabb et al[19]	7	Ependymoma (grade not specified)	11–20*	Salvage	0
Jawahar et al[20]	22 (adults and children)	Anaplastic ependymoma	16.1	Salvage	62.3
Hodgson et al[16]	28	Ependymoma	12.5	Salvage and boost	29†
	3		Not specified	Boost	67
Stafford et al[21]	12 (adults and children)	Ependymoma	18	Salvage	68
Lo et al[18]	5 (2 children)	Ependymoma§	12–20	Salvage	60‡
	2		12–14	Boost	100

* Dose range for the whole group of 25 children (including those with other histologies).
† Local control for all 29 patients.
‡ Local control for all 5 patients.
§ One patient had anaplastic ependymoma.

not achieved, chemotherapy is often given in young children to delay the need for immediate postoperative radiation therapy because of great concerns of collateral damage to the developing brain. However, if gross total resection or subtotal resection can be achieved, those children may be observed. SRS has been used in the treatment of low-grade astrocytoma in children in various settings, but the data in the literature are limited.

The data from the University of Pittsburgh represent one of the largest bodies of experience in the use of SRS in pediatric low-grade astrocytomas. In their early series, SRS was used as adjuvant treatment for growing and unresectable deep-seated pilocytic astrocytoma in nine children (two failed prior external beam radiation therapy). The mean prescribed dose was 15 Gy. With a median follow-up of 19 months, none of the patients treated developed progression (five had marked tumor shrinkage, and four had stable findings).[23] None of the patients experienced any acute or late toxicity. In a subsequent study from the same institution, 37 patients (25 pediatric patients) with recurrent or unresectable pilocytic astrocytoma were treated with SRS. The prescribed dose was 15 Gy. Eighteen patients had brainstem tumors. Out of the 37 patients treated, 10 had complete response, 8 had partial response, 7 had stable findings, and 12 had delayed tumor progression on imaging studies.[24] There was no treatment-related mortality. At a median follow-up of 28 months, the crude survival rate was 89%.[24] The researchers also reported their treatment outcomes of SRS for WHO grade II fibrillary astrocytoma. A total of 12 patients (4 children) with progressive disease were treated with SRS to a median dose of 16 Gy. Four of the 12 patients had tumors in the brainstem. Tumor volumes ranged from 1.2 to 45.1 mL. At a median follow-up of 52 months, all patients were alive.[25] Five patients had tumor shrinkage (one complete and four partial responses), three had stable findings, and four had delayed progression. The crude freedom from progression (FFP) rate was 67%.[25]

One of the largest series of SRS for low-grade astrocytoma was from Japan. A total of 51 adult and pediatric patients with low-grade astrocytomas were treated with Gamma Knife radiosurgery. Out of the 51 patients, 12 had WHO grade I astrocytomas around the optic pathway or hypothalamus. The remaining patients had WHO grade II astrocytomas. The mean age for patients with grade I astrocytomas was 9.8 years. The mean prescribed doses for grades I and II tumors were 12.5 and 15.7 Gy, respectively. The respective tumor diameters were 2.54 and 2.37 cm. With a median follow-up period of 27.6 months, the response rates for grades I and II astrocytomas were 50.0 and 46.2%, respectively.[26] The corresponding tumor control rates were 91.7 and 87.2%, respectively.[26] There was a significantly better response for patients 10 years of age or older with grade I tumors and those with a follow-up period of more than 24 months. Radiation-induced edema occurred in 18 (35.3%) patients, cyst formation or enlargement in 5 (9.8%), and transient tumor enlargement in 3 (5.9%).[26]

In a study from Spain, Barcia et al reported the treatment results of 16 patients with low-grade gliomas treated with SRS. Six patients had prior conventional radiation therapy. The mean dose given was 21.7 Gy. Complete response and partial response or stabilization were observed in 50 and 31% of the tumors treated, respectively.[27] Three patients with tumors located in the brainstem died of tumor progression. Another study from Europe reported favorable treatment outcomes. Nineteen patients (16 children) from a Swedish institution were treated with SRS for pilocytic astrocytoma. The median tumor volume and the median prescribed dose were 2.2 mL and 10 Gy, respectively. Out of the 19 patients treated, 18 achieved tumor control at a median follow-up of 4.7 years.[28] The tumor shrinkage rate was 85%. Increased contrast enhancement and edema attributable to SRS were observed in 25% of the patients.[28] **Table 20.2** summarizes the treatment outcomes of selected series.

As described by Larson et al, low-grade astrocytomas or gliomas are classified as category III targets, which are defined as

Table 20.2 Summary of Treatment Outcomes of Stereotactic Radiosurgery for Low-Grade Astrocytomas in Children

Study	No. of Patients	Histology	Marginal Dose (Gy)	Setting of Treatment	Local Control (%)
Somaza et al[23]	9	JPA	15	Adjuvant or salvage	100
Hadjipanayis et al[24]	25	JPA	15	Primary or salvage	89*
Hadjipanayis et al[25]	12 (4 children)	Well-circumscribed WHO grade II astrocytoma	16	Primary or salvage	67†
Kida et al[26]	51 (adult and children)	WHO grade I astrocytoma	12.5	Not specified	91.7
		WHO grade II astrocytoma	15.7		87.2
Barcia et al[27]	16	Low-grade glioma	21.7	Primary or boost	81
Boëthius et al[28]	16	JPA	10	Adjuvant	94‡

* Local control of 37 patients, including 12 adults.
† Local control for all 12 patients.
‡ Local control of 19 patients, including 3 adults.
Abbreviations: JPA, juvenile pilocytic astrocytoma; WHO, World Health Organization.

targets that are early-responding tissue intermingled with normal brain parenchyma, which is late-responding tissue.[6] It is more common to have normal brain parenchyma intermingled with the target tissue in WHO grade II than in WHO grade I astrocytomas. Based on the radiobiological characteristics described by Larson et al, low-grade astrocytomas are not regarded as ideal targets for SRS.[6] Furthermore, as opposed to WHO grade I or pilocytic astrocytomas, WHO grade II tumors are usually less well demarcated from the normal brain parenchyma. Data in the literature regarding the use of SRS in children with newly diagnosed or recurrent low-grade astrocytomas are relatively limited. Despite the notion that low-grade astrocytomas are not ideal targets for SRS, data from various series have demonstrated good local control and acceptable toxicity profile. **Figure 20.2** shows the treatment plan of a WHO grade I astrocytoma treated with SRS. It appears that SRS is safe and efficacious in the management of pediatric patients with low-grade astrocytoma and is especially useful in cases where there is a prior history of external beam radiation therapy and complete surgical resection is not possible. Currently, there are not enough data to support the routine use of SRS in children with newly diagnosed low-grade astrocytoma, and this is best tested in a clinical trial setting.

High-Grade Gliomas

High-grade gliomas constitute 15% of primary brain tumors in children and usually carry a dismal prognosis despite the improvement in treatments in the past 2 decades.[2] They have a propensity to spread microscopically beyond the extent of tumor demonstrated on diagnostic imaging, but the main pattern of failure is still within 2 cm of the original tumor.[29] In adults, prospective trials and studies have been done using hyperfractionation or addition of a boost with brachytherapy.[30–32] Because of its favorable

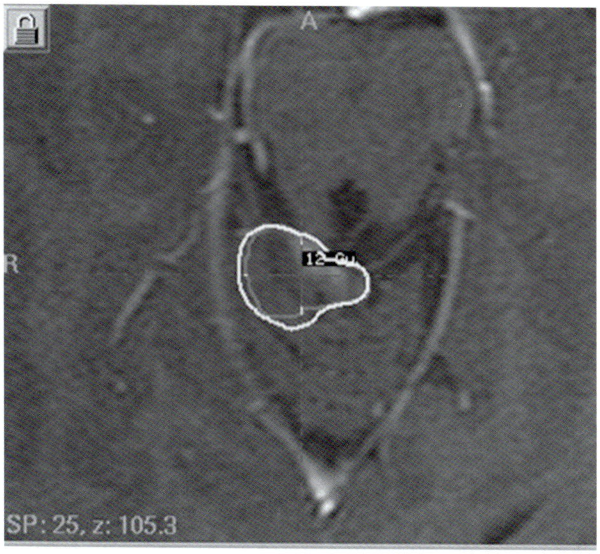

Fig. 20.2 A 5-year-old patient with WHO grade I (pilocytic) astrocytoma in the posterior fossa treated with Gamma Knife radiosurgery to a prescribed marginal dose of 12 Gy.

dosimetric characteristics, SRS has also been used as a boost therapy for dose escalation in adults with high-grade gliomas.[33] SRS has also been used in patients with recurrent high-grade gliomas after prior external beam radiation therapy. However, data regarding the use of SRS for children with high-grade gliomas are very limited.

In a series from Harvard University, 18 patients with glioblastoma multiforme or anaplastic astrocytoma received SRS. Out of the 18 patients treated, only 4 of them, all of whom received SRS as boost therapy, survived, with progression after 50 to 119 months.[16] The overall median survival time was 12 months after SRS. Other series showed similar dismal outcomes. In a study from the University of California, San Francisco, 11 children with high-grade gliomas were treated with SRS. Out of the 14 tumors treated, only 5 (36%) were controlled.[34] In the study from the University of Pittsburgh, 12 children with malignant glial tumors (malignant astrocytoma or ependymoma) were treated with Gamma Knife radiosurgery. Ten of the children had prior external beam radiation therapy. Five of them were alive 12 to 72 months after SRS, with three remaining disease free.[19] The remaining seven children died of their disease, with a median survival of 6 months.

As in adults, high-grade gliomas carry a very poor prognosis in children. SRS has been used in children with high-grade gliomas as primary or adjuvant treatment, boost therapy, and salvage treatment for recurrent disease with uniformly poor survival outcomes. Based on the very limited data available, it is very difficult to draw any meaningful conclusions regarding the role of SRS in the management of high-grade gliomas in children. Attempts have been made by the Children's Cancer Study Group (CCG) and the Pediatric Oncology Group (POG) to conduct prospective trials to test the use of SRS in recurrent pediatric brain tumors, but both trials were closed because of poor accrual. If data are extrapolated from adult literature, there does not seem to be enough evidence to support the routine use of SRS as the sole treatment or as boost therapy after external beam radiation therapy in children with high-grade gliomas. Radiation Therapy Oncology Group (RTOG) has conducted a phase III randomized trial (RTOG 9305) comparing no boost and SRS boost after external beam radiation therapy and carmustine (BCNU) chemotherapy for adult patients with glioblastoma multiforme but has not resulted in any improvement of survival outcomes.[33] However, SRS may have a role in the recurrent setting when there is a history of prior external beam radiation therapy, when the patient is not responding to chemotherapy, or when complete surgical resection is not achievable. An evidence-based review by the American Society for Therapeutic Radiology and Oncology (ASTRO) arrived at the same conclusions mentioned above.[35]

Medulloblastomas

Medulloblastomas constitute 15 to 20% of all childhood primary brain tumors.[1,2] Secondary to the high propensity for spinal axis dissemination, craniospinal irradiation followed by a posterior fossa boost with or without chemotherapy after maximal safe resection of the tumor is the standard therapy. Like other malignant brain tumors, a radiation dose response has been demonstrated in medulloblastomas.[1,2] SRS can potentially be used as boost therapy to escalate the radiation dose to residual disease after external beam radiation therapy. It can also be used as salvage therapy for children who develop recurrence after radiation therapy.

There are very scarce data on the use of SRS for the treatment of children with medulloblastomas. Two series came from Harvard University. In the earlier series, 11 children with recurrent and 3 with newly diagnosed medulloblastomas were treated with SRS to a median dose of 12 Gy as salvage treatment and as boost therapy, respectively. Those three patients who received SRS as boost therapy were alive without evidence of recurrence at a median follow-up interval of 27 months.[36] Out of the 11 children with recurrent disease, 6 developed distant failure and eventually died of their disease, but none of the 11 patients developed any local failure. Their median survival time was 10 months.[36] In their subsequent study with more patients included and longer follow-up interval, Hodgson et al reported a median progression-free survival time of 11 months. The 3-year local control rate was 57%.[16] Again, the main pattern of failure was distant. In a smaller study by Woo et al, the reported local control rate of the four patients (two children) treated with SRS as boost therapy after craniospinal and posterior fossa irradiation was 100%.[37] The prescribed dose ranged from 4.5 to 10.0 Gy.

SRS has been used as boost or salvage therapy for medulloblastomas in children. Based on the very limited data available, it is very difficult to draw meaningful conclusions regarding the role of SRS in this disease. The standard treatment for newly diagnosed medulloblastoma is maximal safe resection and combined chemotherapy and craniospinal followed by posterior fossa irradiation. The amount of residual tumor after surgical resection affects disease control. Although using SRS as boost therapy appears to be a sound approach for radiation dose escalation to residual tumor, there is insufficient evidence to support its routine use in children with residual medulloblastoma after surgical resection. In the recurrent setting, SRS provides a noninvasive option for ablative local therapy. Based on the very limited data from the literature, SRS can provide reasonable local control, although it does not address the high risk of distant failure, which is to be tackled with chemotherapy.

Meningiomas

Meningiomas are rare in children and account for 1 to 3% of all childhood intracranial tumors.[1,2] The standard treatment is complete surgical extirpation. If a gross total resection is achieved, no further treatment is required. However, complete resection of skull base meningiomas is not always achievable even with modern microsurgical techniques.

In adults, SRS has become one of the standard treatments for meningiomas. There are abundant data in the literature documenting the efficacy and safety of SRS in the treatment of meningiomas in adults, and this is discussed elsewhere in this textbook. Radiobiologically, meningiomas are category II targets (tumor composed of late-responding tissue with no intermingling normal brain tissue) and have a sharp demarcation from normal brain parenchyma.[6] These characteristics lend themselves well to SRS. However, the data on the use of SRS for the treatment of children with meningiomas are very limited. Eder et al reported the treatment results of two pediatric patients treated with Gamma Knife radiosurgery for skull base meningioma. Tumor shrinkage after treatment was demonstrated in both patients.[38] Im et al reported tumor control at 2.5 years in a 15-year-old patient who underwent Gamma Knife radiosurgery after subtotal resection for a meningioma.[39] Other reports included both adult and pediatric patients, and the results were collectively reported. In a series of 121 adult and pediatric patients treated with Gamma Knife radiosurgery, DiBiase et al reported a crude local control rate of 91.7%.[40]

Data from the large body of experience in adults and limited data in children suggest that SRS is a safe and efficacious treatment for meningiomas. It appears that similarly favorable outcomes in adults can be reproduced in children. Based on the description by Larson et al, meningiomas are category II targets.[6] Coupled with their sharp demarcation from normal brain parenchyma, they are regarded as excellent targets for SRS. The typical prescribed dose for meningiomas in adults is 12 to 18 Gy, and similar guidelines should apply to children. **Figure 20.3** shows the treatment plan of a prepontine meningioma treated with SRS.

Vestibular Schwannomas

Vestibular schwannomas (VSs) are typically slow-growing benign tumors that usually occur in adults. In children, VSs are usually associated with neurofibromatosis type 2 (NF2).[1,2] Treatment options include observation, surgery, SRS, and fractionated radiation therapy. VSs are regarded as category II targets, and they have very sharp margins of demarcation from the surrounding normal tissue.[6] These characteristics render them excellent targets for SRS.

SRS has emerged as one of the standard treatments for VS. There is a large body of experience in the use of SRS in adults, but the data on its use in pediatric patients are scarce.[41,42] In the earlier adult series where the prescribed

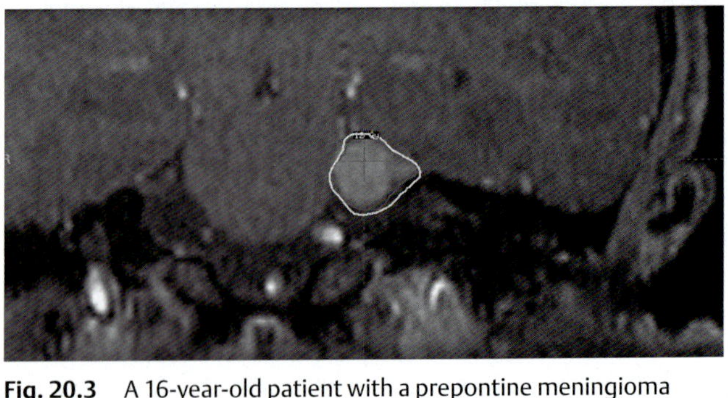

Fig. 20.3 A 16-year-old patient with a prepontine meningioma treated with Gamma Knife radiosurgery to a prescribed marginal dose of 12 Gy.

marginal dose was 16 to 20 Gy, there was a substantial incidence of hearing loss and cranial nerve deficits.[41,43] These have prompted dose reduction to minimize those risks. Utilization of reduced doses of 12 to 13 Gy in modern series has resulted in a much higher rate of preservation of serviceable hearing and also a lower incidence of trigeminal and facial nerve injury from SRS.[41,42]

In a series from the University of Pittsburgh, five children with NF2 were treated with Gamma Knife radiosurgery. Tumor shrinkage or stabilization was achieved in all patients at a mean follow-up of 23 months, although one patient required surgical resection for recurrence.[44] In a subsequent series from the same institution, 62 adult and pediatric patients with 74 VSs were treated with Gamma Knife radiosurgery for VS associated with NF2. Patients with bilateral VSs were treated with staged SRS. The median marginal dose was 14 Gy. Thirty-two tumors were associated with complete deafness, whereas the remaining tumors were associated with some hearing function (26 of them associated with serviceable hearing). The local control rates were 85, 85, and 81%, respectively, at 5, 10, and 15 years.[45] The rates of preservation of serviceable hearing were 73, 59, and 48% at 1, 2, and 5 years, respectively, if MRI-based image-guided treatment planning and a prescribed dose of $\leq$ 14 Gy were used.[45] Other studies including both adults and children treated with SRS for VS associated with NF2 showed similarly favorable tumor control rates but worse hearing preservation rates.[46,47] **Table 20.3** summarizes the treatment outcomes of selected series.

In children, VS is usually associated with NF2, and special considerations have to be taken in regard to treatment recommendation. Preservation of serviceable hearing is of particular importance in children because hearing deficits can result in speech and learning problems. Compared with sporadic VS, a higher risk of treatment-related complications is observed in NF2-associated VS.[45] Furthermore, patients with the latter may develop multiple central nervous system tumors. Therefore, the goals of therapy are preservation of function and maintenance of quality of life, rather than complete tumor ablation. For children with asymptomatic NF2-associated VSs, close observation is the most reasonable option. Treatment is indicated only when there is evidence of progressive tumor growth, progressive hearing loss, or large symptomatic tumors. SRS provides a minimally invasive method to control those tumors.

Malignant transformation of VS has always been a concern after SRS.[48] It has been postulated that radiation might predispose NF2 patients who have loss of one allele of a tumor suppressor gene to late secondary malignant transformation. However, there is no conclusive evidence in the literature suggesting that the malignant transformation rates are higher in NF2-associated VSs than the very low rate reported in sporadic VSs.[45]

Craniopharyngiomas

Craniopharyngiomas are benign brain tumors that commonly occur in children. They can be purely solid, purely cystic, or mixed solid and cystic. If feasible, maximal safe resection is the standard treatment. However, complete surgical resection is not always achievable, and postoperative radiation therapy is often offered to improve local control.[2] Occasionally, primary external beam radiation therapy or intralesional brachytherapy is offered. Similar to other extra-axial benign tumors in childhood, craniopharyngiomas have sharp margins of demarcation from the surrounding structures, including the brain parenchyma.[2] Furthermore, based on the description by Larson et al, they should be regarded as category II targets.[6] All these characteristics lend themselves well to SRS, which allows for a rapid fall-off of radiation dose beyond the target volume and therefore can be potentially beneficial in pediatric patients with craniopharyngiomas. However, the typically close proximity of the optic apparatus from tumor poses a challenge in the use of SRS for treatment.[1,2]

There is a moderate amount of data from the literature on the use of SRS for craniopharyngiomas in adults and children. In a study from Sweden, the treatment outcomes of 21 patients (11 children) with 22 craniopharyngiomas were reported. The prescribed dose ranged from 3 to 25 Gy. Some patients who had craniopharyngiomas with a cystic component received SRS for the solid component and intralesional brachytherapy for the cystic component. The mean tumor volume was 7.8 mL. With a mean follow-up time of 7.5 years (range 0.5–29.0 years), 5 tumors shrank in size, 3 were unchanged, and 14 enlarged.[49] Eleven (85%) of 13 tumors that

Table 20.3 Summary of Treatment Outcomes of Stereotactic Radiosurgery for Vestibular Schwannoma Associated with Neurofibromatosis Type 2 in Children

Study	Age Range (years)	No. of Patients/ Tumors	Dose (Gy)	Tumor Control (%)	Hearing Preservation (%)	Complications (%)
Kida et al[47]	7–71	20/20	13 (10–15)	100	33.3	VII nerve: 20%
Rowe et al[46]	11–59	96/122	Mostly 10–16, with 30 tumors receiving 17.5–25.0	79	40	VII nerve: 8% V nerve: 2%
Mathieu et al[45]	11–79	60/72*	14 (11–20)	88	53	VII nerve: 8% V nerve: 4%

* Two patients were lost to follow-up.

received a dose < 6 Gy to the margin enlarged compared with only 3 (33%) of 9 tumors that received ≥ 6 Gy.[49] Nine (82%) of 11 tumors in children ultimately enlarged after SRS, compared with 5 (50%) of 10 in adults. Eight patients developed visual deterioration, which was attributed to tumor enlargement in all but one case.[49] Four patients developed pituitary deficiencies. In a study from Taiwan, Chung et al treated 31 patients (9 children younger than 16 years) who had craniopharyngioma with SRS. Ten tumors were purely cystic, 5 purely solid, and 16 mixed cystic and solid. Two patients had external beam radiation therapy. Although the tumor marginal doses ranged from 9.5 to 16.0 Gy (mean 12.2 Gy), the dose delivered to the optic apparatus was limited to 8 Gy (range 7.2–12.5 Gy). Three patients underwent stereotactic aspiration to decompress the cystic component before SRS. The mean target volume was 8.94 mL. The tumor response and tumor control rates were 64.6 and 87.2%, respectively.[50] The complete response rate was 32.7%.[50] Tumors that were purely cystic or solid had better local control than tumors with mixed components. Smaller tumors had better tumor control than larger ones. Three patients developed cystic enlargement of their tumor that compressed the adjacent structures at 5, 8, and 17 months after SRS, respectively.[50] They all required further intervention for decompression.[50] Mokry from Austria reported on 23 patients (11 children younger than 15 years) who had craniopharyngiomas treated with SRS. Ten patients underwent cyst aspiration and intracystic instillation of bleomycin prior to SRS. The mean dose was 10.8 Gy (range 8–15 Gy). Tumor control was 56%.[51] Five patients with multicystic residual or recurrent tumors developed tumor progression.

Amendola et al reported on the outcomes of 14 patients (12 children) who had craniopharyngiomas treated with Gamma Knife radiosurgery. The mean dose was 14 Gy. The maximum doses to the optic apparatus and brainstem were limited to 8 and 14 Gy, respectively. One patient had prior external beam radiation therapy. A progression-free survival rate of 100% was achieved at follow-up times ranging from 6 to 86 months.[52] Isaac et al also reported a 100% local control rate in five patients treated with SRS for primary or salvage treatment of craniopharyngiomas, with follow-up times ranging from 7 to 29 months.[53] In the series from the University of Pittsburgh, 10 patients (mostly children) received Gamma Knife radiosurgery for the treatment of recurrent or residual craniopharyngiomas. Twelve SRS procedures were performed to treat the solid component of the tumor. The median marginal dose was 16.4 Gy (range 12.5–20.0 Gy), the mean target volume was 1.7 mL, and the median follow-up was 63 months. Six patients noticed improvement of their vision, and one developed further visual deterioration. Two patients had stable vision. Seven of the 12 tumors treated with SRS showed complete or partial response after SRS within a median of 8.5 months.[54]

The largest body of experience was reported by a group in Japan. Kobayashi et al reported the treatment outcomes of 107 patients (38 patients younger than 15 years) who had craniopharyngiomas treated with Gamma Knife radiosurgery. Among those patients, 13 had prior external beam radiotherapy. Ninety-eight patients had follow-up information. The tumor diameter and volume were 1.88 cm and 3.5 mL, respectively. The prescribed dose was 11.5 Gy. With a median follow-up of 65.5 months, the tumor control rate was 79.6%, with a complete response rate of 19.4%.[55] The 5- and 10-year survival rates were 94.1 and 91%, respectively.[55] The progression-free survival rates were 60.8 and 53.8%, respectively.[55] Among the 91 patients with evaluable information on neurologic and endocrinologic symptoms, symptomatic deterioration occurred in 16.5% of the patients.[55] **Table 20.4** summarizes the treatment outcomes of selected series.

Data in the literature show reasonable local control with the use of SRS for craniopharyngiomas as primary treatment or adjunctive treatment alone or combining with intralesional brachytherapy (for cystic lesions or components) or salvage treatment for recurrence.[49–55] The close proximity of the optic apparatus to craniopharyngiomas in many cases can create technical issues in treatment planning.[2] Typically, the dose constraint for the optic apparatus

Table 20.4 Summary of Treatment Outcomes of Stereotactic Radiosurgery for Craniopharyngioma in Children

Study	No. of Patients	Dose (Gy)	Other Treatment Received	Local Control (%)
Ulfarsson et al[49]	21 (11 children)	3–25	Intralesional brachytherapy in some patients with cystic component	< 6 Gy: 15% ≥ 6 Gy: 67% Children: 18%
Chung et al[50]	31 (9 children < 16 years)	9.5–16.0	3 children had stereotactic aspiration	87.2% CR: 32.7%
Mokry[51]	23 (11 children < 15 years)	8–15	10 patients with cystic component received cystic aspiration and intracystic bleomycin	56%
Amendola et al[52]	14 (12 children)	14	1 patient had prior external beam radiation therapy	100%
Chiou et al[54]	10 with 12 tumors (mostly children)	12.5–20.0	Some patients received radiation therapy	58%
Kobayashi et al[55]	107 (38 children < 15 years)*	11.5	13 had prior external beam radiation therapy	79.6

* Only 98 patients had follow-up.
Abbreviation: CR, complete response.

is set at 8 Gy. This is based on a seminal study by Tishler et al from Harvard University.[56] This will entail limiting the prescribed marginal dose to 8 Gy if the tumor is very close to or abutting the optic apparatus. An analysis by Stafford et al from the Mayo Clinic showed that even with a maximum point dose of 10 to 12 Gy in the optic apparatus, no optic neuropathy was observed.[57] The risk of optic neuropathy was 1.7% for patients receiving < 8 Gy, 1.8% for patients receiving between 8 and 10 Gy, and 6.9% for patients receiving > 12 Gy.[57] This dataset suggests that the marginal dose can be safely increased to 10 to 12 Gy even when the tumor is abutting the optic apparatus. Data in the literature suggest that 12 Gy might be an adequate dose to achieve local control of craniopharyngioma.[49,50,52,55] A highly conformal plan is desirable to minimize the risk of optic neuropathy by limiting the amount of optic apparatus receiving the maximum tolerated dose. For Gamma Knife treatments, this can be achieved using smaller shots and plugging/blank sectors. Cystic enlargement of craniopharyngiomas can occur after SRS; this can result in compression of the optic apparatus, leading to visual deterioration.[50] This possibility has to be kept in mind when a child develops visual deterioration after SRS.

Pituitary Adenomas

Pituitary adenomas are a heterogeneous group of tumors arising from the pituitary and are relatively rare in children.[2] They can be secretory or nonsecretory. Maximal safe resection is the mainstay of treatment in most cases, especially when the tumor is encroaching on the optic pathway. However, complete surgical resection may not always be achieved. Furthermore, in cases of secretory pituitary adenomas, persistent hypersecretion may still occur after a complete surgical resection. Postoperative radiation therapy is often offered for tumor or endocrine control. There are data in the literature to suggest that SRS may produce a quicker normalization of hypersecretion compared with fractionated radiation therapy in patients with secretory pituitary adenomas.[2,58]

There is a fair amount of literature on the use of SRS for pituitary adenomas in adults.[58] However, data on the use of SRS for pituitary adenoma in children are much more limited. In a study from the Karolinska Institute in Sweden, Thoren et al reported excellent outcomes in eight children with Cushing disease treated with Gamma Knife radiosurgery. The observation time ranged from 2.60 to 6.75 years. Among the eight patients treated, seven showed complete endocrine remission.[59] All patients exhibited deficiencies of growth hormones after SRS.[59] In a study from Japan, Kobayashi et al also reported excellent results in terms of endocrine response in two children with Cushing disease treated with Gamma Knife radiosurgery.[60] Castinetti et al from France reported the results of 40 patients (4 patients 18 years or younger) with Cushing disease treated with Gamma Knife radiosurgery after surgery. Out of the four children treated, two achieved normalization of their cortisol levels at an average of 12 months.[61] The median dose given was 25 Gy at the 50% isodose line. Both pediatric patients who did not achieve an endocrine cure were on ketoconazole at the time of SRS.[61] In the study from Harvard University, 18 patients (including adults and children) with pituitary adenomas were treated with linac-based SRS. The prescribed dose ranged from 10 Gy at the 85% isodose line to 15 Gy at the 65% isodose line. Although the tumor control rate was 100%, the rate of normalization of hormonal activity was only 33%.[62] The 3-year freedom from central nervous system adverse effects rate was 72.2%.[62]

Limited data in the literature in children suggest that the treatment outcomes are similar to those in adults.[59–62] Typically, the tumor control rates are uniformly excellent, whereas the endocrine control rates are lower. The adverse effect of antisecretory medications on endocrine normalization is also demonstrated in children.[61] One major challenge in the use of SRS in the treatment of pituitary adenomas is the proximity of the target volume to the optic pathway.[1,2] Unlike SRS for craniopharyngiomas, a much higher prescribed dose to the target volume is needed in secretory pituitary adenomas for endocrine cure.[58] Therefore, an adequate gap between the optic apparatus and the pituitary tumor is needed to avoid injury to the optic apparatus. Different maneuvers, such as plugging and adjustment of the gamma angle (to align with the long axis of the optic apparatus), can be used to avoid the optic apparatus.[58] Typically, the dose to the optic apparatus is kept < 8 Gy. If the patient has a pituitary adenoma that is encroaching on the optic pathway, a transsphenoidal resection should be offered because significant shrinkage of the tumor after SRS is not expected. If there is residual disease that is far enough (3–5 mm) from the optic pathway, SRS may be offered as an adjuvant treatment.[2] As in adults, if SRS is used in children with secretory pituitary adenomas, a dose of at least 25 to 30 Gy is required if the dose to the optic apparatus permits. For nonsecretory tumors, a lower dose (15–20 Gy) is required. If the distance between the target volume and the optic apparatus is too narrow so that dose reduction for SRS is necessary, fractionated radiation therapy is more suitable.[2]

Pineal Tumors

Pineal tumors represent a wide spectrum of histologies and are relatively rare. Common histologies include germ cell and pineal parenchymal tumors.[2] Primitive neuroectodermal tumor (PNET) can also occur in the pineal gland.[2] Specific treatment depends highly on histology. Overall, the data in the literature on the use of SRS for pineal tumors are limited.

In an early series from France, 11 patients (adult and children) with pineal tumors of various histologies, including pineocytoma, tectal astrocytoma, germinoma, pineoblastoma, and meningioma, were treated with SRS. The marginal doses ranged from 12 to 20 Gy. None of the 11 patients received external beam radiation therapy. At a median follow-up of 12.3 months (range 2–34 months), all tumors responded to SRS.[63] No significant complications were observed. In another series from France, 13 patients (5 children) were treated with Gamma Knife radiosurgery for pineal parenchymal tumors. Among the five children treated, three had pineocytomas, and two had pineoblastomas. None of them received external beam radiation therapy. The central doses ranged from 24 to 40 Gy. Out of the five pediatric patients treated, one with pineocytoma was lost to follow-up. Both patients with pineoblastoma had either complete response or 90% partial response, but one developed brain metastasis at 23 months, and one died at 10 months.[64] For the remaining two patients with pineocytoma, one achieved a complete response at 72 months and one a partial response after SRS at 12 months.[64]

In the study from the University of Pittsburgh, Hasegawa et al reported the results of 16 patients (adults and children) with pineal parenchymal tumors treated with Gamma Knife radiosurgery as the primary or an adjuvant treatment after surgery. There were six patients in the pediatric age group. Three of them had pineocytoma, two had pineoblastoma, and one had mixed pineal parenchymal tumor. The prescribed dose ranged from 14 to 16 Gy. The two patients with pineoblastoma also received craniospinal irradiation. The local control was 100% for the 14 patients with imaging follow-up.[65] Both pediatric patients with pineoblastoma died 18 and 47 months after SRS.[65] The other four pediatric patients survived.[65] Complications were not observed in the six pediatric patients. In another study from the University of Pittsburgh, four patients (aged 9, 18, 18, and 21 years) with pineal nongerminomatous germ cell tumors were treated with Gamma Knife radiosurgery. All patients received chemotherapy and fractionated radiotherapy, and SRS was used as a boost. The marginal dose ranged from 12 to 16 Gy. At a mean follow-up time of 25 months, local control was obtained in three of the four patients treated.[66]

In a study from Japan, Kobayashi et al reported the outcomes of 30 patients (both adult and pediatric) with pineal and related tumors treated with Gamma Knife radiosurgery. Out of the 30 patients, 19 received previous radiotherapy. There were 21 pineal tumors, including 4 germinomas, 7 malignant germ cell tumors, 2 syncytiotrophoblastic giant cell tumors, 3 pineocytomas, and 2 pineoblastomas. Pineal tumors were treated to a mean dose of 15.7 Gy. Pineocytomas and pineoblastomas were treated to a mean dose of 16.6 Gy. The complete response rate was 26.7%, and the overall response rate was 73.3%.[67] The local control in germinomas and pineocytomas was 100%.[67] Pineoblastomas and malignant germ cell tumors responded poorly to SRS.[67] In another series from Japan, three patients with pineal germinomas were treated with Gamma Knife radiosurgery to a dose of 10 to 12 Gy, followed by whole ventricular irradiation of 24 Gy. All patients had solitary pineal tumors measuring $\leq$ 3 cm. Complete response was obtained in all three patients.[68]

Amendola et al from the Miami Neuroscience Center reported their outcomes of 20 patients (14 patients in the pediatric age group) with pineal tumors of various histologies, including 13 germ cell tumors, 2 pineoblastomas, 2 low-grade gliomas, 1 primitive neuroectodermal tumor, 1 teratoma, and 1 pineocytoma treated with SRS. The median dose was 11 Gy (range 8–20 Gy). The mean target volume was 3.1 mL. Five patients underwent chemotherapy, and four received adjuvant external beam radiation therapy. Seventeen (85%) patients were alive after treatment, with a median follow-up of 30.4 months.[69] Lekovic et al from the Barrow Neurological Institute reported their experience with 17 patients (2 pediatric patients) with pineal tumors treated with Gamma Knife radiosurgery. One of the pediatric patients had malignant teratoma, which was treated with a dose of 13 Gy, with a partial response at 15 months; the other had a nongerminomatous germ cell tumor, which was treated with a dose of 15 Gy, with a complete response maintained at 73 months.[70] Both patients survived without complications.[70]

The lack of good data in both the adult and pediatric literature on the use of SRS for the treatment of pineal tumors renders it very difficult to draw any meaningful conclusions regarding its role in these tumors. Most series have a small number of patients with various histologies. The most important factor in determining the treatment strategy is histology, which governs the biologic behavior. Tumors such as germ cell tumors and pineoblastomas have a high propensity for neuraxis dissemination and require more than local treatment of the tumor alone.[2] Based on the limited literature available and the knowledge of the patterns of failure for germ cell tumors and pineoblastomas, it is probably appropriate to consider SRS as a boost therapy in some cases. SRS can also be used as a salvage therapy for recurrent germ cell tumors and pineoblastomas. For pineocytomas, which have a low propensity for neuraxis dissemination, SRS appears to be an appropriate treatment modality for selected patients.

The pineal gland is located immediately adjacent to the tectal plate of the midbrain, where the superior colliculi are located. Larger pineal tumors can also involve the interstitial nuclei of Cajai, which control downward gaze. A highly conformal SRS plan is desirable to minimize the risk of damage to those structures; this may be achieved by using smaller shots if the Gamma Knife is used or by using an intensity-modulated radiosurgical system with micromultileaf collimation if a linac-based system is used. There are no well-defined guidelines regarding the dosing for SRS for pineal tumors, but 12 to 16 Gy appears to be a reasonable dose range based on the limited data in the literature.

◆ Summary

The dosimetric characteristics of SRS render it an attractive treatment for pediatric patients with brain tumors in various settings. Although treatment outcomes from prospective trials are lacking in the literature, experience with the use of SRS for pediatric brain tumors accumulated at various major radiosurgical centers across the globe have provided useful data that can guide neurosurgeons and radiation oncologists in their treatment decisions. With the accumulation of more data and longer follow-up, it is hoped that more information will be available on which to make even better management decisions. Prospective trials testing the role of SRS in pediatric brain tumors are desperately needed.

References

1. Suh JH, Barnett GH. Stereotactic radiosurgery for brain tumors in pediatric patients. Technol Cancer Res Treat 2003;2(2):141–146
2. Lo SS, Fakiris AJ, Abdulrahman R, et al. Role of stereotactic radiosurgery and fractionated stereotactic radiotherapy in pediatric brain tumors. Expert Rev Neurother 2008;8(1):121–132
3. Giller CA, Berger BD, Pistenmaa DA, et al. Robotically guided radiosurgery for children. Pediatr Blood Cancer 2005;45(3):304–310
4. Lo SS, Chang EL, Sloan AE. Role of stereotactic radiosurgery and fractionated stereotactic radiotherapy in the management of intracranial ependymoma. Expert Rev Neurother 2006;6(4):501–507
5. Kleihues P, Cavenee W. Ependymoma. In: Kleihues P, Cavenee W, eds. World Health Organisation Classification of Tumours: Pathology and Genetics. Tumours of the Nervous System. Lyon, France: IARC; 2000:72–77
6. Larson DA, Flickinger JC, Loeffler JS. The radiobiology of radiosurgery. Int J Radiat Oncol Biol Phys 1993;25(3):557–561
7. Foreman NK, Love S, Thorne R. Intracranial ependymomas: analysis of prognostic factors in a population-based series. Pediatr Neurosurg 1996;24(3):119–125
8. Pollack IF, Gerszten PC, Martinez AJ, et al. Intracranial ependymomas of childhood: long-term outcome and prognostic factors. Neurosurgery 1995;37(4):655–666, discussion 666–667
9. Horn B, Heideman R, Geyer R, et al. A multi-institutional retrospective study of intracranial ependymoma in children: identification of risk factors. J Pediatr Hematol Oncol 1999;21(3):203–211
10. Rousseau P, Habrand JL, Sarrazin D, et al. Treatment of intracranial ependymomas of children: review of a 15-year experience. Int J Radiat Oncol Biol Phys 1994;28(2):381–386
11. Merchant TE. Current management of childhood ependymoma. Oncology 2002;16(5):629–642
12. Marks JE, Adler SJ. A comparative study of ependymomas by site of origin. Int J Radiat Oncol Biol Phys 1982;8(1):37–43
13. Goldwein JW, Leahy JM, Packer RJ, et al. Intracranial ependymomas in children. Int J Radiat Oncol Biol Phys 1990;19(6):1497–1502
14. Healey EA, Barnes PD, Kupsky WJ, et al. The prognostic significance of postoperative residual tumor in ependymoma. Neurosurgery 1991; 28(5):666–671, discussion 671–672
15. Aggarwal R, Yeung D, Kumar P, Muhlbauer M, Kun LE. Efficacy and feasibility of stereotactic radiosurgery in the primary management of unfavorable pediatric ependymoma. Radiother Oncol 1997;43(3):269–273
16. Hodgson DC, Goumnerova LC, Loeffler JS, et al. Radiosurgery in the management of pediatric brain tumors. Int J Radiat Oncol Biol Phys 2001;50(4):929–935
17. Mansur DB, Drzymala RE, Rich KM, Klein EE, Simpson JR. The efficacy of stereotactic radiosurgery in the management of intracranial ependymoma. J Neurooncol 2004;66(1–2):187–190
18. Lo SS, Abdulrahman R, Desrosiers PM, et al. The role of Gamma Knife radiosurgery in the management of unresectable gross disease or gross residual disease after surgery in ependymoma. J Neurooncol 2006;79(1):51–56
19. Grabb PA, Lunsford LD, Albright AL, Kondziolka D, Flickinger JC. Stereotactic radiosurgery for glial neoplasms of childhood. Neurosurgery 1996;38(4):696–701
20. Jawahar A, Kondziolka D, Flickinger JC, Lunsford LD. Adjuvant stereotactic radiosurgery for anaplastic ependymoma. Stereotact Funct Neurosurg 1999;73(1–4):23–30
21. Stafford SL, Pollock BE, Foote RL, Gorman DA, Nelson DF, Schomberg PJ. Stereotactic radiosurgery for recurrent ependymoma. Cancer 2000; 88(4):870–875
22. Statistical report. Primary Brain Tumor in the United States. Chicago: CBTRUS; 2005. Central Brain Tumor Registry of the United States, 1998–2002; 2006
23. Somaza SC, Kondziolka D, Lunsford LD, Flickinger JC, Bissonette DJ, Albright AL. Early outcomes after stereotactic radiosurgery for growing pilocytic astrocytomas in children. Pediatr Neurosurg 1996;25(3):109–115
24. Hadjipanayis CG, Kondziolka D, Gardner P, et al. Stereotactic radiosurgery for pilocytic astrocytomas when multimodal therapy is necessary. J Neurosurg 2002;97(1):56–64
25. Hadjipanayis CG, Niranjan A, Tyler-Kabara E, Kondziolka D, Flickinger JC, Lunsford LD. Stereotactic radiosurgery for well-circumscribed fibrillary grade II astrocytomas: an initial experience. Stereotact Funct Neurosurg 2002;79(1):13–24
26. Kida Y, Kobayashi T, Mori Y. Gamma Knife radiosurgery for low-grade astrocytomas: results of long-term follow-up. J Neurosurg 2000;93 (Suppl 3):42–46
27. Barcia JA, Barcia-Salorio JL, Ferrer C, Ferrer E, Algas R, Hernandez G. Stereotactic radiosurgery of deeply seated low-grade gliomas. Acta Neurochir Suppl (Wien) 1994;62:58–61
28. Boëthius J, Ulfarsson E, Rahn T, Lippittz B. Gamma Knife radiosurgery for pilocytic astrocytomas. J Neurosurg 2002;97(5, Suppl):677–680
29. Hochberg F, Grossman SA, Mikkelsen T, Glantz M, Fisher JD, Piantadosi S. Lack of efficacy of 9-aminocamptothecin in adults with newly diagnosed glioblastoma multiforme and recurrent high-grade astrocytoma: NABTT CNS Consortium. Neuro-oncol 2000;2(1):29–33
30. Laperriere NJ, Leung PM, McKenzie S, et al. Randomized study of brachytherapy in the initial management of patients with malignant astrocytoma. Int J Radiat Oncol Biol Phys 1998;41(5):1005–1011
31. Laperriere N, Zuraw L, Cairncross G. Radiotherapy for newly diagnosed malignant glioma in adults: a systematic review. Radiother Oncol 2002;64(3):259–273
32. Selker RG, Shapiro WR, Burger P, et al. The Brain Tumor Cooperative Group NIH Trial 87–01: a randomized comparison of surgery, external radiotherapy, and carmustine versus surgery, interstitial radiotherapy boost, external radiation therapy, and carmustine. Neurosurgery 2002;51(2):343–355, discussion 355–347
33. Souhami L, Seiferheld W, Brachman D, et al. Randomized comparison of stereotactic radiosurgery followed by conventional radiotherapy with carmustine to conventional radiotherapy with carmustine for patients with glioblastoma multiforme: report of Radiation Therapy Oncology Group 93–05 protocol. Int J Radiat Oncol Biol Phys 2004;60(3):853–860
34. Baumann GS, Wara WM, Larson DA, et al. Gamma Knife radiosurgery in children. Pediatr Neurosurg 1996;24(4):193–201
35. Tsao MN, Mehta MP, Whelan TJ, et al. The American Society for Therapeutic Radiology and Oncology (ASTRO) evidence-based review of the role of radiosurgery for malignant glioma. Int J Radiat Oncol Biol Phys 2005;63(1):47–55
36. Patrice SJ, Tarbell NJ, Goumnerova LC, Shrieve DC, Black PM, Loeffler JS. Results of radiosurgery in the management of recurrent and residual medulloblastoma. Pediatr Neurosurg 1995;22(4):197–203
37. Woo C, Stea B, Lulu B, Hamilton A, Cassady JR. The use of stereotactic radiosurgical boost in the treatment of medulloblastomas. Int J Radiat Oncol Biol Phys 1997;37(4):761–764
38. Eder HG, Leber KA, Eustacchio S, Pendl G. The role of Gamma Knife radiosurgery in children. Childs Nerv Syst 2001;17(6):341–346, discussion 347
39. Im SH, Wang KC, Kim SK, et al. Childhood meningioma: unusual location, atypical radiological findings, and favorable treatment outcome. Childs Nerv Syst 2001;17(11):656–662
40. DiBiase SJ, Kwok Y, Yovino S, et al. Factors predicting local tumor control after gamma knife stereotactic radiosurgery for benign intracranial meningiomas. Int J Radiat Oncol Biol Phys 2004;60(5):1515–1519
41. Lunsford LD, Niranjan A, Flickinger JC, Maitz A, Kondziolka D. Radiosurgery of vestibular schwannomas: summary of experience in 829 cases. J Neurosurg 2005;102(Suppl):195–199
42. Flickinger JC, Kondziolka D, Niranjan A, Maitz A, Voynov G, Lunsford LD. Acoustic neuroma radiosurgery with marginal tumor doses of 12 to 13 Gy. Int J Radiat Oncol Biol Phys 2004;60(1):225–230
43. Kondziolka D, Lunsford LD, McLaughlin MR, Flickinger JC. Long-term outcomes after radiosurgery for acoustic neuromas. N Engl J Med 1998;339(20):1426–1433
44. Kondziolka D, Lunsford LD, Flickinger JC. Stereotactic radiosurgery in children and adolescents. Pediatr Neurosurg 1990;16(4–5):219–221
45. Mathieu D, Kondziolka D, Flickinger JC, et al. Stereotactic radiosurgery for vestibular schwannomas in patients with neurofibromatosis type 2: an analysis of tumor control, complications, and hearing preservation rates. Neurosurgery 2007;60(3):460–468, discussion 468–470
46. Rowe JG, Radatz MW, Walton L, Soanes T, Rodgers J, Kemeny AA. Clinical experience with Gamma Knife stereotactic radiosurgery in the management of vestibular schwannomas secondary to type 2 neurofibromatosis. J Neurol Neurosurg Psychiatry 2003;74(9):1288–1293
47. Kida Y, Kobayashi T, Tanaka T, Mori Y. Radiosurgery for bilateral neurinomas associated with neurofibromatosis type 2. Surg Neurol 2000; 53(4):383–389, discussion 389–390
48. Plowman PN, Evans DG. Stereotactic radiosurgery: 11. Acoustic neuroma therapy and radiation oncogenesis. Br J Neurosurg 2000;14(2):93–95
49. Ulfarsson E, Lindquist C, Roberts M, et al. Gamma Knife radiosurgery for craniopharyngiomas: long-term results in the first Swedish patients. J Neurosurg 2002;97(5, Suppl):613–622

50. Chung WY, Pan DH, Shiau CY, Guo WY, Wang LW. Gamma Knife radiosurgery for craniopharyngiomas. J Neurosurg 2000;93(Suppl 3):47–56
51. Mokry M. Craniopharyngiomas: A six year experience with Gamma Knife radiosurgery. Stereotact Funct Neurosurg 1999;72(Suppl 1):140–149
52. Amendola BE, Wolf A, Coy SR, Amendola MA. Role of radiosurgery in craniopharyngiomas: a preliminary report. Med Pediatr Oncol 2003;41(2):123–127
53. Isaac MA, Hahn SS, Kim JA, Bogart JA, Chung CT. Management of craniopharyngioma. Cancer J 2001;7(6):516–520
54. Chiou SM, Lunsford LD, Niranjan A, Kondziolka D, Flickinger JC. Stereotactic radiosurgery of residual or recurrent craniopharyngioma, after surgery, with or without radiation therapy. Neuro-oncol 2001;3(3):159–166
55. Kobayashi T, Kida Y, Mori Y, Hasegawa T. Long-term results of Gamma Knife surgery for the treatment of craniopharyngioma in 98 consecutive cases. J Neurosurg 2005;103(6, Suppl):482–488
56. Tishler RB, Loeffler JS, Lunsford LD, et al. Tolerance of cranial nerves of the cavernous sinus to radiosurgery. Int J Radiat Oncol Biol Phys 1993;27(2):215–221
57. Stafford SL, Pollock BE, Leavitt JA, et al. A study on the radiation tolerance of the optic nerves and chiasm after stereotactic radiosurgery. Int J Radiat Oncol Biol Phys 2003;55(5):1177–1181
58. Witt TC. Stereotactic radiosurgery for pituitary tumors. Neurosurg Focus 2003;14(5):e10
59. Thoren M, Rahn T, Hallengren B, et al. Treatment of Cushing's disease in childhood and adolescence by stereotactic pituitary irradiation. Acta Paediatr Scand 1986;75(3):388–395
60. Kobayashi T, Kida Y, Mori Y. Gamma Knife radiosurgery in the treatment of Cushing disease: long-term results. J Neurosurg 2002;97(5, Suppl):422–428
61. Castinetti F, Nagai M, Dufour H, et al. Gamma Knife radiosurgery is a successful adjunctive treatment in Cushing's disease. Eur J Endocrinol 2007;156(1):91–98
62. Mitsumori M, Shrieve DC, Alexander E III, et al. Initial clinical results of linac-based stereotactic radiosurgery and stereotactic radiotherapy for pituitary adenomas. Int J Radiat Oncol Biol Phys 1998;42(3):573–580
63. Manera L, Regis J, Chinot O, et al. Pineal region tumors: the role of stereotactic radiosurgery. Stereotact Funct Neurosurg 1996;66(Suppl 1):164–173
64. Reyns N, Hayashi M, Chinot O, et al. The role of Gamma Knife radiosurgery in the treatment of pineal parenchymal tumours. Acta Neurochir (Wien) 2006;148(1):5–11, discussion 11
65. Hasegawa T, Kondziolka D, Hadjipanayis CG, Flickinger JC, Lunsford LD. The role of radiosurgery for the treatment of pineal parenchymal tumors. Neurosurgery 2002;51(4):880–889
66. Hasegawa T, Kondziolka D, Hadjipanayis CG, Flickinger JC, Lunsford LD. Stereotactic radiosurgery for CNS nongerminomatous germ cell tumors: report of four cases. Pediatr Neurosurg 2003;38(6):329–333
67. Kobayashi T, Kida Y, Mori Y. Stereotactic gamma radiosurgery for pineal and related tumors. J Neurooncol 2001;54(3):301–309
68. Endo H, Kumabe T, Jokura H, Tominaga T. Stereotactic radiosurgery followed by whole ventricular irradiation for primary intracranial germinoma of the pineal region. Minim Invasive Neurosurg 2005;48(3):186–190
69. Amendola BE, Wolf A, Coy SR, Amendola MA, Eber D. Pineal tumors: analysis of treatment results in 20 patients. J Neurosurg 2005;102(Suppl):175–179
70. Lekovic GP, Gonzalez LF, Shetter AG, et al. Role of Gamma Knife surgery in the management of pineal region tumors. Neurosurg Focus 2007;23(6):E12

Index

Note: Page numbers followed by *f* and *t* indicate figures and tables, respectively.

D

E

N

O

P

U

V

W